"If you are what you eat, I want to be Robin Arzón! The same infectious energy that whips us into shape translates seamlessly into delicious, healthy recipes that will help each of us live our best lives."
—**KATIE COURIC**

"Arzón dismantles the myth that plant-based eating is bland or limiting. In *Eat to Hustle*, she proves it can be powerful fuel. These recipes are simple, full of flavor, and packed with protein—built to support the layered realities of life: workouts, family, and everything in between."
—**ARASH HASHEMI**, author of *Shred Happens: So Easy, So Good*

"*Eat to Hustle* is a radiant celebration of strength, motherhood, and flavor—all wrapped into one empowering cookbook. Arzón's wisdom is something I have leaned on for years, and now she shares her vibrant recipes that remind us that confidence begins with how we nourish ourselves."
—**EVA LONGORIA**, actor, director, and author of *My Mexican Kitchen*

"This cookbook delivers high-protein, high-fiber fuel for the hustle—whether it's pre-run, post-run, or when moving through your day. As a fellow athlete and mom, I'm inspired by how Arzón powers both performance and family."
—**ALLYSON FELIX**, Olympian and cofounder of Saysh

"Arzón rewrites the script on powerful eating. *Eat to Hustle* proves you don't need meat to fuel peak performance—every recipe is nutrient-dense, thoughtfully crafted, and built for endurance. A must-read for anyone looking to align food with fitness and purpose."
—**RICH ROLL**, author of *Finding Ultra*

"*Eat to Hustle* is a smart, purposeful guide to eating well and living with intention. Arzón's approach to food reflects her leadership—focused, driven, and inspiring. These recipes do more than nourish—they support the energy, clarity, and balance needed for a full and ambitious life."
—**CANDICE KUMAI**, author of *Kintsugi Wellness* and host of the *Wabi Sabi* podcast

EAT TO HUSTLE

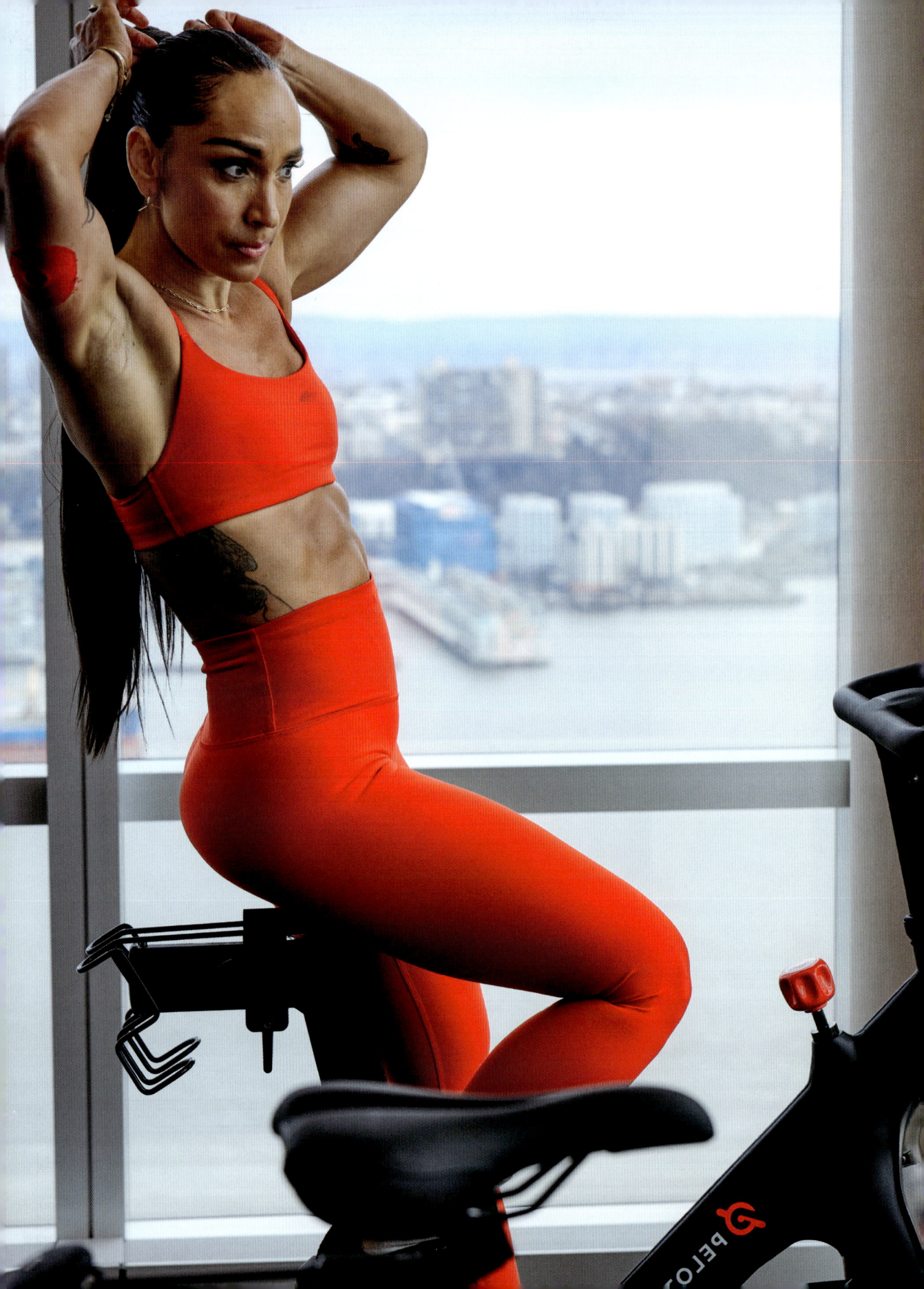

75 HIGH-PROTEIN PLANT-BASED RECIPES

EAT TO HUSTLE

ROBIN ARZÓN

PHOTOGRAPHY BY JOHNNY MILLER

Little, Brown and Company
New York Boston London

FOR MY SISTER, MOM, ABUELAS,
AND THE DYNASTY OF WOMEN
WHO BUILT ME.

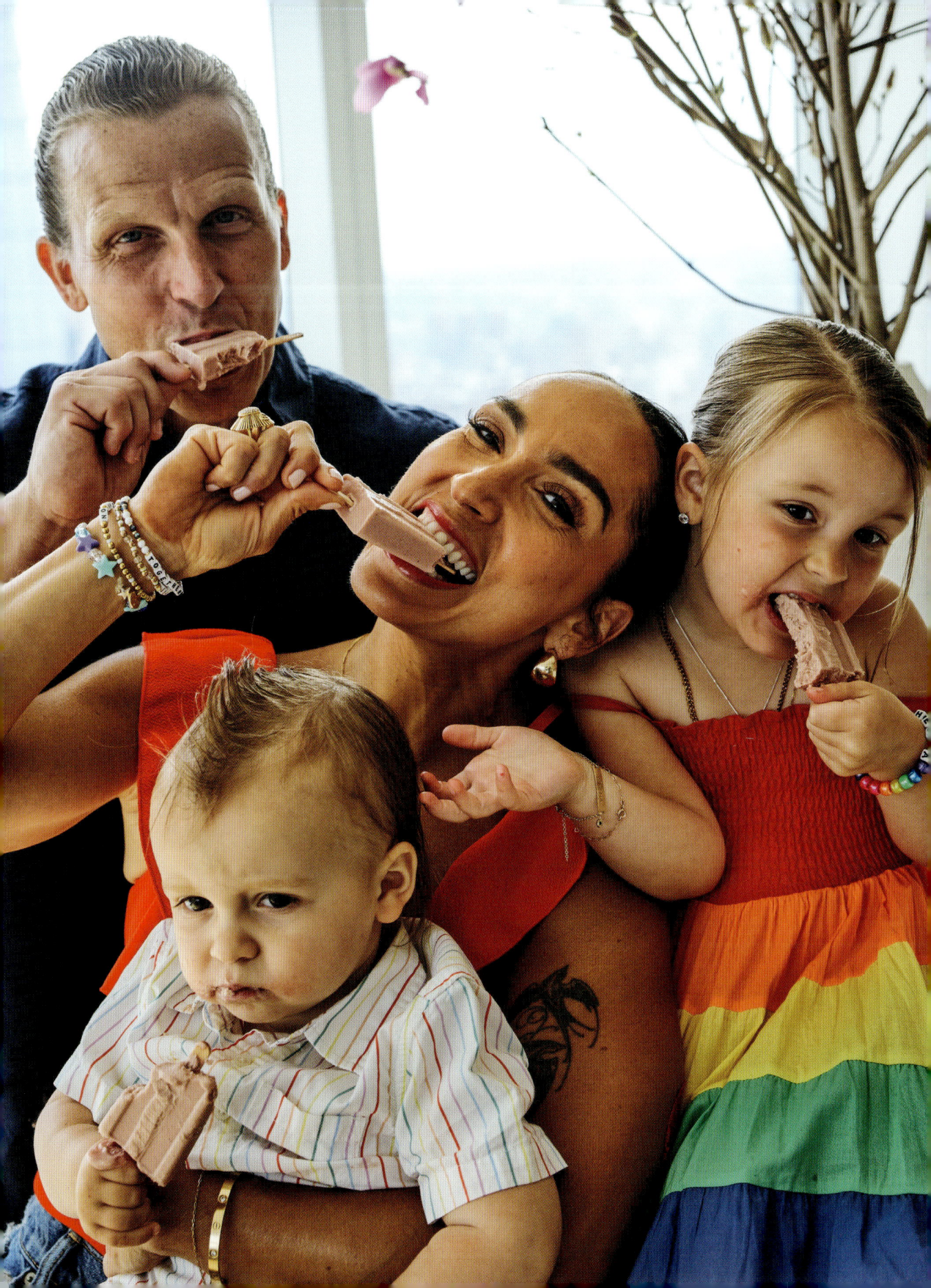

CONTENTS

Introduction
How to Use This Book 8
.... 12
UNDERSTANDING MACROS 14
THE PROTEIN PRINCIPLE 16
SHOP SMARTER, NOT HARDER 18
TOOLS OF THE TRADE 22
FACT CHECK: VEGAN MYTHS 24
HEALTH MATTERS 30

Morning Routines
A Weekend Jewish Deli Breakfast 37
Acorn Squash Breakfast Bowls 41
Anything-But-Basic Avo Toast 42
Buckwheat & Berry Parfaits 46
Drew's Famous Smoothie 49
Lentil Waffle Mix (and Pancakes, Too!) 50
Peppermint Hot Chocolate 53
Protein Matcha Latte 54
Savory Oats & Lentil Porridge 57
Shakshuka-Style Tofu Scramble 58
Sweet Bean–Stuffed French Toast 61
Veggie & Pesto Frittata 62

Skip the Lunch Salad
Chickpea Pozole 67
Chorizo Burrito Bowl 68
Creamy Alfredo Pasta 71
Creamy Mac and Cheese 72
Mushroom & Lentil Bolognese 75
Red Lentil Curry 76
Seitan Reuben Bowl 79
Three-Bean Chili 80

I ♥ Sandwiches
Bodega Chopped Cheese 87
Classic Chi*ken Salad 88
Fried No-Chick Deluxe 91
I'm from Philly Cheesesteak 95
Lentil Sloppy Joes 99
Plant-Powered Bean & Chile Burritos 100
Vegan Big Stack 105
Fully Loaded Crunchy Wrap 109

Eat Your Veggies

Kimchi Ginger Poke Bowl	114
Loaded Cobb Salad	120
Tofu Ranch Dressing	121
Med Chopped Salad	123
The Big (Kale) Salad with Tempeh "Croutons"	124
Vegan Hand Rolls	129
Sriracha Mayo	130

Sit-Down Dinners

Creamy Ziti & Broccoli	134
Lentil Shepherd's Pie	137
Lupini Pot Pie	138
Protein-Packed Lasagna	141
Seitan Fajitas	145
Vegan Sour Cream	146
Vegan Pernil Plate	149
Arroz con Gandules (Rice with Pigeon Peas)	150
Maduros (Fried Sweet Plantains)	151

Keep Calm and Snack On

Sweet Crispy Treats	154
Mini Energy Muffins	157
Seasoned Kale Chips	158
Tofu Chicharrones	161
Vegan Candy Bar Bites	162

Couch Potato Cravings

Air Fryer Artichoke Wings with Lemony Hummus Dip	166
Crispy Air-Fried Tofu Nuggets	169
Pizza Bites	170
Stacked Nacho Fries	173
Tempeh Buffalo Dip	174

Desserts with Muscle

Apple Chocolate "Nachos"	178
Black Bean Brownies	181
Chickpea Choco-Chip Cookies	182
Coco-licious Cream Pie	185
Gooey Cinnamon Rolls	186
Oatmeal Raisin Power Cookies	189
PB&J Swirl Nice Cream	190
Power-Packed Rice Pudding	193
Pumpkin Spice Mousse with Maple Brittle	194
Chocolate Silk Pie	198
Silky Caramel Flan	201
Strawberry Protein Pops	202
Sweet Potato Pie Bars	205

Sundays Are for Meal Prep

Bagels with a Boost	211
Bread of Champions	215
Packed Pizza Dough	219
Cashew Parm	220
DIY Seitan	222
TVP MVP	224
Fire Veggies	225
Grains for Days	229
Best Basic Beans	232
Lentils on Lock	233
Vegan Whip	234
Liquid Gold	235

RECIPES BY EFFORT	*236*
RECIPES BY TIME	*238*
SOURCES	*240*
ACKNOWLEDGMENTS	*244*
INDEX	*246*

Nutritional Disclaimer

The material in this book is for informational purposes only and not intended as a substitute for the advice and care of your physician—you should always consult with your physician to make sure any wellness program is appropriate for your individual circumstances. Keep in mind that nutritional needs vary from person to person. The information contained in this book is based upon sources that the author believes to be reliable. However, the author and publisher make no representations or warranties with respect to the accuracy or completeness of the information published herein and disclaim responsibility for any adverse effects that may result from the use or application of the information contained in this book.

INTRODUCTION

THE NUMBER ONE QUESTION I GET ASKED IS: How do you fuel? People assume that because I'm an athlete, I must be loading up on steak and eggs, and when I tell them I'm plant-based, their jaws drop. But here's the deal: I train hard. I lift heavy. I run marathons, crush HYROX competitions, and push my body to its limits. And I do it all powered by plants — and yes, I get enough protein.

I didn't grow up eating this way, and I'm not about to pretend I stepped into the world with a quinoa bowl in one hand and a kale smoothie in the other. My background, my culture, my family — none of it was inherently plant-based. My mom, Carmen, is a Cuban refugee. My dad, Ruddy, grew up in Puerto Rico before moving to the Bronx. We're Jewish on my mom's side, with Sephardic roots. I grew up in Philly, and we are a multifaith, multicultural household where food is everything. Philly cheesesteaks, Puerto Rican pernil, Jewish deli spreads — I loved it all. At first, I thought going plant-based meant saying goodbye to those flavors, but I quickly realized it just meant getting creative with how I re-created them.

And then there was Drew. When I met my husband, he was running purely on protein shakes and slabs of meat — a true bachelor diet. I wasn't about to be that pushy vegan girlfriend — but I also wasn't going to let this man go another day without a vegetable! So I did what any good strategist would do: I played the long game. I started making him massive, flavorful salads with lots of textures and hearty vegan meals that didn't feel like stereotypical "health food." The shift was immediate. He felt stronger and he recovered from training faster. And within a few months, he was plant-based, too. Now, our kids, Athena and Atlas, are growing up fueled by plants from day one — strong, thriving, and yes, getting all the protein they need (because that's always the first question, right?).

But let's back up because this shift was not planned. I was working as a corporate litigator in Midtown Manhattan, and every single day I grabbed the same overpriced, uninspired grilled chicken salad from the bodega near my office. And then one fateful day, I took a big bite of a piece of chicken that was raw and cold in the center—it was so nasty! I cut out meat on the spot, starting with sending that salad straight to the trash.

That snap decision kicked off a gradual and deeply personal food journey. My younger sister, Margaret, was a huge influence on my decision to cut out meat. She was in college while I was grinding away at my law firm, and she was already deep into plant-based eating. Margaret introduced me to the fact that vegan food wasn't just "good" for being vegan — it could actually be pretty delicious, too. She taught me a new way of cooking and looking at food that made me feel like I wasn't missing out on anything. But the shift wasn't overnight. In the beginning I took small steps — I still ate dairy and eggs for a while. I experimented, found some go-to recipes like simple black bean burritos and a morning smoothie — and relied heavily on Thai and Indian takeout — and learned to build a plate that worked for me. There were no rigid rules — just a curiosity to see what felt best for my body. And my body noticed the difference.

At the same time that I was cutting out meat, I was getting more serious about endurance running. The impact was immediate: after I dropped meat, I

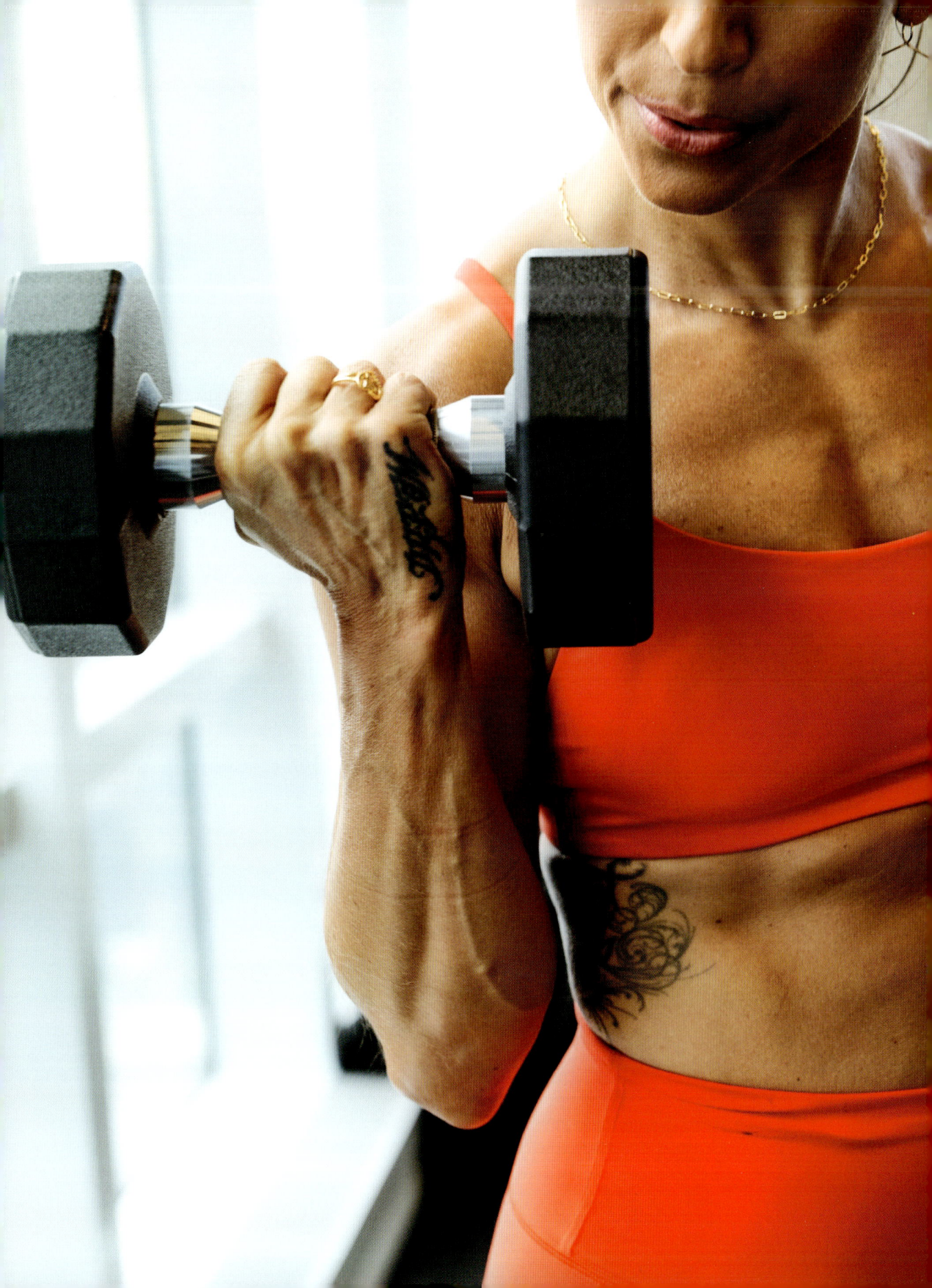

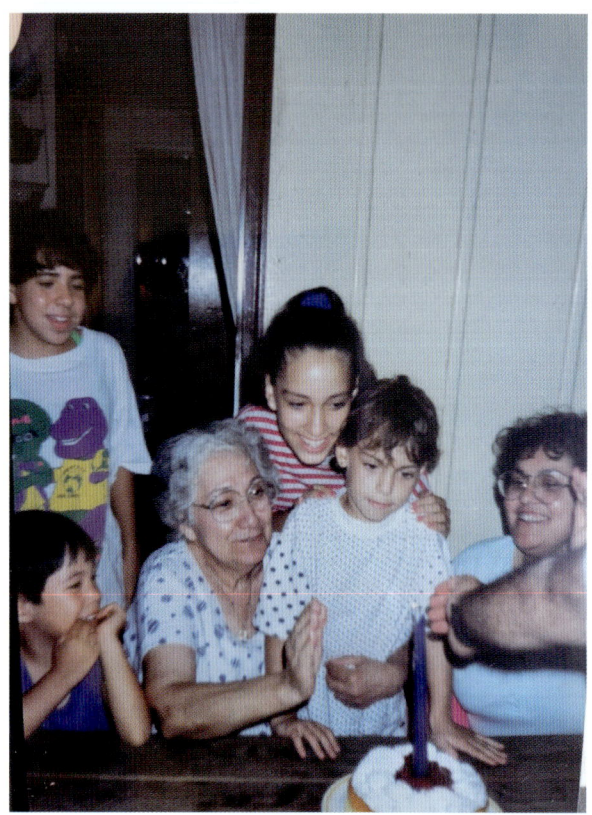
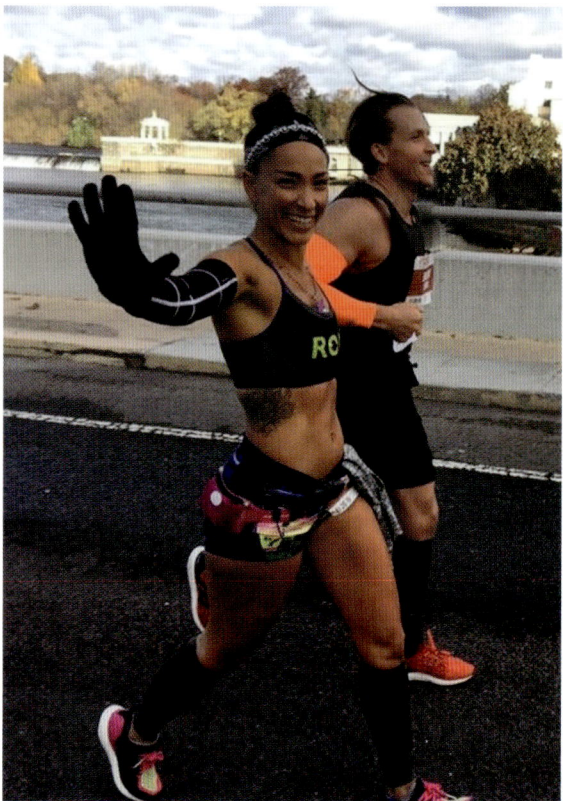
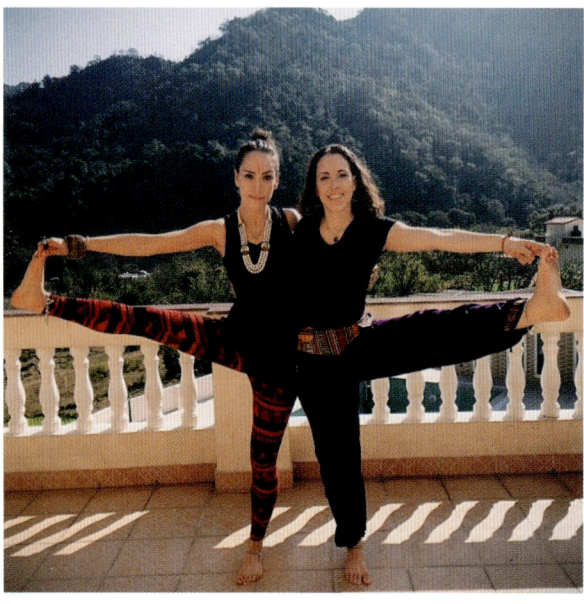
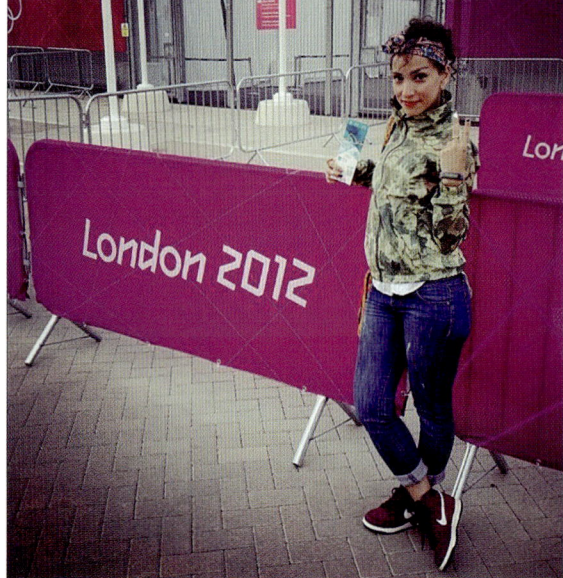

> I see every meal as an opportunity to fuel my body with intention, to eat in a way that keeps me strong, steady, and ready for whatever comes next.

was running harder, recovering faster, and feeling unstoppable. And it wasn't just in training — I saw it at work, too. That afternoon slump, the one we all just accept as normal when we feel like we're running on fumes? It simply went away. It made me realize that just because something is common doesn't mean it's normal, and once I figured that out, there was no going back.

By 2012, my whole life was shifting. I had spent years grinding in corporate law, thinking that success meant following the path I had laid out for myself. But deep down, I knew I wanted more than just a good-on-paper career — I wanted something that lit me up. So I did something radical: I bet on myself. I left my law job, flew to London for the Olympics, and started vlogging, interviewing athletes, and chasing a career in fitness. That immediately led to a job in social media for Nike Women where I created content for the brand. And then I read about this new fitness company called Peloton. I sent a cold email, auditioned, and became one of their first instructors. Getting on that bike for the first time was incredible. The moment I clipped in, I knew — I was done telling someone else's story. It was time to write my own. What I didn't know was that I was stepping into something so much bigger than just a job. I was about to help build a movement, one ride, one class, one community at a time.

My life was moving at full speed, and then — right before I started at Peloton — life threw me a curveball. I had been feeling off for a while, noticing extreme thirst and lots of fatigue. One week before my first day, my doctor realized my pancreas wasn't producing insulin and I was diagnosed with type 1 diabetes. It was a lot to take in, but I was grateful I had already built a strong foundation of fueling with intention. I fine-tuned my nutrition even further, learning how to regulate my insulin management through macros (more on that on page 14) and keep my energy steady by pairing complex carbs with protein and fiber.

That experience reshaped the way I think about food — not just as something to enjoy, but as fuel with a purpose. I needed meals that worked as hard as I did, ones that kept me steady, strong, and ready for whatever the day threw at me. While meat-based foods can cause sharp blood sugar spikes and crashes, plant-based foods are nutrient dense to help you digest better and recover faster. So, in true Virgo fashion, I did what I do best — I made a plan. And that plan slowly turned into this book! I wanted a record of my favorite high-protein, flavor-loaded meals designed to fuel every kind of movement — whether that's running a marathon, crushing a Peloton workout, or just getting through a long workday without face-planting onto your keyboard at 3 p.m. Food can be so much more than just something to enjoy — I see every meal as an opportunity to fuel my body with intention, to eat in a way that keeps me strong, steady, and ready for whatever comes next.

If you think this means bland, boring "health food" — you know what I mean (steamed vegetables and brown rice, I'm looking at you) — you'll be pleasantly surprised. In this book, I dive into hearty, satisfying, eat-with-intention meals that keep you energized and ready to go. My journey to plant-based eating wasn't about rigid meal plans, or a pressure to go all-in, so I wrote this book to provide options and to meet you where you are — I don't want to hit you over the head with rules or restrictive eating. I learned over time to take what serves me and leave what doesn't, and this book is about giving you the tools to fuel your body in a way that feels good. If you're just dipping your toes into plant-based eating, I hope these recipes will become your encouragement to explore deeper. If you're already deep in the game, I hope they become part of your regular rotation. Either way, I'm here to shut down the myth that a plant-based diet won't support strength, muscle, and high performance. So, let's get cooking. And don't forget to crank up the music — because good food deserves a good soundtrack!

HOW TO USE THIS BOOK

This book is built for action. Whether you're meal prepping for the week, grabbing a quick bite between meetings, or fueling up before a workout, every recipe is designed to fit your hustle. Here's how to navigate it and make the most of every meal.

Eat What You Want, When You Want

You'll find recipes grouped by meal type — from morning fuel-ups to power-packed lunches, sit-down dinners, snacks for every craving, and even desserts. But you make the rules. If you're craving a breakfast-for-dinner moment or want a hearty lunch for a post-workout meal, go for it. Every recipe is designed to be flexible, so you can mix and match based on what your body needs.

Your Secret Weapon

If you want to stay ahead of the game, the Sundays Are for Meal Prep chapter (page 207) will get you set up for the week. Batch-cooking key ingredients, prepping proteins, and making sure your fridge is stocked with plant-powered fuel will make hitting your goals effortless.

Food for Thought

I want to introduce you to my friend Dalina Soto, MA, RD, LDN, who shares her expert take on all things nutrition throughout this book. Dalina is a bilingual registered dietitian, a proud Dominican-American, and the author of the genius book *The Latina Anti-Diet* (it's a must-read). She's also the founder of the website Your Latina Nutritionist, where she helps people ditch diet culture and embrace their cultural foods without guilt. Whether you're looking to understand your body, navigate a health diagnosis, or fuel your workouts, a consultation with a nutritionist can be a game-changer. Dalina's superpower is blending real talk with real science, and I'm so excited for you to learn from her.

Timing Made Simple

Every recipe also includes a **Start the Clock** estimate, so you know exactly what you're signing up for:

⏱️ **Under 30 Minutes:** Fast, no-fuss meals for when time is tight.

⏱️⏱️ **30 to 60 Minutes**: Balanced meals that don't take all day but deliver on flavor.

⏱️⏱️⏱️ **1 Hour +:** Recipes that require a little more patience (or an overnight rest) but pay off in a big way.

At the back of this book (page 236), you'll find every recipe organized by effort and time for easy reference!

Know Your Effort Level

Each recipe comes with a **Dumbbell Score**, giving you a quick idea of the effort required. Think of it like a workout rating:

🏋️ **Easy Lift:** Quick, simple, and foolproof. These recipes come together fast with minimal effort — perfect for busy days, post-workout meals, or when you need to eat *now*.

🏋️🏋️ **Moderate Lift:** Some chopping, sautéing, and multitasking involved, but nothing too intense. These are your go-to weekday meals when you've got a little extra time.

🏋️🏋️🏋️ **Heavy Lift:** These recipes take time, technique, and maybe a little patience, but the results are worth it. Perfect for weekends or when you're ready to flex your cooking skills.

Built with Purpose

This book isn't just about what's on your plate—it's about the bigger picture. The recipes in these pages lean into plant-powered ingredients, not only to support your performance but also to tread more lightly on the planet. Choosing more plants, even just a few times a week, is a powerful way to reduce your environmental impact—and it's a choice that shows care for animals, too. You don't have to be fully vegan to make mindful moves that matter. Every flex counts. So whether you're going meatless on Mondays or diving into plant-based cooking full throttle, know that your choices here fuel more than just your body. They fuel change.

Macros Made Easy

No guesswork, no complicated calculations. Each recipe includes a macronutrient breakdown per serving so you can track your protein, carbs, and fats at a glance. (See page 14 for a deeper dive into macros.) Whether you're bulking, maintaining, or just staying mindful of your intake, these numbers help you fuel smarter.

Turn Up the Heat (and the Volume)

Cooking is more fun when there's a beat behind it—and for me, that tradition started with my dad. Some of my earliest memories are of us dancing in the kitchen while dinner was on the stove, and now I keep that energy alive with my own kids. We turn up the volume, dance it out while we stir things up, and keep the joy flowing right into the food. I even have a sign in the kitchen that says, "This kitchen is for dancing," because—facts—it is.

I made you a Kitchen Dance Party playlist packed with high-energy tracks to keep your vibe right while you're chopping, sautéing, or straight-up vibing in your slippers. Scan the QR code to open it up and hit play when it's go time. Whether you're in the mood to groove or just need a little push to get the meal prep started, this is your soundtrack.

UNDERSTANDING MACROS

IN THE WORLD OF NUTRITION, macros are the heavy hitters, and understanding how they work can completely change your approach to food. Macronutrients are the three major nutrients your body needs in large amounts: protein, carbohydrates, and fats. There's no need to become a registered dietitian or obsess over every calorie — just learning to balance these "big three" will help fuel your body and make every bite count.

Protein: The MVP of muscle growth, recovery, and overall strength. Protein helps rebuild tissue, support your immune system, and keep you fuller for longer.

Carbohydrates: Your body's primary fuel source. Whether you're crushing a workout or just getting through the workday, carbs keep your energy levels stable.

Fats: Essential for brain function, hormone balance, and absorbing key vitamins. Healthy fats, like those found in avocados, nuts, and seeds, are crucial for long-term health.

And while **fiber** isn't technically a macro, I like to include it in my tracking because it's a powerhouse. Aim for 30 grams a day to support digestion, gut health, and even better blood sugar control.

```
Dalina Says...
As a dietitian, I like to think of macros—protein,
carbs, and fat—not as things to track obsessively,
but as tools to help you feel nourished, full, and
energized throughout the day.
    Protein supports muscle repair, fullness, and
hormone health. Carbs give your body and brain
their favorite form of energy—especially important
if you're active, stressed, or just human. And fats?
They're essential for hormones, brain function, and
satisfaction with your meals.
    You don't need to count or measure every gram to
benefit from understanding macros. Just having a
basic sense of how they show up in your food (and
show up for you) can help you build balanced meals
that actually work for your body, especially when
recovering from exercise.
```

How to Read a Nutrition Label

Flip to the back of any packaged food, and you'll see a nutrition facts panel. Here's what to focus on:

Serving Size: Everything on the label is based on this amount. If you eat double, you're getting double the macros.

Calories: A general guide, but don't let it dictate everything. Focus on what makes up those calories — specifically protein.

Protein: The most important macro in this book. There's no one-size-fits-all recommendation, but many experts suggest aiming for anywhere from 1.6 to 2.2 grams of protein per kilogram of lean body mass. These numbers vary depending on your health status, goals, and especially your lean body mass — which many people don't know offhand. Always consult a medical or nutrition professional before making big dietary changes, especially if you have kidney or metabolic concerns.

Carbs & Fiber: Not all carbs are created equal. Prioritize whole food sources that come with fiber, like beans and legumes, whole grains (such as quinoa, oats, farro, and brown rice), and veggies. Fiber slows digestion, keeping you full and fueled.

Fats: Look for healthy fats from natural sources — like avocados, olive oil, nuts, and seeds — and avoid trans fats and ultraprocessed oils where possible.

The recipes in this book also list these major categories so you can plan, track, and power up on your macro intake through the week.

How to Use Macros Without Losing Your Mind

I recommend tracking everything you naturally eat — and the macros you're getting — for two weeks. Don't change your habits, just get a picture of where you're at. You might be surprised by which macros you're excelling at, and it's totally fine if you're surprised by where you're falling behind. The goal is to start getting a clear picture of what you're eating, kind of like creating a nutritional budget!

From there, start focusing on protein. Don't stress over carbs and fats — if you're hitting your daily protein goals, you'll naturally start eating enough whole foods to keep everything else balanced. Protein keeps you full and satisfied, which means you'll crowd out the junk without even trying. And here's my hot take: don't stress about calories! It'll just drive you crazy and encourage unhealthy obsessing.

If you want to hone in, call in an expert for extra guidance informed by your needs. I started working with a nutritionist, Amanda Sangiacomo, when I was postpartum with Atlas to ensure that I was getting enough fuel while training and breastfeeding. Macros are super individual and they will change as your lifestyle and body changes, but the big goal is to get yourself in alignment and listen to what's working for your body. The rest will take care of itself!

How to Track Your Macros

If you're using a tracker app, the easiest way to get accurate numbers for what you're eating is to weigh your serving on a digital kitchen scale and enter the weight in grams into the app. Most apps let you search for the food or ingredient, and once you've found the closest match, you can adjust the serving size by weight to match what you're eating. Keep in mind that macros can vary depending on the brand or type of ingredient — like protein powder or yogurt — and even the size of produce (a large squash will have different macros than a medium one).

The macros listed in this book are calculated using common or average values for each ingredient, so your own totals might be a bit different depending on what you use. The best way to get as close as possible is to weigh your specific ingredients and check their nutrition labels or the app's database for exact numbers. Tracking macros is a tool to guide you, not a strict rulebook — use it to learn, adjust, and fuel your body in a way that works for you.

The Protein Principle

Whether you're training hard, rebuilding strength, or just trying to stay steady in a chaotic world, protein is your ride-or-die. It rebuilds muscle, supports your immune system, fuels your hustle, and keeps you full and focused between meals.

So how much protein do you actually need? That's where things get a little less one-size-fits-all. You've probably heard the old-school "0.8 grams per kilogram of body weight" recommendation. That's not wrong — it's just the minimum to avoid deficiency — but we're not here to scrape by. We're here to thrive. If you're lifting, running, cycling, chasing toddlers, or coming back from an injury or big life shift, your body's demand for protein is higher — and you've got to meet it.

Most sports nutrition experts suggest aiming for somewhere between 1.6 to 2.2 grams of protein per kilogram of lean body mass (see Sources, page 240). That's different from total body weight — lean body mass refers to everything in your body that isn't fat: muscle, bone, organs, water. Unless you've had a DEXA scan or worked with a dietitian, you probably don't know that number offhand. That's okay! You can still get in the right ballpark by using your weight in kilograms and adjusting based on your goals.

For most people, 1.2 grams of protein per kilogram of body weight is a solid place to start. Especially if you're over 40, staying on top of your protein can help fight off muscle loss as you age.

If you train regularly, 1.6 grams will give you what you need to recover and get stronger. And if you're going hard — lifting heavy, logging miles, pushing your limits — 2.2 grams per kilogram puts you in high-performance territory. (See Sources, page 240.) Use the chart at right to find your protein target based on your weight and lifestyle.

Now, a quick reality check: if you have kidney issues, diabetes, or a metabolic condition, don't guess — get guidance. A registered dietitian or medical provider can help you figure out what's right for your body. Same goes if you're on weight-loss medication, underweight, or overweight — working with a pro ensures you're calculating needs based on lean mass, not total mass, so you're not over- or underdoing it.

If you're just starting out, don't stress over every gram. This isn't about being perfect. It's about being intentional. Build meals around protein — whether that's tofu, tempeh, lentils, seitan, edamame, or a protein shake — and spread it out over the day. Your body doesn't store protein the way it stores carbs or fat, so spacing it out keeps your muscles fueled and your energy steady. (Think of it like charging your phone throughout the day instead of letting it run low.)

Bottom line: Show up for your body with the fuel it needs to meet you at your level of ambition. Protein is a non-negotiable for performance, strength, and staying ready for whatever life throws at you. Let's fuel up with purpose!

Robin Says...

I personally go higher than the chart—around 2.4 grams of protein per kilogram. But remember, I train like a pro athlete and work with a nutritionist to dial in exactly what my body needs. Use this chart as proof that protein goals flex with your lifestyle, your grind, and your support team.

Dalina Says...

Most people will land in the lower ranges of the chart, especially if you're just starting to get serious about macros and fitness. As you push higher, it's smart to check in with a nutrition expert to be sure you're not crowding out other key nutrients in the chase for protein—balance matters as much as the grams.

Protein Goals by Body Weight

Body Weight (lb)	Body Weight (kg)	Active Lifestyle 1.2g protein/kg	Train & Sustain 1.6g protein/kg	High-Performance Athlete 2.2g protein/kg
100 lb	45 kg	54 g	73 g	100 g
110 lb	50 kg	60 g	80 g	110 g
120 lb	54 kg	65 g	87 g	120 g
130 lb	59 kg	71 g	94 g	130 g
140 lb	64 kg	77 g	102 g	140 g
150 lb	68 kg	82 g	109 g	150 g
160 lb	73 kg	88 g	116 g	160 g
170 lb	77 kg	92 g	123 g	170 g
180 lb	83 kg	100 g	131 g	180 g
190 lb	86 kg	103 g	138 g	190 g
200 lb	91 kg	109 g	145 g	200 g
210 lb	95 kg	114 g	153 g	210 g
220 lb	100 kg	120 g	160 g	220 g
230 lb	104 kg	125 g	167 g	230 g
240 lb	109 kg	131 g	174 g	240 g
250 lb	113 kg	136 g	181 g	250 g
260 lb	118 kg	142 g	189 g	260 g
270 lb	123 kg	148 g	196 g	270 g
280 lb	127 kg	153 g	203 g	280 g
290 lb	132 kg	158 g	210 g	290 g
300 lb	136 kg	163 g	218 g	300 g

SHOP SMARTER, NOT HARDER

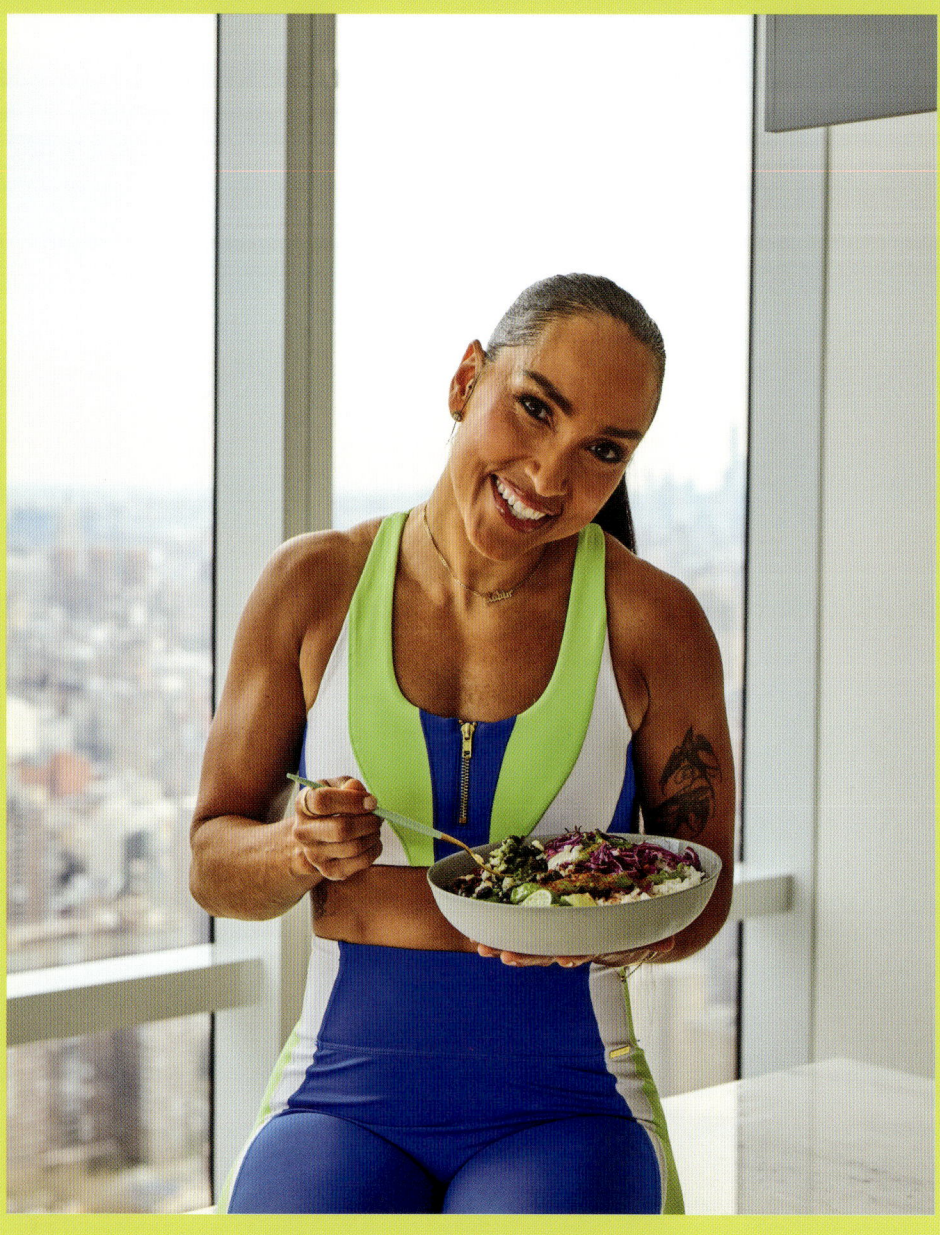

Stocking your kitchen should feel like setting yourself up for success, not running an obstacle course through endless grocery aisles like a contestant on *Supermarket Sweep*. The right staples mean you're always just a few steps away from a solid, protein-packed meal. These are the ingredients I rely on and keep on hand to ensure my energy is steady, my meals exciting, and my macros on point.

Beans
Black beans, chickpeas, cannellini, kidney, pinto — you name it, I've got it stocked. These little powerhouses are packed with protein, rich in fiber, and ready to fuel you up. See page 232 to cook your own from scratch, but I always keep a few cans in the pantry for backup. Fast, easy, no excuses.

Lupini Beans
Lupini beans get their own shout-out because they're absolute protein machines. They've got more protein per bite than any other bean, and they're an easy addition to almost anything savory when I need a quick macro boost. Plus, their firm, hearty texture makes them a great gateway legume for anyone who thinks they're "not into beans" — no mush, no fuss, just straight-up power.

Lentils
Lentils are one of the all-time unsung heroes — high in protein, loaded with fiber, and they cook quickly. While green, brown, and black lentils hold their shape beautifully for salads, soups, or grain bowls, red and yellow lentils shine as thickeners in soups, stews, and curries. See page 233 for the breakdown on how to cook them to perfection.

Tofu
Silken, firm, extra firm — each kind of tofu has a job to do. Silken makes a creamy base for sauces or sneaks extra protein into pastries (like my Chocolate Silk Pie on page 198). Firm and extra firm are where you get a hearty bite that makes plant-based meals feel extra satisfying and filling.

Seitan
Seitan is *the* protein MVP — meaty texture, crazy high protein, and endlessly versatile. It's made from vital wheat gluten and while you can buy it in the store for easy meal prep, you can make your own (page 222). Either way, it's a plant-based game changer offering 31 grams of protein per serving.

TVP (Textured Vegetable Protein)
TVP is the ultimate shape-shifter — it starts out dry and crumbly, but once you hydrate it, it transforms into a toothsome bite and is the perfect swap for ground meat in tacos, burgers, or Bolognese. Plus, it soaks up flavor like crazy and brings serious protein — 23 grams per serving. Keep a bag in your pantry, and you'll never be more than a few minutes away from an easy high-protein meal.

Protein Pasta
Protein pasta is my secret weapon for keeping carbs working hard. Kaizen is my go-to brand — their pasta cooks up perfectly al dente and packs serious protein to keep you full and focused. Keep some in your pantry, and you'll always have a powerhouse meal ready in minutes.

Protein Powder

I like to keep a few flavors — vanilla, chocolate, and strawberry — for drinks (Peppermint Hot Chocolate, page 53, or Drew's Famous Smoothie, page 49) and sneaking into desserts (like Gooey Cinnamon Rolls, page 186, and Sweet Potato Pie Bars, page 205). I also keep one made with pea protein, which carries a neutral flavor that slides into recipes totally unnoticed. There are a million options out there, so do your homework — look for brands that back up their claims with research and also use third-party testing to check for heavy metals and other contaminants.

Nondairy Milk

I stick with unsweetened soy milk because it's got the best protein punch — about 8 grams per cup. But any plant-based milk will work in these recipes — just keep an eye on the protein content if that's your focus.

Vegan Butter

A good vegan butter makes all the difference, whether I'm spreading it on toast or using it to bring richness to baked goods. Go for one with a creamy texture for the best results.

Vegan Greek Yogurt

Thicker, tangier, and higher in protein than regular plant-based yogurt, vegan Greek yogurt is my go-to for everything. Look for one with an almond base and a creamy and rich texture, just like the real deal. If you can't find it near you, any unsweetened vegan yogurt will work in a pinch (strain in a cheesecloth-lined sieve set over a bowl overnight in the fridge for a thicker consistency). Heads up: always check your yogurt labels — some plant-based yogurt brands have a lot more protein than others.

Sweeteners

Coconut sugar is my go-to, but I also love maple syrup and agave syrup when I need a liquid sweetener. I try to avoid refined sugar where I can. Honey is a personal choice, but if you use it, it works as a 1:1 swap for agave.

Oils

I keep three on rotation:

- **Avocado oil** for high-heat cooking and a boost of healthy fats
- **Extra-virgin olive oil** for finishing, dressings, and low-heat cooking
- **Refined coconut oil** when I need a neutral flavor for baking

Tamari or Soy Sauce

Both add serious umami. Tamari is gluten-free, while soy sauce is not. Use whichever works for you — just don't skip it. A splash makes everything taste better.

Nutritional Yeast

Cheesy flavor, packed with protein, and rich in B vitamins (we're talking up to 8 grams of protein and a full day's worth of B_{12} per serving!)? Nutritional yeast — made from deactivated yeast that's grown on molasses — earns its place in my pantry. I sprinkle it on everything from popcorn to pasta and use it in all of my cooking.

Spices

A well-stocked spice rack makes plant-based cooking anything but boring. My essentials:

- **Dried oregano** — piney, herby backbone
- **Ground cumin** — deep, warm, and earthy
- **Smoked paprika** — a little smoke, a lot of sweet pepper depth
- **Red pepper flakes** — for when you need a spicy kick
- **Sazón** — an instant, all-over flavor upgrade made from a blend of spices like coriander, cumin, garlic, and annatto (for that signature orange hue). It's a pantry shortcut that packs a punch in proteins, rice, and stews.

Kosher Salt

I use Diamond Crystal for the recipes in this book. If you're using Morton or table salt, cut the amount in half — Morton is denser, and adding too much can derail a dish real quick.

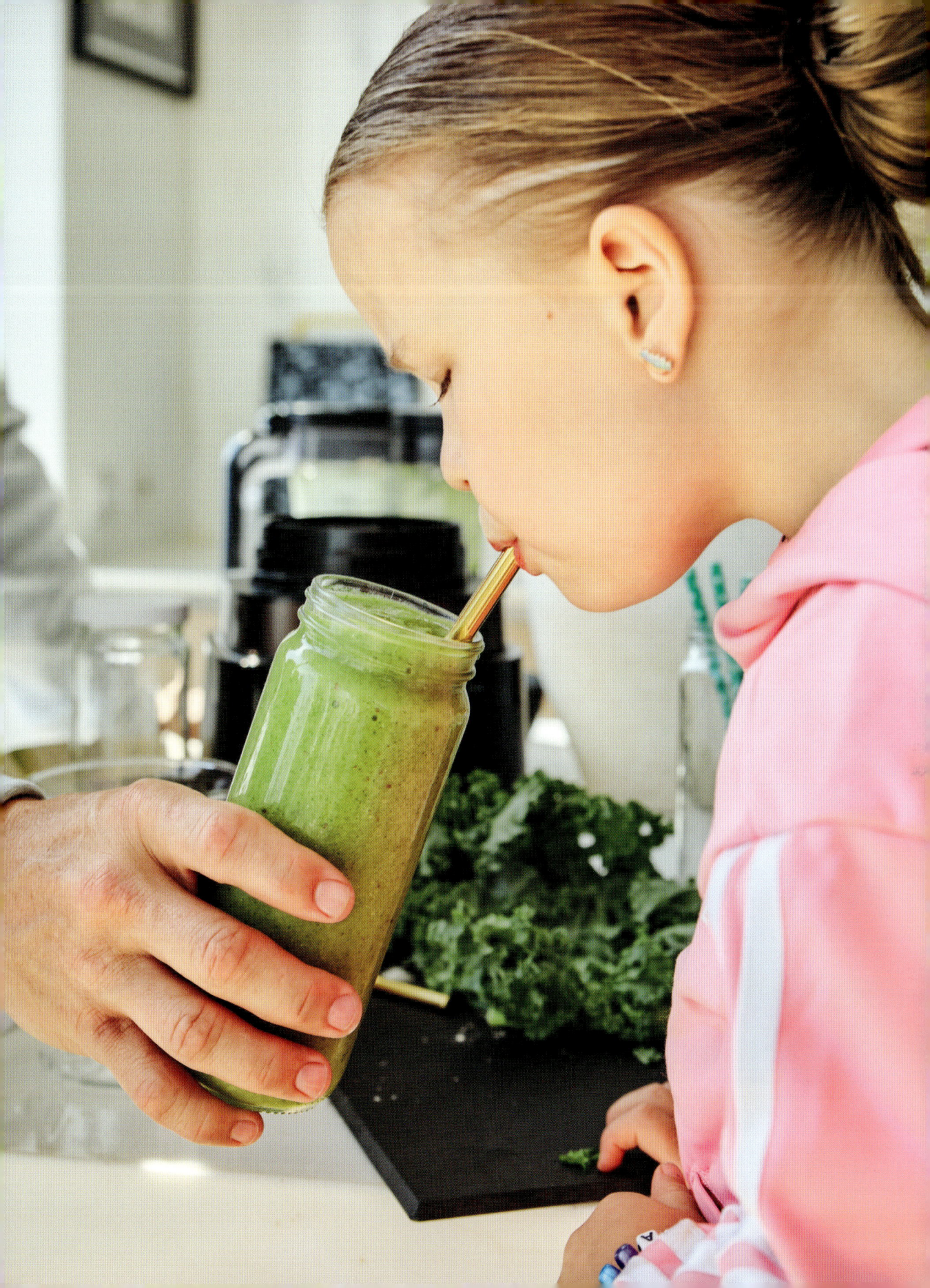

TOOLS OF THE TRADE

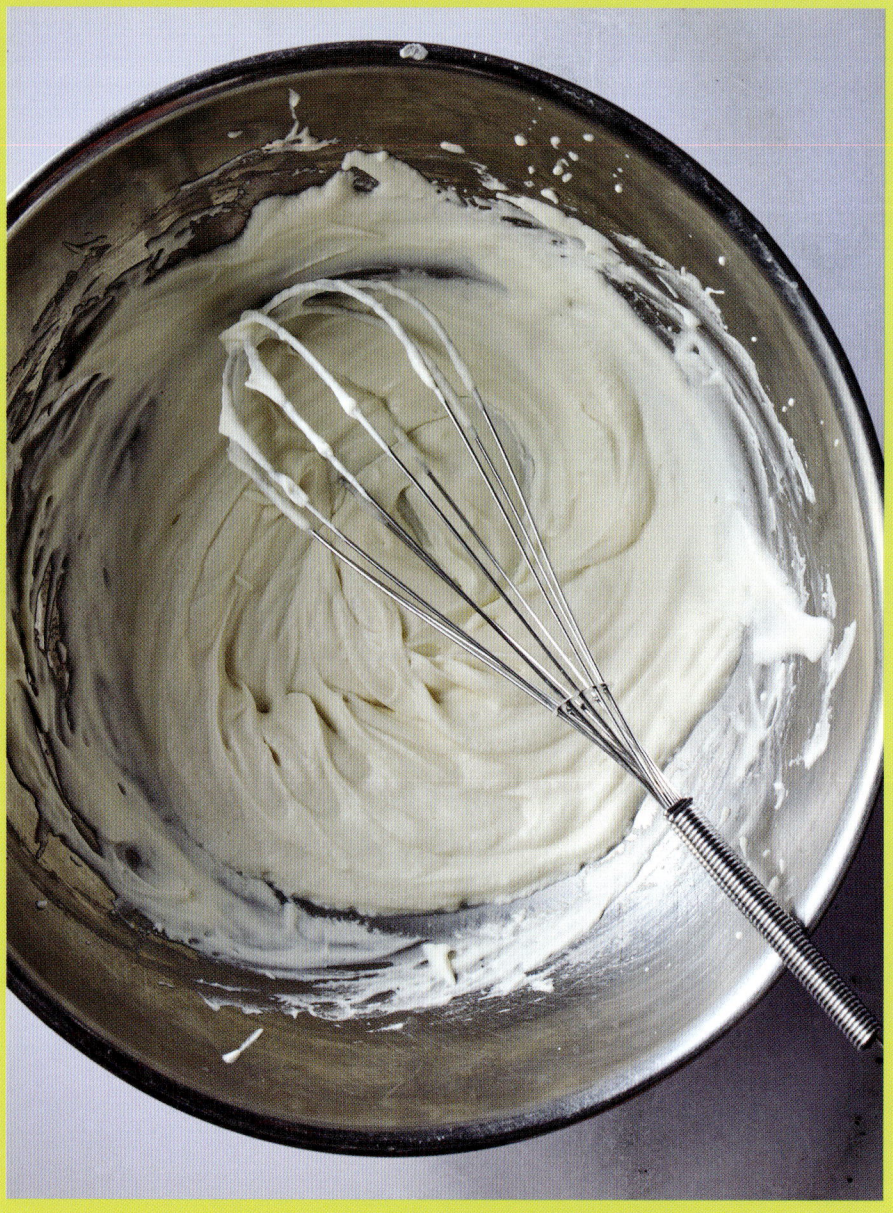

You don't need a kitchen packed with every gadget under the sun—just a few solid tools that make cooking easier, faster, and more fun. This section covers the essentials I use to whip up everything in this book. Stock your kitchen with the right gear, and you'll be ready to tackle any recipe like a pro!

Blender and Food Processor
A solid blender is a kitchen must for smoothies, sauces, and batters. If you get a high-powered one like a Ninja, it can sometimes pull double duty as a food processor for slicing, dicing, and whipping up dips in seconds (and saving you precious counter space).

Cast-Iron Skillet
This pan goes everywhere — on the stove, in the oven, and even on the grill. It holds heat like a champ, gives the best sear, and lasts forever (as long as you treat it right: wash it gently, dry it completely, and keep it seasoned with a little neutral oil). And they're pretty inexpensive, too.

Nonstick Skillet
For those moments when you don't feel like scrubbing. Essential for quick stovetop cooking — think pancakes, scrambled tofu, and anything that benefits from an easy release.

Dutch Oven
If soups, stews, and braises are in your rotation, this is your best friend. Heavy, sturdy, and built to handle long, slow cooking for maximum flavor.

Rimmed Baking Sheet
Don't sleep on a good sheet pan — it's not just for cookies. Whether you're roasting veggies, making pizza, or just getting your prep organized, this is the (cheap) workhorse that does it all.

Mixing Bowls
Get a set of metal or glass bowls in various sizes — you'll thank yourself later. Whether you're tossing a salad, mixing batter, or marinating protein, having options keeps things moving.

Measuring Cups and Spoons
Because eyeballing works — until it doesn't. Precise measurements make sure your bakes rise, your seasonings are balanced, and your macros stay on point.

Chef's Knife
An 8-inch chef's knife is your ride-or-die. A good one makes chopping faster, easier, and way more satisfying. Keep it sharp, and it'll do the work for you.

Whisk, Spatula, Wooden Spoon, and Tongs
The kitchen dream team. Whisk for sauces and batters, spatula for flipping and scraping, wooden spoon for stirring, and tongs for grabbing, turning, and plating like a pro.

Storage Containers
Meal prep, leftovers, snacks on the go — you need somewhere to stash it all. Look for glass or BPA-free plastic with airtight lids that are stackable for maximum cupboard efficiency.

FACT CHECK: VEGAN MYTHS BUSTED

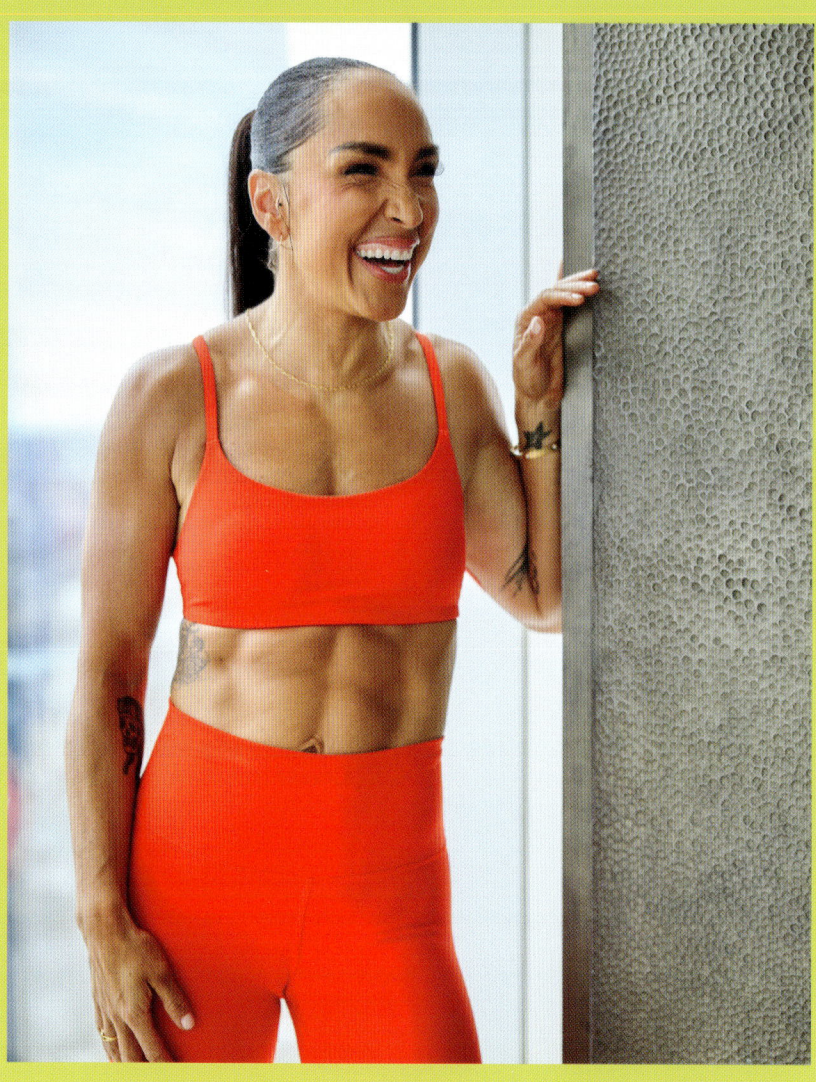

The myths around plant-based diets just won't quit, so let's put these outdated misconceptions to rest, once and for all.

MYTH: Vegans Don't Get Enough Protein

Everyone's favorite question is "But where do you get your protein?" Listen up: Plants have protein! Beans, lentils, tofu, tempeh, quinoa, nuts, seeds — even veggies like broccoli and Brussels sprouts are great sources. A cup of lentils has 18 grams of protein. That's equal to three scrambled eggs. According to recent studies (see Sources, page 242), people who eat only plants build muscle just as well as people who eat meat.

Need some real-life proof? Venus Williams, seven-time Grand Slam singles champion and four-time Olympic gold medalist. Deatrich Wise Jr., Super Bowl champion and defensive end for the New England Patriots. Kyrie Irving, NBA champion and eight-time All-Star. Scott Jurek, ultra-endurance legend. Lewis Hamilton, Formula 1 driver. Rich Roll, ultra-endurance athlete and bestselling author. I train 2 to 3 hours a day, most days of the week, from riding at Peloton to weightlifting to race prep. We're all thriving on plants and seeing long-lasting results in our careers.

Fact Check: Next time someone asks where you get your protein, hit them with "From plants, obviously."

Dalina says: Lentils, beans, tofu, tempeh, soy milk, whole grains, and nuts/seeds provide all the amino acids your body needs to form proteins. The goal is to eat a variety of foods and to make sure your aminos come from various sources throughout the day.

MYTH: Being Vegan Is Expensive

One of the biggest myths about plant-based eating is that it requires a trust fund to make it through the week. In reality, it's a diet based on some of the most affordable, accessible foods — legumes, grains, and in-season produce. A pound of dried beans is a fraction of the cost of a pound of ground meat and it'll last you way longer — both in your fridge and pantry.

Think about the layout of a grocery store. The perimeter — the place where all the fresh produce, whole grains, and staple ingredients live — is usually cheaper than the processed, packaged foods in the center aisles or prepared foods in the freezer sections. When you build meals around whole foods at the perimeter, you're not just getting more nutrition per dollar — you're also skipping the mystery ingredients and unnecessary additives that you really don't want to be eating anyway.

Now, let's be real: If your shopping cart is full of artisan nut cheeses, mock meats, and prepackaged vegan snacks, your bill *will* add up. All those things are fine, but they're accessories, not essentials (and you should limit the processed stuff anyway). This book sticks to recipes that build whole foods into satisfying meals that won't break the bank.

Fact Check: Eating plant-based won't just fuel your body — it'll fuel your bank account, too.

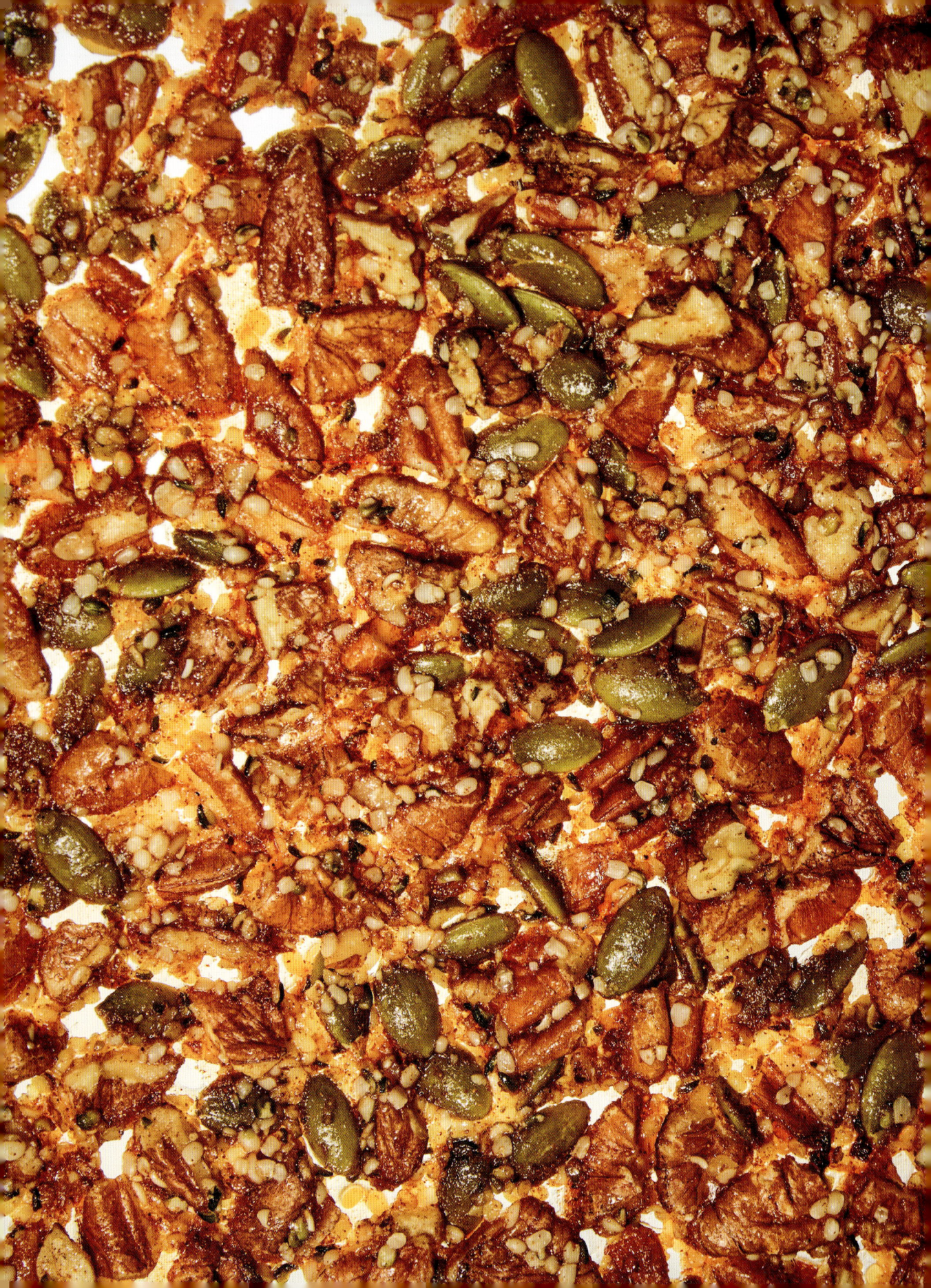

MYTH: Soy Will Mess with Your Hormones

People love throwing around that one outdated study, and I'm here to say the "soy is bad for you" narrative needs to be put to bed. I get my blood work done a few times a year — iron, B_{12}, vitamin D, and especially hormones. All solid. Entire continents have been eating soy for centuries without any epidemic of hormone imbalances.

Soy contains isoflavones, a type of plant compound that can bind to estrogen receptors, but they do not act like human estrogen. Studies have debunked the myth that soy lowers testosterone or messes with hormones (see Sources, page 242). What soy *does* do is provide a high-quality, complete protein that supports muscle growth, recovery, and long-term health. That said, it's important to opt for organic soy whenever possible — soybeans are one of the worst crops for pesticide and GMO use, which can have a big impact on your health. And remember, as with anything, diversity is the best mantra, so make sure soy is working with an array of plant proteins in your diet.

Fact Check: Soy is too busy fueling your body to bother with your hormones.

Dalina Says: This myth is rooted in fear. Soy contains phytoestrogens—not estrogen—and phytoestrogens do not interfere with hormone levels in the way people may think they do. Many Asian cultures consume soy daily (and in larger amounts than most Western diets) with no negative hormonal effects. In fact, soy may even support heart and bone health.

MYTH: Vegans Can't Get Enough Nutrients

Yes, vegans need to be mindful — just like everyone else because nutrition gaps aren't exclusive to vegans — but you can get almost everything you need from plants. My morning routine includes my nonnegotiables:

B_{12}: Since it's harder to get from plants, supplementation is a must (see Sources, page 242). (And fun fact: Even farmed animals get B_{12} supplements, so really, we're just cutting out the middleman.)

Vitamin D: Because sunshine isn't always enough, and deficiency is common across *all* diets (see Sources, page 242).

Creatine: The holy grail for muscle retention, brain function, and energy, and some studies show it can even combat symptoms of depression. Creatine is moving past the gym bro reputation into one of the most widely studied and beneficial supplements. (It's especially beneficial for women looking to hold on to muscle as they age.) (See Sources, page 240.)

Remember, vegans actually get *more* of many essential nutrients than the average nonvegan. We're talking fiber, antioxidants, vitamins A, C, and E, magnesium, and potassium (see Sources, page 242). So, when it comes to health, vegans are often walking around with the nutritional upper hand.

Fact Check: The next time someone asks you where you get your nutrients, go ahead and ask them where they get their fiber.

Dalina Says: While it's true that some nutrients—like B_{12}, iron, omega-3s, and zinc—need to be supplemented when on a vegan diet, it's very possible to meet your body's needs with eating fortified foods and taking supplements as needed. A vegan plate can be just as rich in flavor, fiber, and nourishment as any other.

MYTH: Carbs Are the Enemy

We need to stop villainizing carbs because they are literally your body's fuel. As a type 1 diabetic, I learned early on to make my carbs work for me — I plan them, time them, and use them throughout the day when I need to be at peak performance. For example, I wouldn't load up on a carb-heavy dinner right before comfy pants couch mode, but starting my day with a carb-fueled breakfast powers me straight through my morning workout and into the start of my day.

Complex carbohydrates — like those found in whole grains, legumes, and vegetables — are some of the best sources of long-lasting energy, gut healthy fiber, and steady performance fuel you can get (see Sources, page 242). The key is to pair carbs with fiber and protein to help keep blood sugar steady, so instead of an energy spike and crash, you get sustained fuel. Eating beans with your rice, protein-rich hummus with whole-grain crackers, and yogurt with a little granola (it's not meant to be eaten like cereal!) are all great examples. Think about it this way: chugging a glass of orange juice spikes and crashes your sugar; eating an orange offers fiber to help with a slow and steady release of energy.

Fact Check: Carbs aren't the enemy. Bad nutrition advice is.

Dalina Says: Carbs are your body's preferred source of fuel. On a vegan or plant-based diet, many carbs come attached to fiber, vitamins, and minerals—think beans, fruits, sweet potatoes, plantains, and rice. These foods support stable energy, digestion, and even blood sugar regulation when paired with protein and fats. Demonizing carbs leaves out their cultural and nutritional importance. Also it is very important to point out that nine out of ten Americans do not eat enough fiber, and incorporating more plant-based proteins in our day can also help us meet our fiber goals.

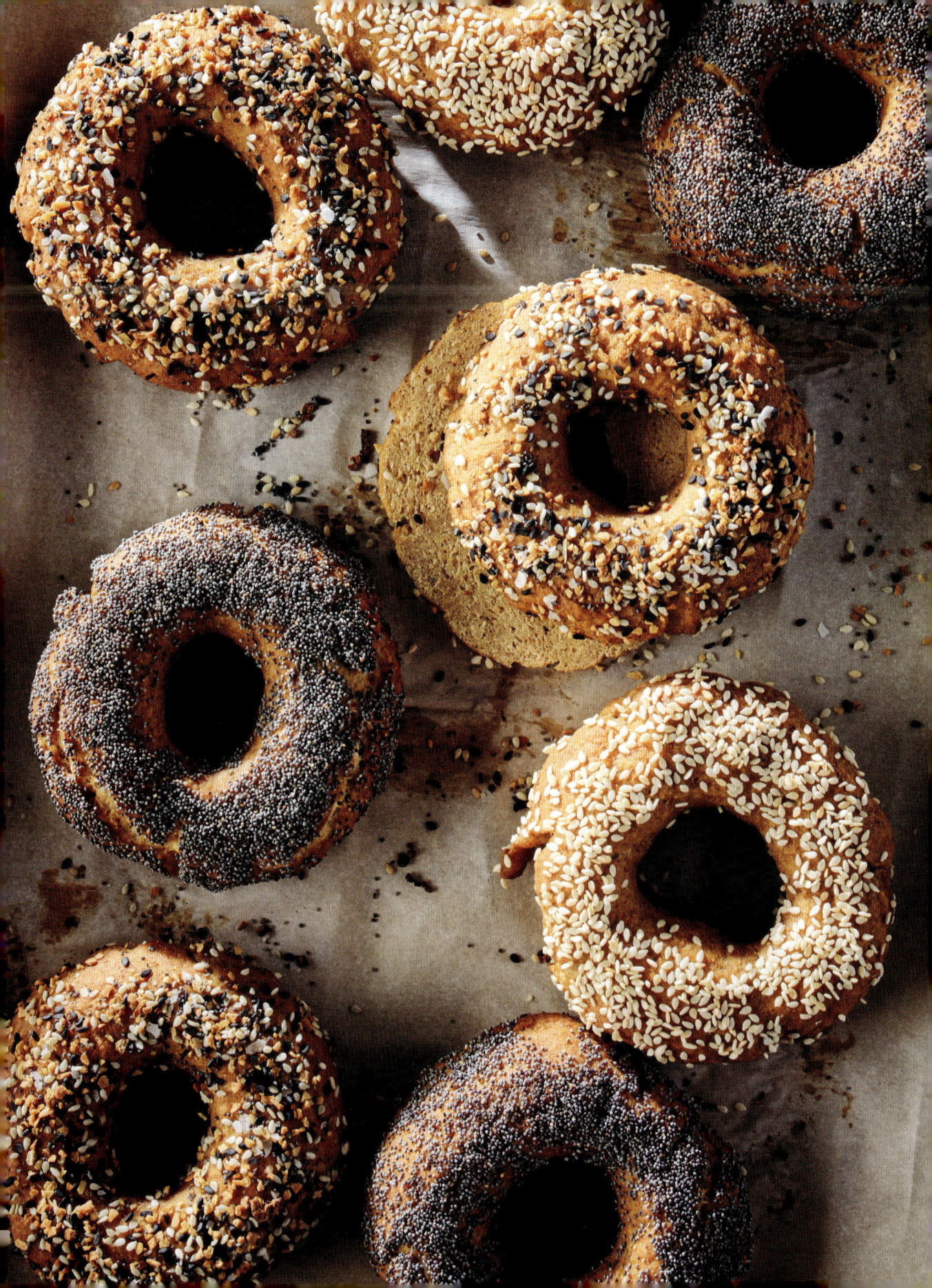

HEALTH MATTERS

The goal isn't to get through life—it's to dominate it. Food is fuel, and every bite is a chance to nourish, strengthen, and elevate. Whether you're managing a health condition, navigating big life transitions, or just looking to level up your recovery game, a plant-based diet is one of the best tools in your arsenal. Let's break it down.

Type 1 Diabetes

A lot of people assume that living with type 1 diabetes means you can't be plant-based. "But what about all the carbs?" they ask, like I haven't been navigating this every day. I've always been health-conscious, and I would live this way no matter what. The key isn't cutting carbs — it's understanding how to balance them with protein, fiber, and energy expenditure so that my blood sugar stays stable. For example, I drink half of my morning smoothie before my workout to fuel myself and half after to recharge, with a snack at the ready in case my sugar drops.

I know how my body responds to food, movement, and macros because I track them — not obsessively, but strategically. I plan my meals so that when I'm fueling up for a workout, my carbs are paired with protein and fiber to prevent spikes and crashes (this can be as simple as a protein-packed smoothie or a yogurt with granola). I time my meals around my training so my energy is sustained — carbs before a workout for fuel, extra protein after for recovery. As I've increased my muscle mass through the years, my insulin management has become easier. Muscle mass and insulin sensitivity are closely related, and higher muscle mass is generally associated with improved insulin sensitivity for all people, not just those with T1D (see Sources, page 243).

Even on my most dialed-in days, I can have unexpected blood sugar highs or lows. That's why I always carry a carb source that also includes protein, like a banana with almond butter or a protein bar made with real ingredients. It helps me correct a low while also giving my body something more substantial than candy or those overly processed 'low' snacks. Living with T1D isn't about restriction; it's about optimization. My diagnosis didn't limit me — it made me sharper, more intentional, and more aware of what my body needs to perform at its best.

Perimenopausal/Menopausal

If you're in perimenopause or menopause, you already know that your body is changing, and that change can hit hard. The old rules don't apply anymore: the types and amount of food you used to eat may no longer work for you because your metabolism has slowed. Even though you're still working out just as hard — or even harder — doing the same routines you've always done, your muscle mass may start to decline. In short, the diet and exercise that worked before aren't delivering the same results. It can be frustrating and overwhelming, but here's the good news: protein is your best friend, and this book is your new secret weapon.

Protein is crucial for preserving and building muscle, which in turn helps support bone health and prevent osteoporosis. More muscle means a stronger metabolism, better energy levels, and greater resilience as you move through this stage of life (see Sources, page 243). I know there's already so much information coming at you about what you "should" be doing, so my goal here isn't to overwhelm you — it's to make things simple. You don't need a complete overhaul. You just need to make informed, empowered choices at mealtime. Check out page 16 for a protein primer that will guide you toward the right amount you need to meet your goals.

Inflammation and Recovery

I couldn't do what I do — hours of training, marathons, ultra races, strength workouts — without a plant-based diet. When you train hard, your muscles break down. Your joints take a beating. Your body is constantly working to recover and rebuild. Plant-based eating fights inflammation like nothing else. Animal products can increase inflammation, but plants do the opposite — they help your body heal faster (see Sources, page 243).

I've seen it firsthand, from my own postpartum recoveries to my ultra-endurance training. And I'm not the only one — elite athletes and Olympians swear by plant-based eating for this exact reason. When your body isn't bogged down by excess inflammation, you move better, recover faster, and stay in the game longer.

The way we fuel ourselves determines how strong, energized, and resilient we feel. Whether you're managing a health condition, navigating menopause, or pushing your body to new limits — or all three! — food is one of the most powerful tools you have. Use it wisely and watch what happens.

Dalina Says...

Your health matters—because how you *feel* matters. Whether you're managing diabetes, inflammation, or going through peri/menopause, nutrition can support your body in real, tangible ways. Having more stable blood sugar, feeling less joint pain, getting better sleep, and experiencing fewer energy crashes are all things that can make day-to-day life feel more manageable—and more joyful. And we need to be eating enough and consistently for our body to feel better.

I'd also like to point out that health is *not* a moral obligation. Some people are born with conditions like type 1 diabetes, and others do all the "right" things and still get sick. That's not a failure—it's part of being human. The goal isn't perfection, it's supporting your body with what you have, and where you are. Moving your body, eating more fiber and plants, and reducing stress can make a difference—but they don't define your worth. Health is personal, it's fluid, and it's not a pass/fail grade.

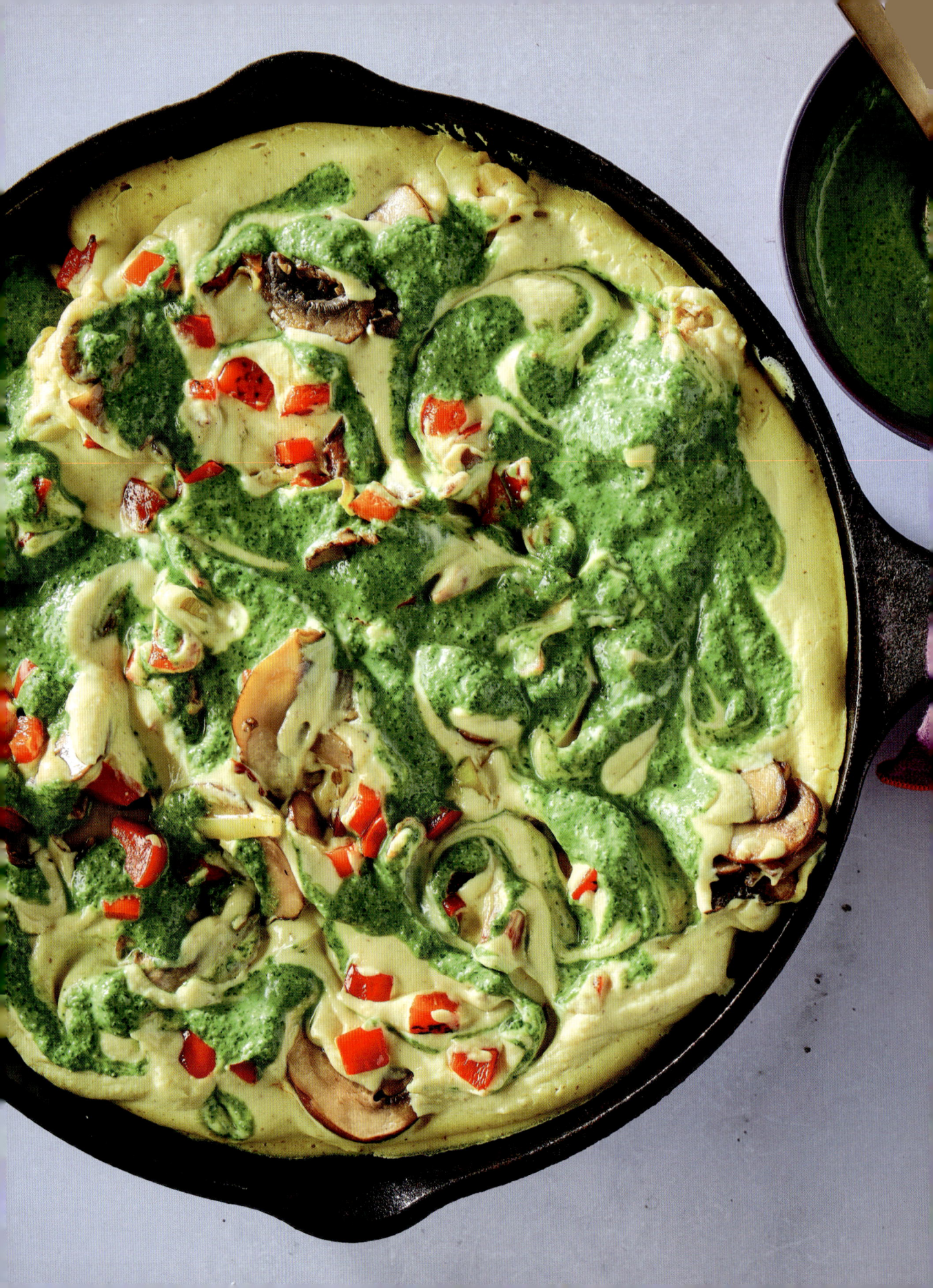

MORNING ROUTINES

Mornings set the tone for everything that follows, and a strong start means a strong finish. I need a breakfast that works as hard as I do — one that fuels my body, keeps me full, and powers me through whatever the day throws my way. On busy weekdays, I try to prep meals with carbs for sustenance and high protein to keep my energy steady and my focus locked in. But life is about balance, and you'll also find a few of my kids' favorites in here — like a smart update on waffles — that we all feel good about enjoying, especially on the weekends. This chapter is packed with high-protein, no-nonsense breakfasts. Whether you're sitting down for a slow morning or grabbing something on the go, these meals make sure you start the day right. When you eat to hustle, breakfast isn't just the first meal — it's the launchpad.

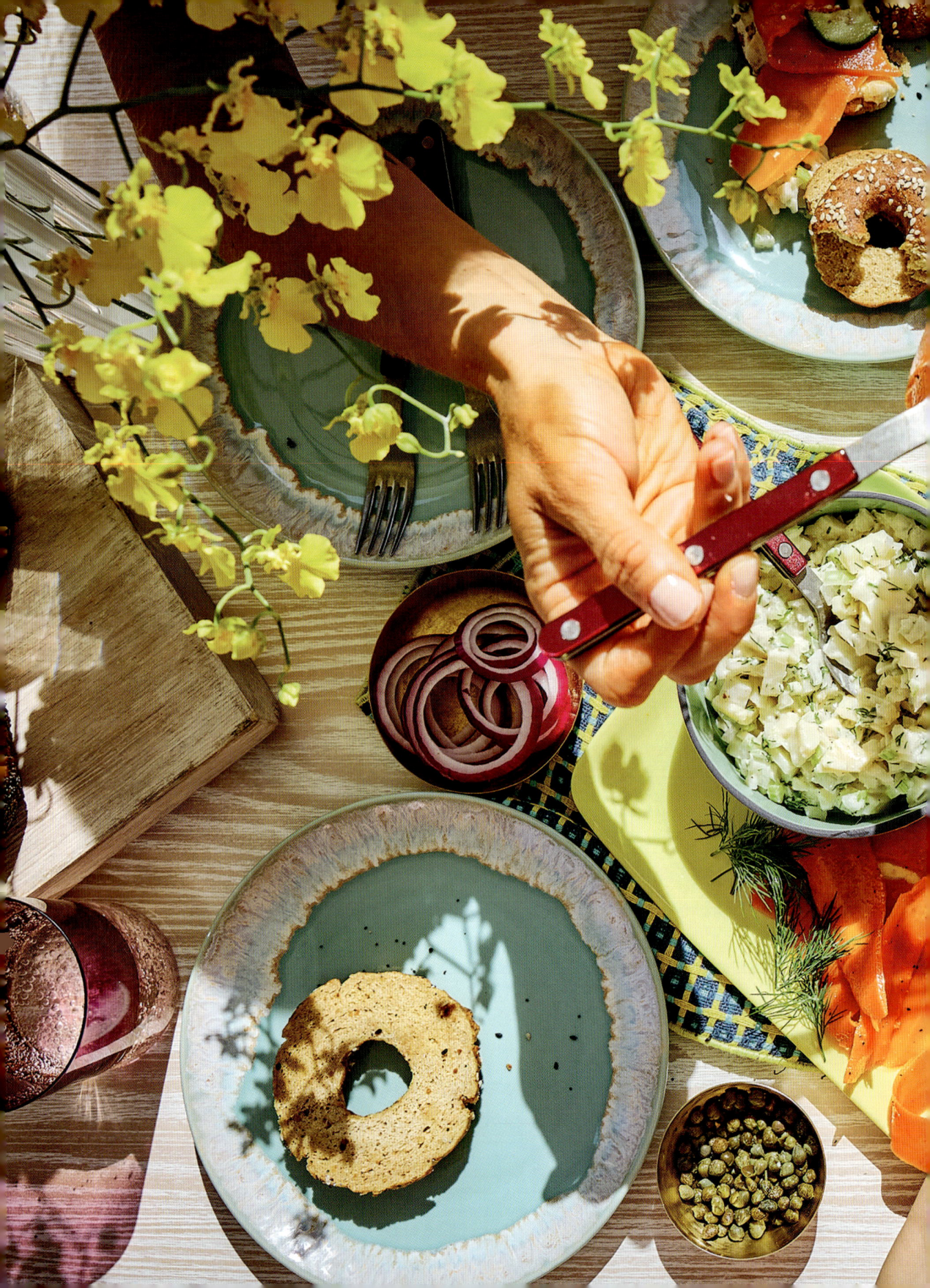

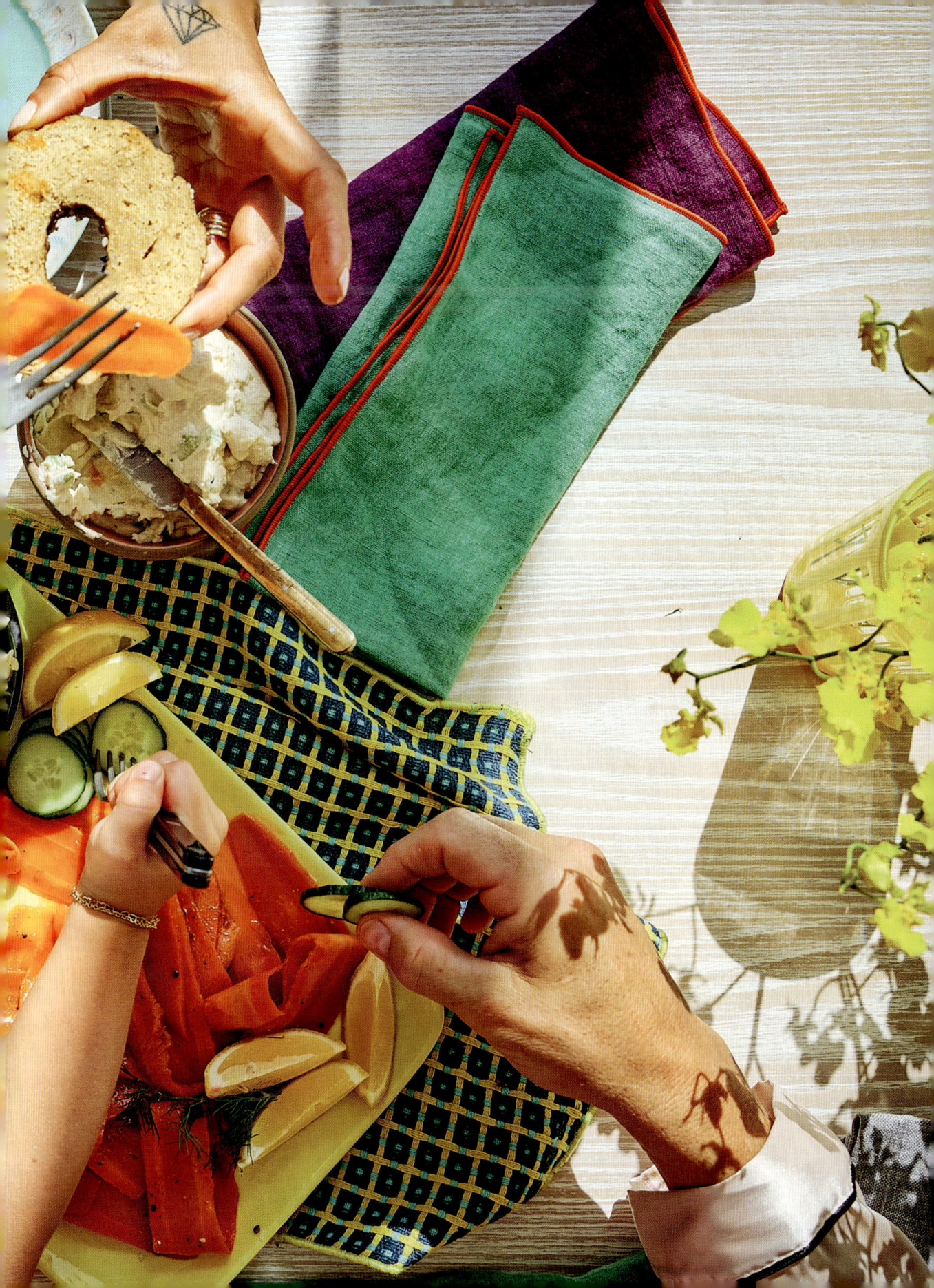

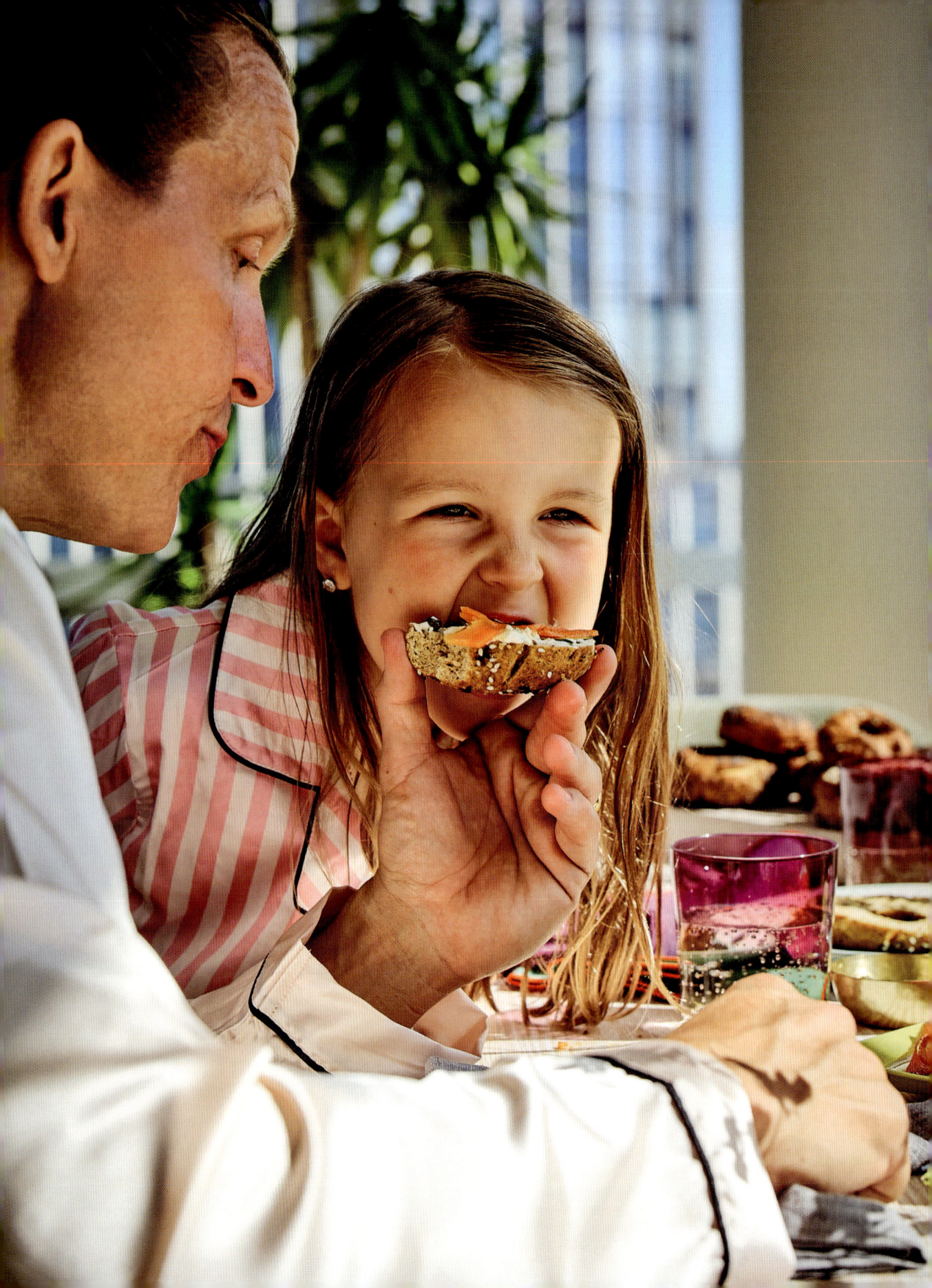

I'm a Jewish-Latina-New Yorker, so bagels and lox are a way of life. This plant-based version has all the hits: silky lox made from carrots, tangy tofu cream cheese, and a vegan whitefish salad so good, you won't believe there's no fish in it (the secret is the meaty hearts of palm). My family has been going strong with this tradition for years, and not just on weekends — we love laying out this spread on Christmas morning, too. Grab a bagel, stack it high, and don't skimp on the capers.

SERVES 8

A WEEKEND JEWISH DELI BREAKFAST

Roast the carrots: Preheat the oven to 400°F. In an 8 by 8-inch baking pan, evenly space the carrots (yes, left whole) and heavily season with salt. Roast the carrots until fork tender, about 40 minutes. Remove from the oven and set aside on a cutting board to cool.

While the carrots roast and cool, make the tofu cream cheese: In a food processor or blender, combine the tofu, yogurt, coconut oil, lemon juice, salt, nutritional yeast, and onion powder. Process, stopping to scrape down the sides, until smooth. Fold in the scallions and taste for seasoning, then transfer to an airtight container. Refrigerate for at least 30 minutes to set, or for up to 1 week.

Carrot Lox
3 medium carrots
Kosher salt
¼ cup extra-virgin olive oil
¼ cup rice vinegar
3 tablespoons caper brine
1 tablespoon soy sauce
1 teaspoon smoked paprika
½ teaspoon freshly ground black pepper

Tofu Cream Cheese
14 ounces firm tofu, drained
½ cup plain vegan Greek yogurt
2 tablespoons refined coconut oil, melted
2 tablespoons fresh lemon juice
1 teaspoon kosher salt
1 teaspoon nutritional yeast
1 teaspoon onion powder
4 scallions, thinly sliced

Bagels with a Boost (page 212) or protein bagels, for serving
Fresh dill fronds, drained capers, and thinly sliced red onion, for serving

Carrot Lox, per serving — Calories: 146 | Fat: 14g | Carbs: 6g | Fiber: 2g | Protein: 1g

Recipe continues...

Morning Routines 37

Make the carrot lox: In a large airtight container, whisk together the olive oil, rice vinegar, caper brine, soy sauce, paprika, and pepper. Rub any excess salt off the cooled carrots. Use a vegetable peeler to carefully shave long, thin strips down the length of each carrot (they'll be soft from roasting, so go slowly and flip to get the other side, too!). Add the carrot strips to the container and toss to coat in the marinade. Cover and refrigerate for at least 30 minutes, but ideally overnight for better texture. The carrot lox can be refrigerated for up to 5 days.

Make the vegan whitefish salad: In a medium bowl, mix the hearts of palm, celery, onion, dill, lemon juice, mayonnaise, salt, liquid smoke, and pepper. Taste for seasoning. The salad can be served immediately or refrigerated in an airtight container for up to 5 days. The flavor only gets better over time.

To arrange breakfast, transfer the cream cheese and whitefish salad to separate bowls. Arrange the lox on a platter with the bagels (toasted or not), dill, capers, and onions. Let everyone dive in and make their own plate!

```
Dalina Says...
You've got carbs for energy, plant-based
satisfying creaminess (hello, tofu cream
cheese), and that smoky, savory carrot
"lox" for fiber and flavor. Plus, those veg-
gies are bringing antioxidants and anti-
inflammatory benefits, too.
```

Vegan Whitefish Salad

1 (14-ounce) can hearts of palm, drained and roughly chopped
1 celery stalk, finely chopped
½ small white onion, finely chopped
1 tablespoon finely chopped fresh dill
Juice of 1 lemon
1 tablespoon vegan mayonnaise, plus more as needed
1 teaspoon kosher salt
½ teaspoon liquid smoke
¼ teaspoon freshly ground black pepper

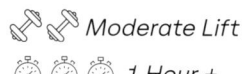 *Moderate Lift*

1 Hour +

Tofu Cream Cheese, per serving — Calories: 175 | Protein: 12g | Fat: 14g | Carbs: 5g | Fiber: 4g

Vegan Whitefish Salad, per serving — Calories: 60 | Protein: 4g | Fat: 2g | Carbs: 9g | Fiber: 4g

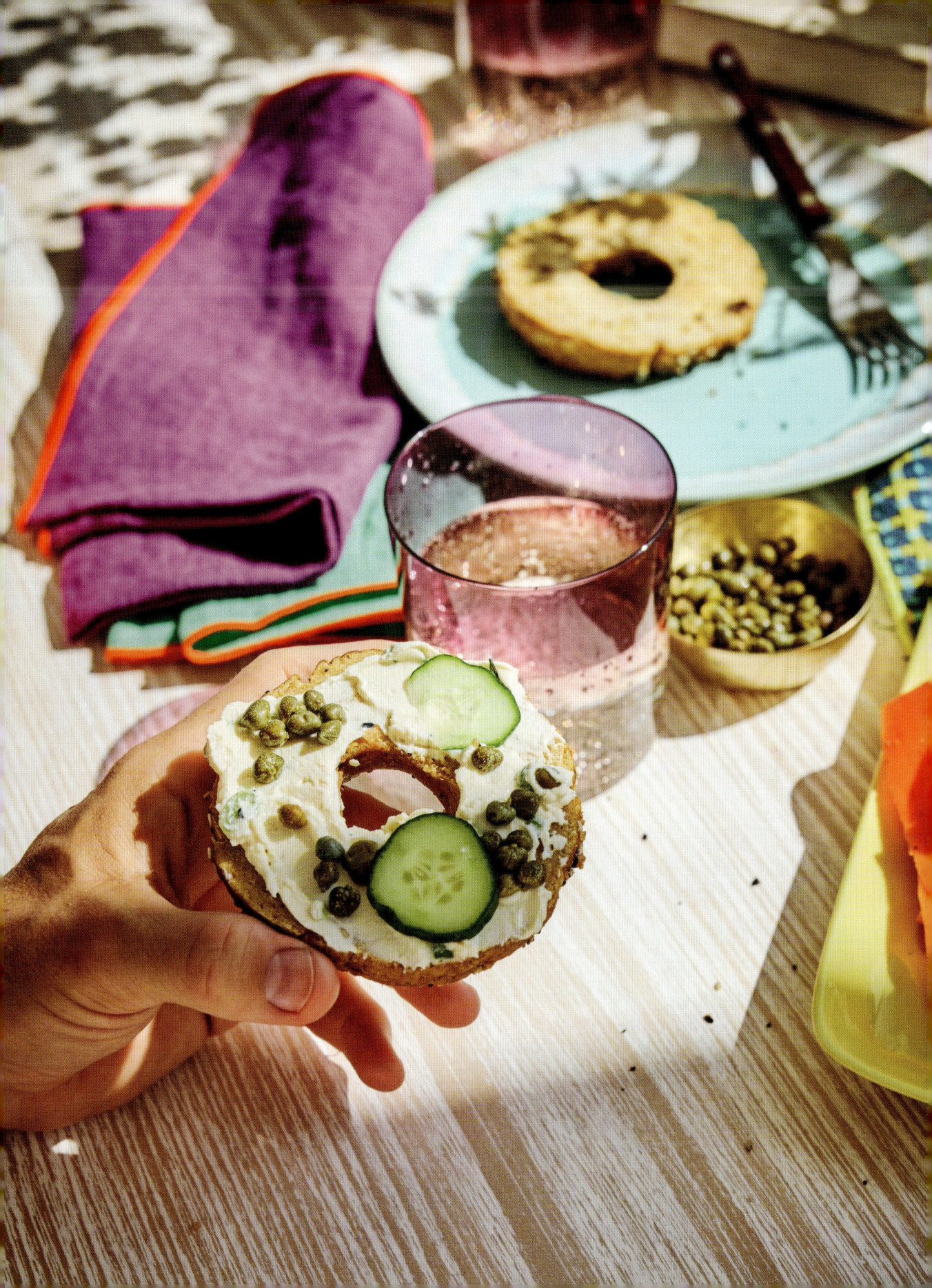

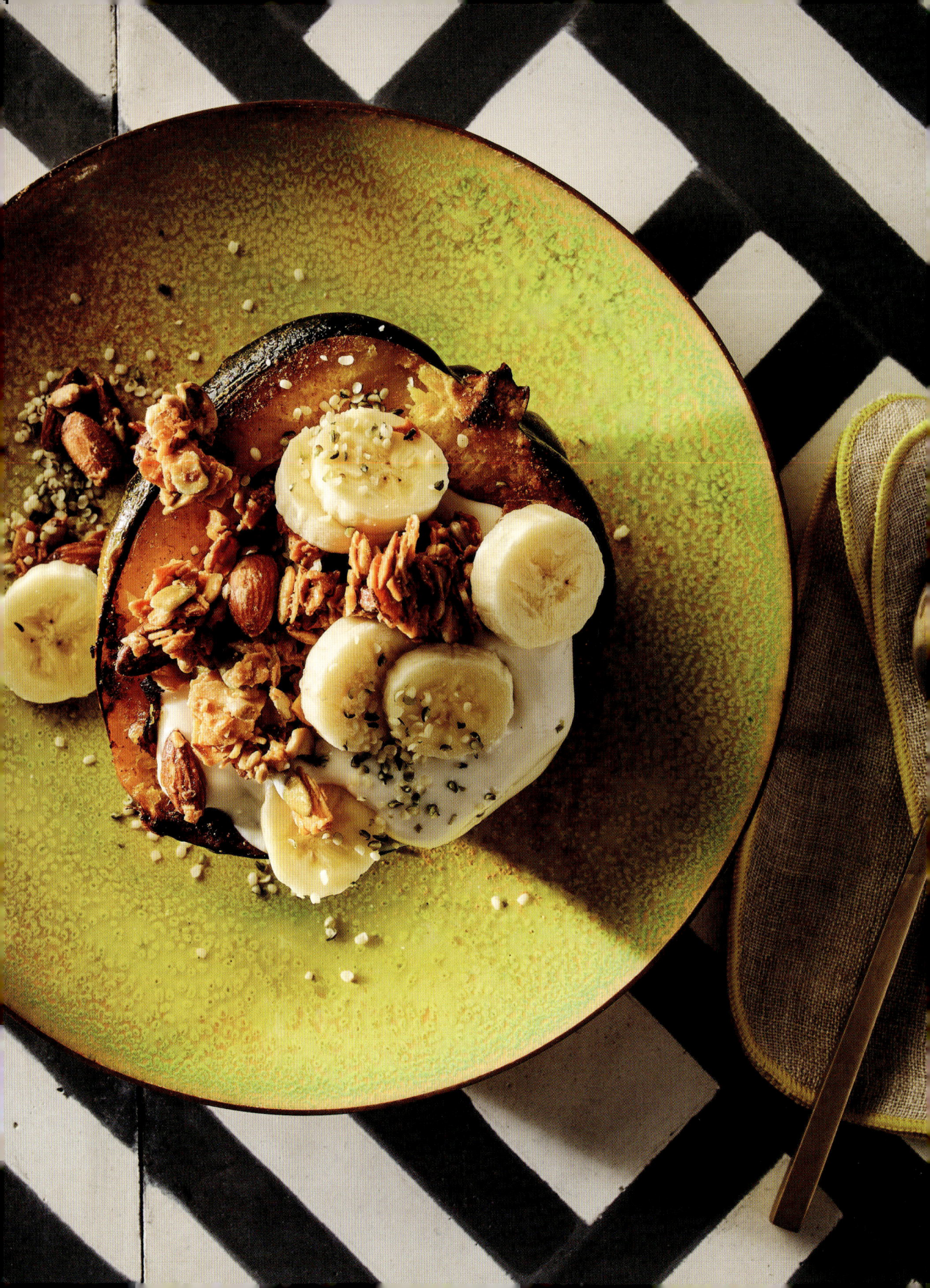

This is your morning meal prep game changer. You've seen acorn squash lurking around the grocery store or farmers' market and most likely wondered what to do with it — and probably only considered it for dinner. That's about to change. Simply roast a few halves at the start of the week, then fill them with whatever flavors you're craving that day. Here they get a scoop of yogurt and granola, a drizzle of maple syrup, and some bananas on top. These bowls are proof that cozy and nutritious food can live in the same bite.

SERVES 4

ACORN SQUASH BREAKFAST BOWLS

Preheat the oven to 400°F. Rub the cut sides of the squash with the olive oil and season with the salt. Arrange the 4 squash halves cut side down in a 9 by 13-inch baking pan. Pour 1 cup of water into the pan. Bake the squash until a knife easily slides into the flesh, about 1 hour. Remove the squash from the pan and let cool completely. The cooled squash can be refrigerated in airtight containers for up to 1 week.

Trim a little off the pointy/rounded side of each squash half so it sits flat like a bowl. Drizzle 1 tablespoon of the maple syrup and sprinkle ½ teaspoon of the cinnamon over the flesh of each, then fill the center with ½ cup of the yogurt, ¼ cup of the granola, and some banana slices, or any other protein-packed ingredients you love. Serve immediately.

Pro Tip: For days when I know I need the extra carbs to power me through, I add a scoop of nut butter and toasted pumpkin and hemp seeds on top.

- 2 medium acorn squash, halved, seeds scooped out
- 2 tablespoons extra-virgin olive oil
- 2 teaspoons kosher salt
- 4 tablespoons pure maple syrup
- 2 teaspoons ground cinnamon
- 2 cups plain vegan Greek yogurt
- 1 cup high-protein granola
- 1 banana, sliced

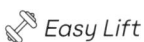 *Easy Lift*

 1 Hour +

Per serving

Calories: 405

Fat: 14g

Carbs: 52g

Fiber: 8g

Protein: 20g

Avocado toast is my go-to safety net when a menu's looking bleak on the vegan front. But let's be real — most places are phoning it in, and we can do better. Smashed edamame adds a protein punch, making the toast way more satisfying and filling. But the real game changers here are the toppings — one sweet, one savory — which take it to the next level. (Sweet on avocado? Trust me, it works.) These upgraded avo toasts will have your macros thanking you.

EACH VERSION MAKES 2 TOASTS, SERVING 1 TOTAL

ANYTHING-BUT-BASIC AVO TOAST

In a medium bowl, use a fork to mash the avocado and edamame into a chunky mixture. Add the lime juice and salt and stir to combine.

Divide the mixture and spread in large swoops on both slices of bread. Add any toppings and serve immediately.

1 ripe avocado, halved, pitted, and peeled
½ cup shelled edamame, thawed if frozen
Juice of 1 lime
½ teaspoon kosher salt
2 slices protein bread, store-bought or homemade (page 215), toasted
Toppings (see page 45)

 Easy Lift

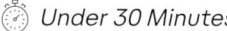 *Under 30 Minutes*

Recipe continues...

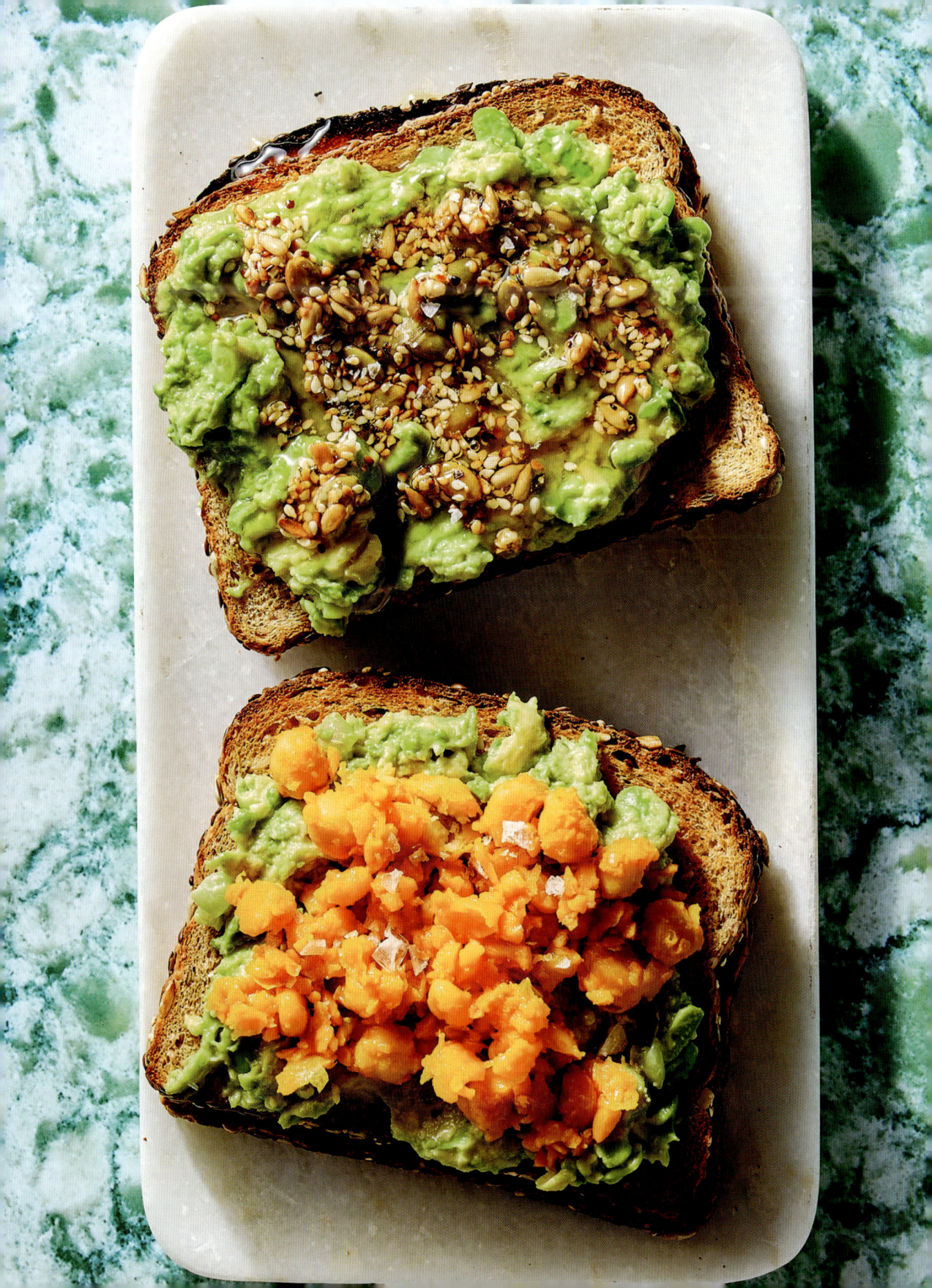

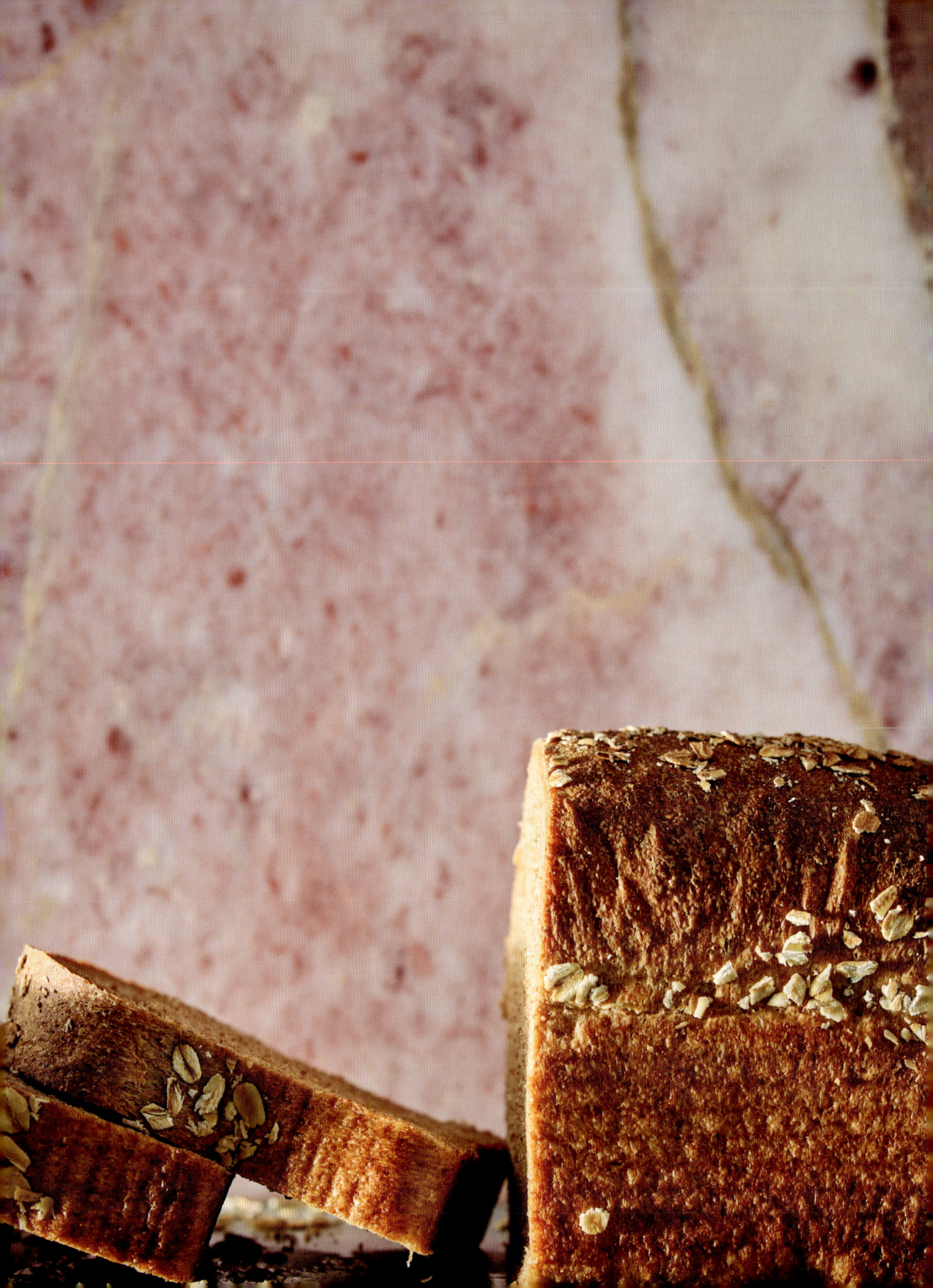

SWEET

In a small skillet, combine the hemp, sesame, pumpkin, and sunflower seeds. Set over low heat and stir frequently until the seeds are lightly toasted, about 5 minutes. Remove from the heat and stir in the agave. Spoon the mixture evenly over the avocado toasts.

1 tablespoon hemp seeds
1 tablespoon sesame seeds
1 tablespoon raw pumpkin seeds
1 tablespoon sunflower seeds
⅓ cup agave syrup

SAVORY

In a small skillet, arrange the chickpeas in an even layer, then use a potato masher to lightly smash them. Stir in ½ cup water and the sazón. Set over low heat and stir often until the water simmers away, about 5 minutes.

Remove from the heat, taste for seasoning, and add a pinch of salt. Spoon the mixture evenly over the avocado toasts.

1 cup drained cooked chickpeas
4 teaspoons sazón or chili powder
Kosher salt

	Sweet + Seedy	Savory Chickpea
Calories	551	480
Fat	23g	19g
Carbs	72g	53g
Fiber	11g	18g
Protein	23g	28g

Overnight oats walked so this parfait could run. It's got everything: creamy yogurt, nutty buckwheat, juicy berries, and a little crunch from chia and hemp seeds. The buckwheat adds a toasty, earthy flavor that plays well with the sweetness of the berries and the creaminess of the yogurt — unexpected in the best way. Plus, it's meal prep royalty — make a batch, stash them in the fridge, and, boom, breakfast (or snack) is handled for the week. Kids love it, adults feel like they've got their life together — it's a win-win. Since these are set up in individual containers, they are great for grab-and-go situations.

SERVES 4

BUCKWHEAT & BERRY PARFAITS

Line up four pint jars with lids. In each jar, layer ¼ cup of the yogurt, ¼ cup of the buckwheat, ¼ cup of the berries, 1 tablespoon of the chia seeds, and 1 tablespoon of the soy milk. The next layer is 2 tablespoons of the yogurt, another ¼ cup buckwheat, ¼ cup of the berries, and 1 tablespoon of the soy milk. The final layer in each is ¼ cup berries, 1 tablespoon maple syrup, 1 tablespoon hemp seeds, and a sprinkle of coconut flakes. Screw the lids on and refrigerate overnight or up to 5 days. Grab a quick and nourishing breakfast that's ready to go!

1 (16-ounce) container plain vegan Greek yogurt
2 cups cooked and cooled buckwheat (see Grains for Days, page 231)
3 cups frozen berries, any combination
4 tablespoons chia seeds
8 tablespoons unsweetened soy milk or other plant-based milk
4 tablespoons pure maple syrup
4 tablespoons hemp seeds
Unsweetened coconut flakes

 Easy Lift

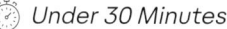 *Under 30 Minutes*

Per serving | Calories: 423 | Fat: 15g | Carbs: 54g | Fiber: 10g | Protein: 22g

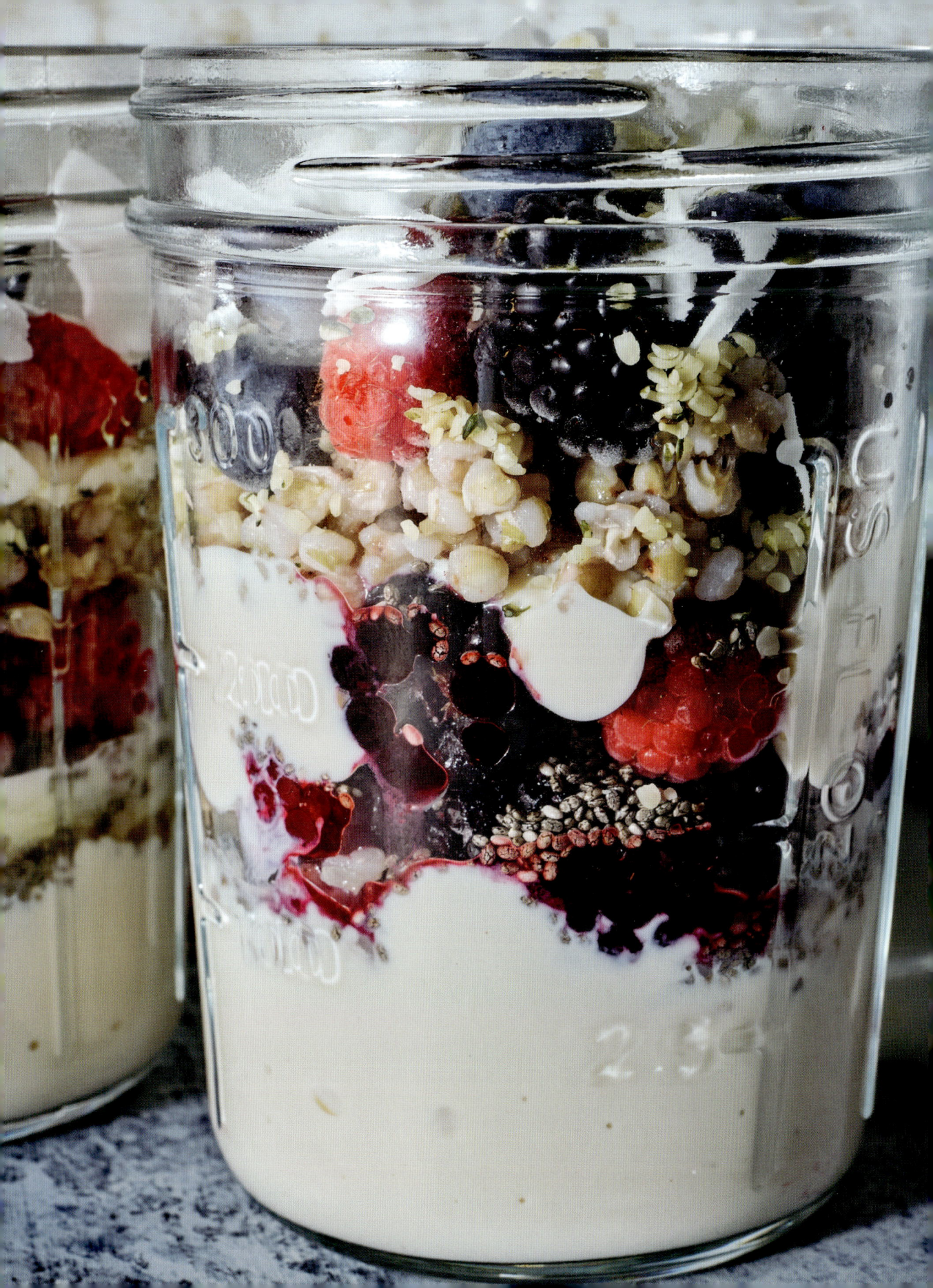

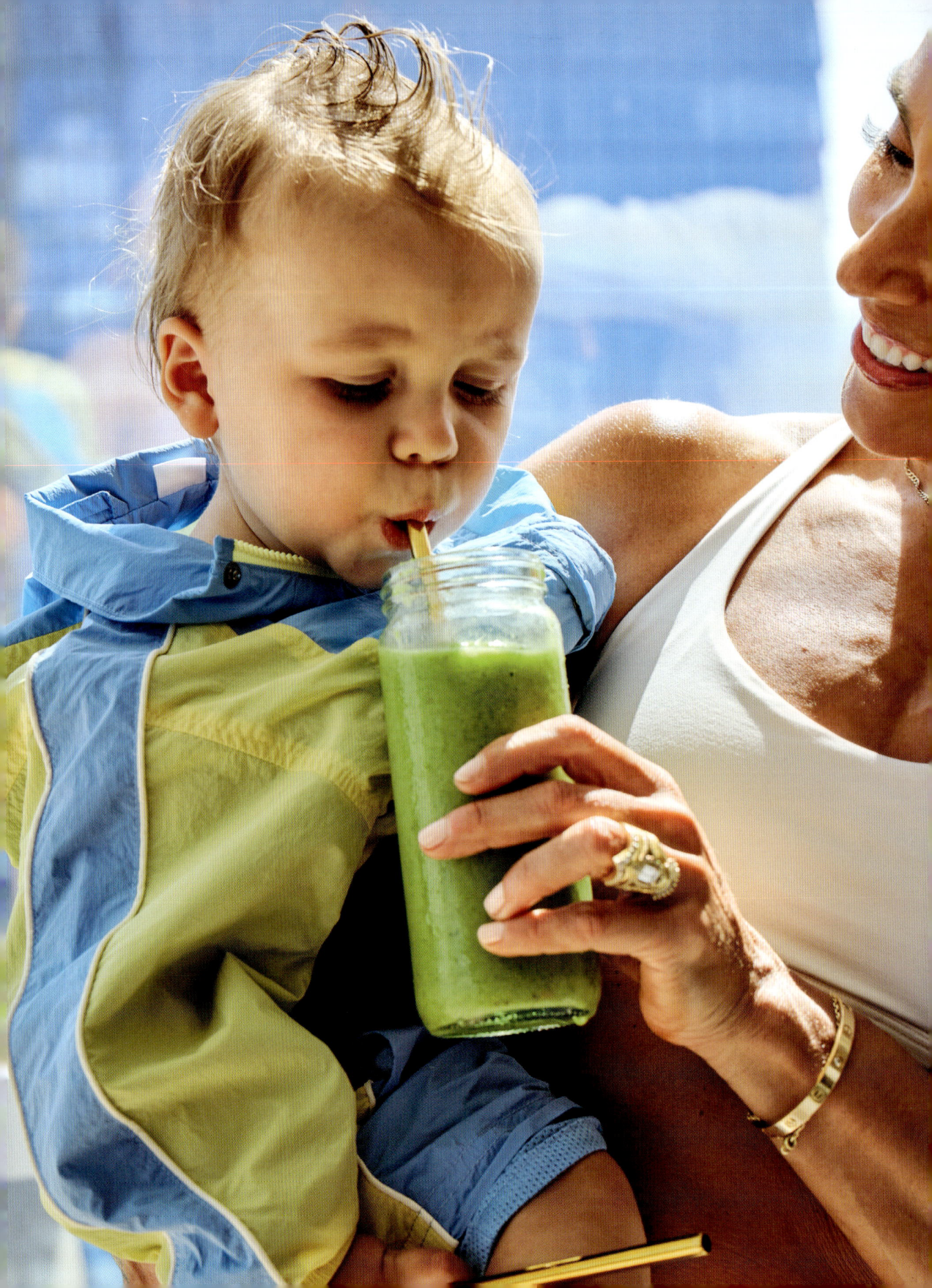

This is my 365, every-day-of-the-year, ride-or-die love of my life. Yes, Drew is too, but right now I'm talking about his famous smoothie. No matter where we are in the world, even in the farthest hotel rooms, this smoothie is happening. It's fueled marathons, book tours, and, let's be real, total parenting chaos. Our kids were practically raised on this — Athena had her first taste before she could even sit up. We load ours with tons of supplements, which is a personal journey of learning your body, so take this bare-bones version and add all the extra things you need to fuel you.

MAKES 1 SMOOTHIE

DREW'S FAMOUS SMOOTHIE

To a blender add 2 cups cold water with the protein powder, mango, kale, hemp seeds, chia seeds, and flaxseed. Blend on high until smooth, about 30 seconds. Pour into your favorite to-go container and hit your workout.

- 1 scoop plant-based protein powder (according to the package), plain or vanilla
- ½ cup frozen mango pieces
- 2 cups packed kales leaves (from about 2 stems)
- 1 teaspoon hemp seeds
- 1 teaspoon chia seeds
- 1 teaspoon ground flaxseed

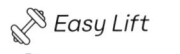 Easy Lift

Under 30 Minutes

Per smoothie

Calories: 290

Fat: 6g

Carbs: 23g

Fiber: 9g

Protein: 34g

This mix is genius — you get fluffy, golden waffles (or pancakes!) with a boost of lentil-powered protein, and you'd never even know. They're so light and fluffy that my kids have no clue. You can make a bigger batch and keep the extra in the fridge for the week, or meal prep and freeze extras. Either way, breakfast is handled. Note that the lentils need to soak overnight, so start the recipe the night before you plan on making the pancakes or waffles.

MAKES 8 WAFFLES OR 16 SILVER DOLLAR PANCAKES

LENTIL WAFFLE MIX (AND PANCAKES, TOO!)

In an airtight container, combine the soy milk, lentils, and dates. Cover and refrigerate for at least 4 hours or overnight.

To a blender, add the lentil mixture, baking powder, cinnamon, and salt. Blend on high until completely smooth.

For waffles: Heat a waffle iron over medium heat and coat both sides with nonstick spray. Pour the batter into the waffle iron and cook until browned and crisp (timing varies according to your waffle maker). Remove from the iron and serve immediately.

For pancakes: Heat a large nonstick skillet over medium heat. Coat with a little nonstick spray and add about ¼ cup of batter per pancake to the pan. Add a few more portions, making sure to not crowd the pancakes so you can easily turn them. Cook until firm on the bottom, about 2 minutes, then flip and cook the other sides until firm, about 2 minutes more. Transfer to a platter and cover with aluminum foil while you cook the remaining batter.

Serve the waffles or pancakes hot with butter and maple syrup, of course!

2⅔ cups unsweetened soy milk or other plant-based milk
1⅓ cups dry red lentils, rinsed and drained
3 medjool dates, pitted
1½ teaspoons baking powder
1½ teaspoons ground cinnamon
1 teaspoon kosher salt
Nonstick cooking spray
Vegan butter and pure maple syrup, for serving

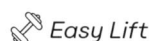 *Easy Lift*

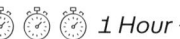 1 Hour +

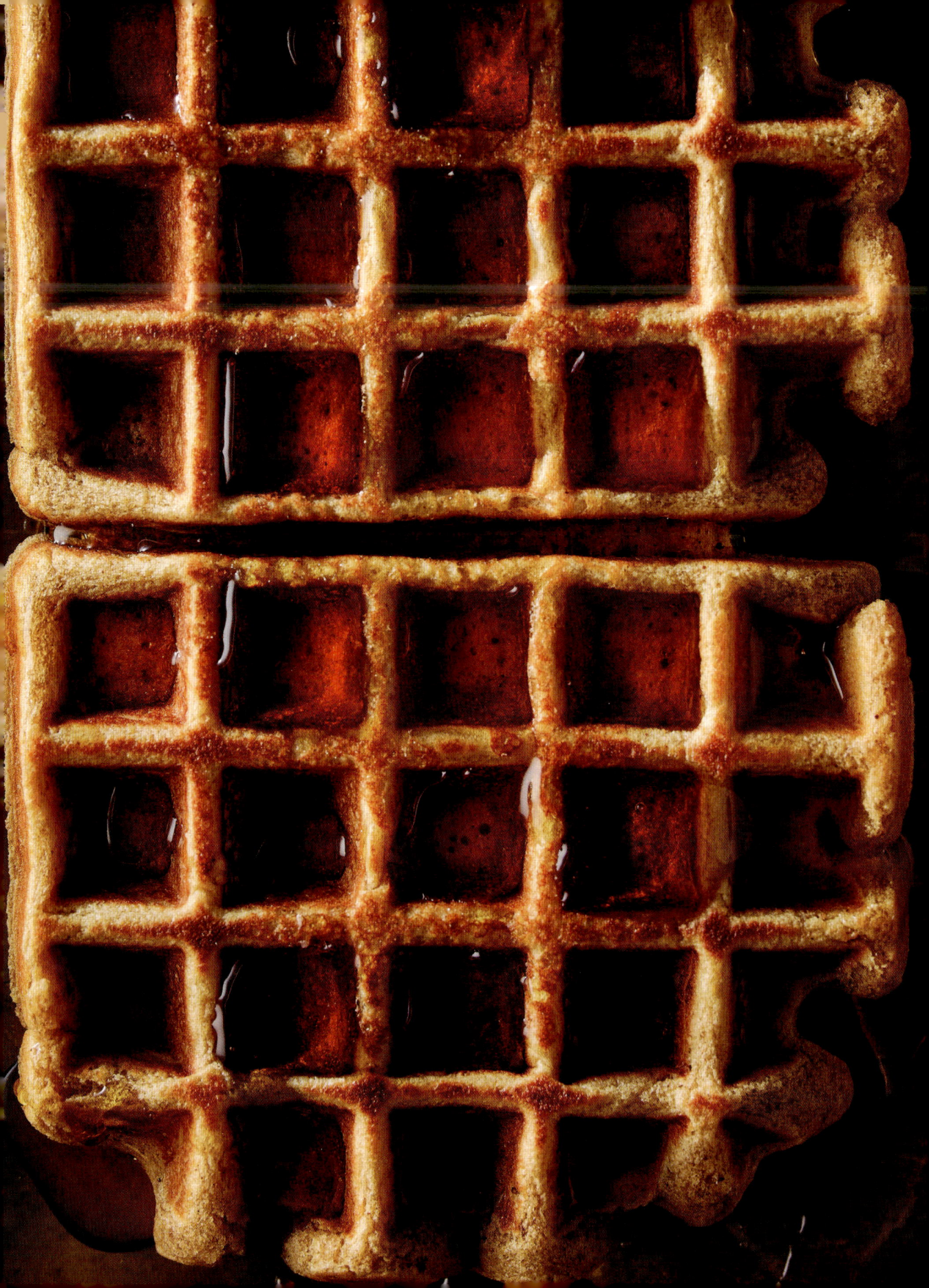

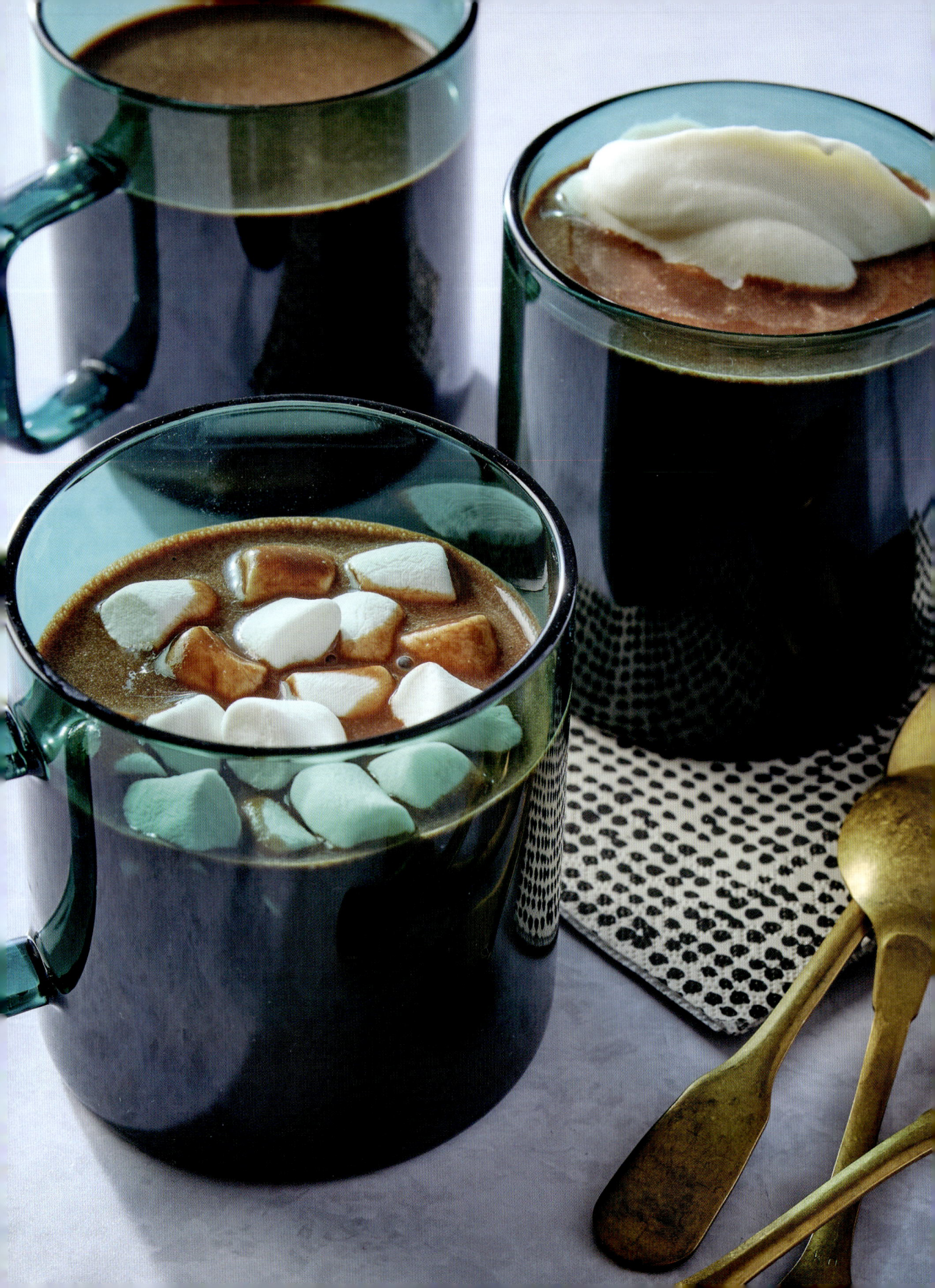

Who says peppermint hot chocolate is just for December? This is a year-round, Hallmark-movie-on-repeat, curl-up-on-the-couch type of situation. It's rich, it's cozy, and, thanks to a sneaky scoop of protein powder, it's also functional. Load up on the (vegan) marshmallows, pile on the vegan whip — this is a cup of pure joy, and you deserve it.

MAKES 1 MUG

PEPPERMINT HOT CHOCOLATE

In a small saucepan, whisk together the soy milk, protein powder, cacao powder, maple syrup, and peppermint extract, if using, until no lumps remain. (If you have a shaker bottle, this step is much faster!)

Set over low heat, whisking often, until the liquid around the edges starts to simmer, about 4 minutes. Immediately pour into a mug, top with mini marshmallows or a dollop of whip, and serve.

- 1 cup unsweetened soy milk or other plant-based milk
- 1 scoop plant-based chocolate protein powder
- 1 tablespoon cacao powder or Dutch-process cocoa powder
- 1 tablespoon pure maple syrup
- ¼ teaspoon pure peppermint extract (optional)
- Vegan mini marshmallows or Vegan Whip (page 234), for topping

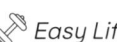 Easy Lift

Under 30 Minutes

Per mug

Calories: 219

Fat: 6g

Carbs: 24g

Fiber: 6g

Protein: 21g

I am not a coffee girlie, I'm a matcha girlie — a matcha-with-protein girlie, to be exact. This is my ultimate pick-me-up — clean energy, no crash, plus a sneaky hit of protein to keep you going. It's smooth, slightly sweet, and just the right amount of earthy. Whether you're powering up for a workout, an early meeting, or just life in general, this is the kind of green energy we love.

MAKES 1 LATTE

PROTEIN MATCHA LATTE

In a blender (or shaker bottle) combine 1 cup of the soy milk with the pea protein powder, agave, and matcha. Blend on medium (or shake) until combined.

Fill a tall glass with ice and pour the remaining ½ cup soy milk into the bottom of the glass. Slowly pour the matcha mixture on top to float. Serve immediately with a straw.

1½ cups unsweetened soy milk or other plant-based milk
1 scoop unflavored pea protein powder
1 tablespoon agave syrup
2 teaspoons matcha powder
Ice

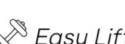 *Easy Lift*
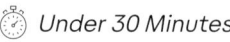 *Under 30 Minutes*

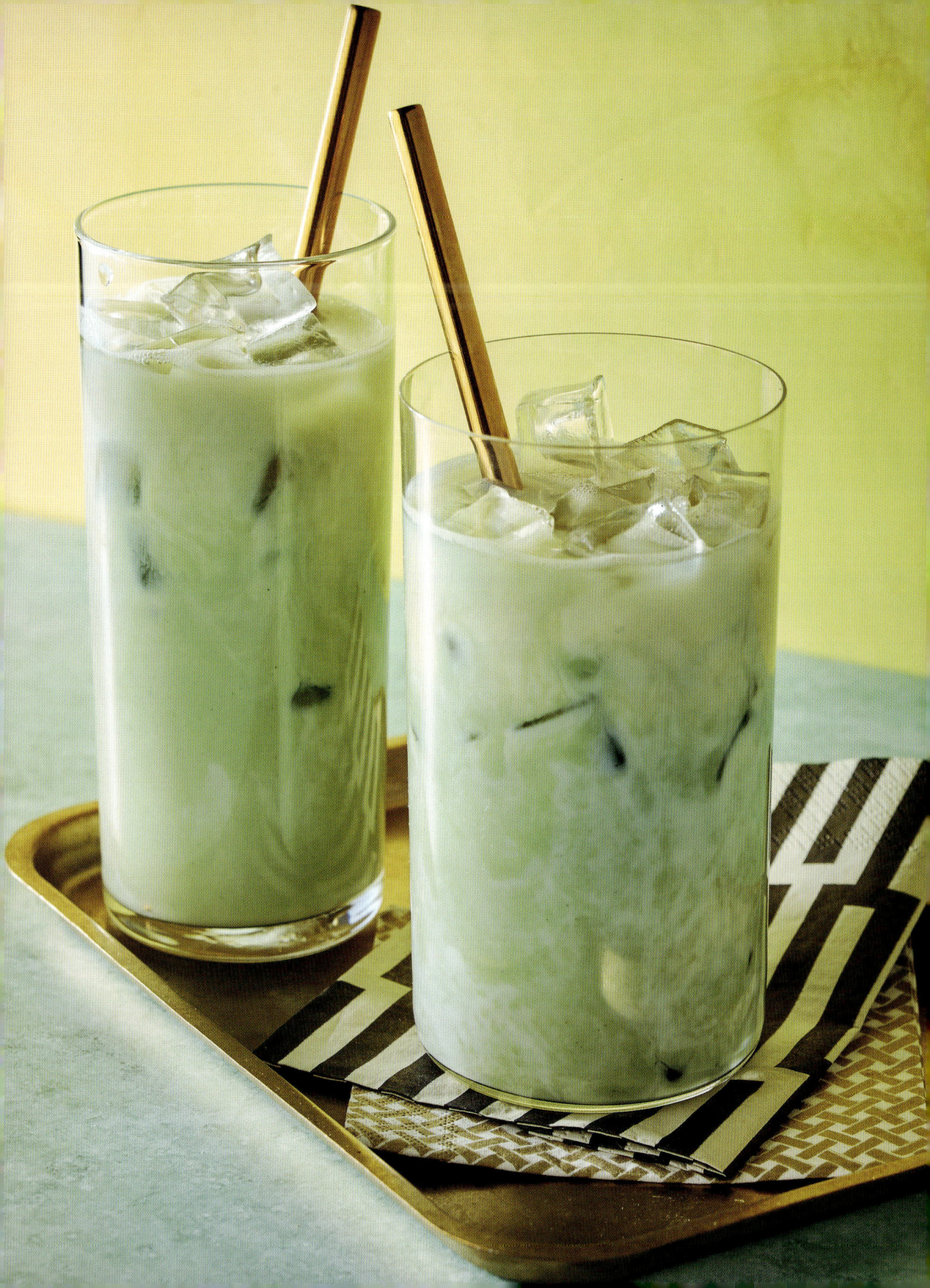

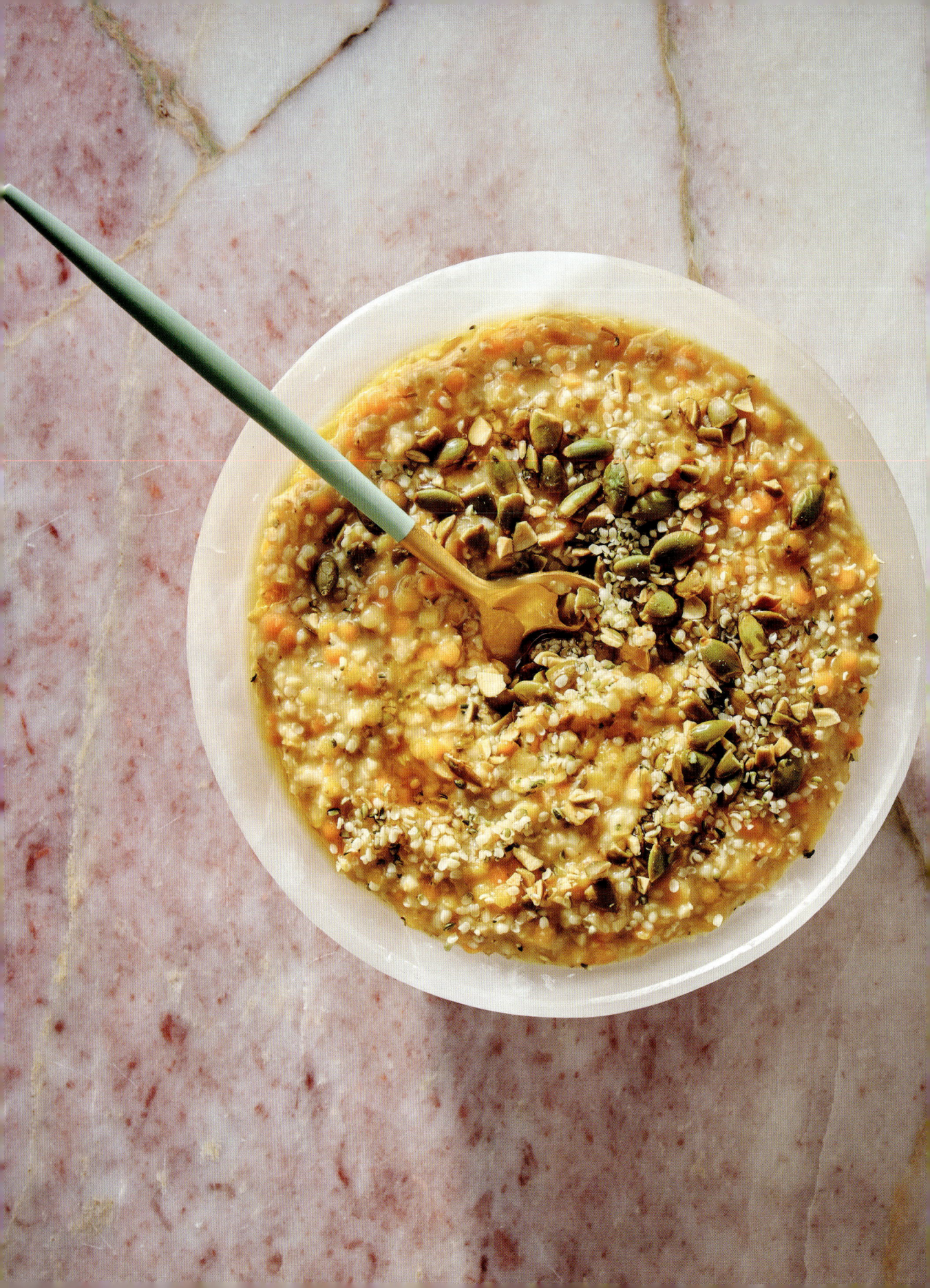

A savory breakfast porridge is such a common thing in many parts of the world, but in the US we always veer a little sweet. This warm bowl invites you to rethink that. It has lots of plant-powered protein, warming umami flavors, and enough texture to keep things interesting — and since you're not topping it with brown sugar, maple syrup, and other "traditional" oatmeal toppers, you won't get that spike/crash effect. Add toasted seeds for crunch, drizzle with sesame oil for depth, and take a deep breath because, yes, you just made a perfect meal.

SERVES 4

SAVORY OATS & LENTIL PORRIDGE

Bring 4 cups water to a boil over high heat in a large saucepan. Stir in the oats and soy sauce. Reduce the heat to low and simmer, stirring occasionally to keep the oats from sticking. After 10 minutes, stir in the lentils. Continue simmering until the water is almost completely absorbed, about 5 more minutes. Remove from the heat, cover, and let sit for 10 minutes to steam.

The porridge can be served immediately, each serving topped with 1 cup of the warmed stock, a drizzle of sesame oil, ¼ cup of the pumpkin seeds, and 1 tablespoon of the hemp seeds. The porridge can also be cooled and refrigerated in an airtight container for up to 5 days (without toppings). To reheat, simmer or microwave a portion of the porridge with a little water to loosen it up, stirring occasionally, until warm.

- 1 cup steel-cut oats
- 2 tablespoons soy sauce or tamari
- 1 cup dry red lentils, rinsed and drained
- 4 cups warmed vegetable stock or Liquid Gold (page 235)
- Toasted sesame oil
- 1 cup toasted pumpkin seeds
- 4 tablespoons hemp seeds

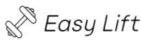 *Easy Lift*

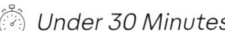 *Under 30 Minutes*

Per serving
Calories: 406
Fat: 9g
Carbs: 71g
Fiber: 16g
Protein: 24g

Per serving — Calories: 430 | Fat: 21g | Carbs: 37g | Fiber: 21g | Protein: 23g

Back in my NYU days, my après late-night move was a recap and a shakshuka with the girls. This version swaps the eggs for a silky tofu scramble (look for black sea salt at spice shops or online for an extra sulfurous, eggy flavor), but keeps everything else: smoky, slow-cooked peppers, tangy tomatoes, and all the fresh herbs. Serve it with warm pita and enjoy — preferably after a good night's sleep.

SERVES 4

SHAKSHUKA-STYLE TOFU SCRAMBLE

Make the shakshuka: In a large skillet, heat the olive oil over medium heat. When the oil is shimmering, add the onion and peppers with a good pinch of salt and pepper. Cook, stirring often, until the vegetables are very soft, about 8 minutes. Stir in the paprika and cumin until fragrant, about 1 minute. Add the tomatoes and reduce the heat to low. Simmer gently until the sauce is thickened and flavorful, about 15 minutes. Stir in the spinach until wilted, about 1 minute. Remove from the heat.

While the shakshuka is simmering, make the tofu scramble: Drain the tofu. In a medium nonstick skillet, heat the olive oil over low heat. When the oil is shimmering, use your hands to crumble the tofu into the skillet in large pieces. Season with the nutritional yeast, turmeric, and a good pinch of salt and pepper. Stir the tofu occasionally as it releases water and starts to firm up, about 3 minutes. Season with a pinch of black salt, if using. Remove from the heat.

When the shakshuka is ready, spoon the tofu scramble evenly around the skillet. Finish with a shower of herbs and serve with warm pitas for dipping.

Shakshuka

- 3 tablespoons extra-virgin olive oil
- 1 medium red onion, thinly sliced
- 2 medium bell peppers, seeded and thinly sliced
- Kosher salt and freshly ground black pepper
- ½ teaspoon smoked paprika
- ½ teaspoon ground cumin
- 1 (28-ounce) can diced tomatoes
- 2 cups baby spinach

Tofu Scramble

- 2 tablespoons extra-virgin olive oil
- 16 ounces extra-firm tofu
- 2 tablespoons nutritional yeast
- 1 teaspoon ground turmeric
- Kosher salt and freshly ground black pepper
- Black salt (optional)

Fresh cilantro, parsley, and/or mint leaves, for serving
4 protein pitas, warmed

 Easy Lift

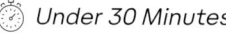 Under 30 Minutes

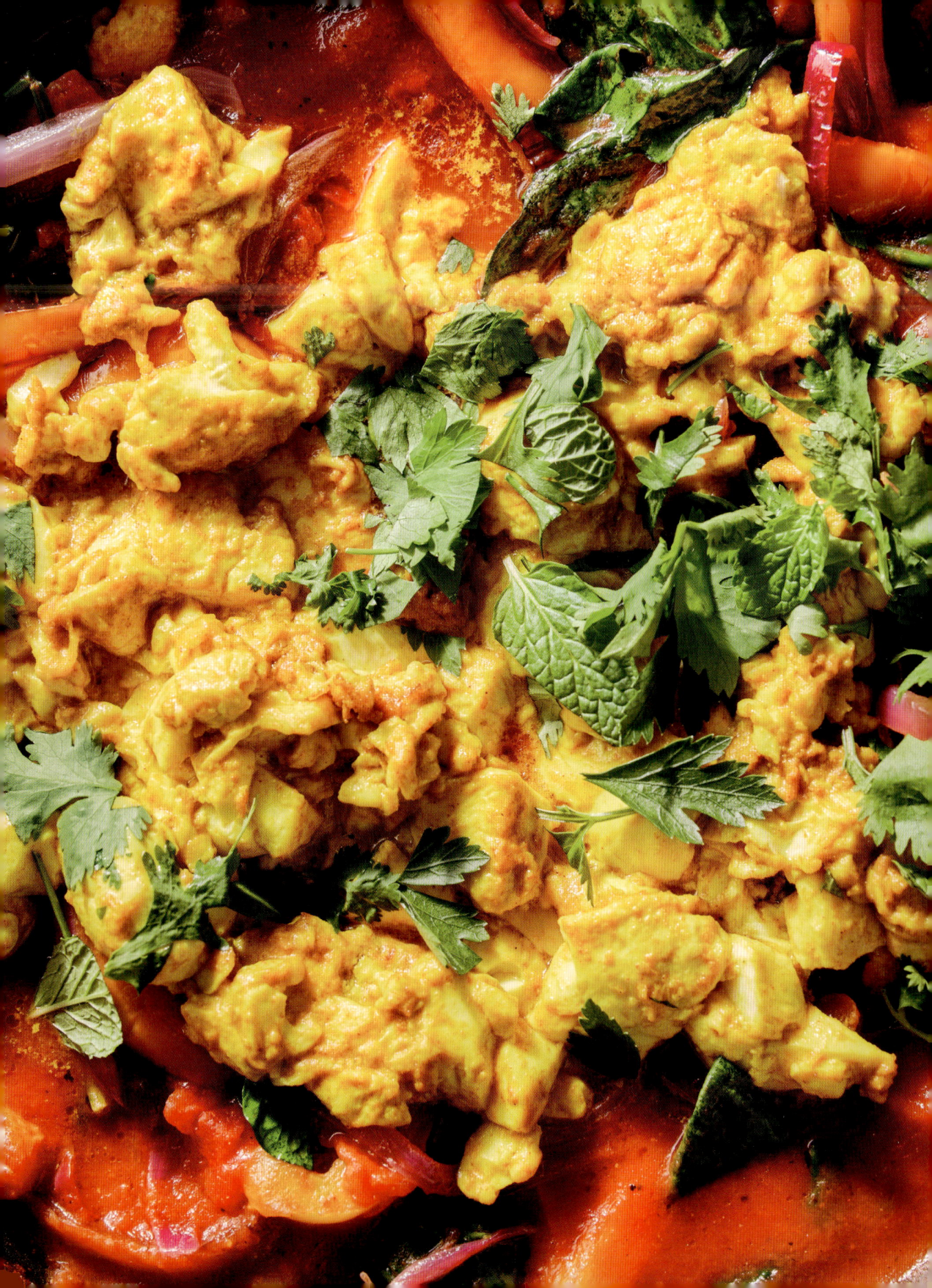

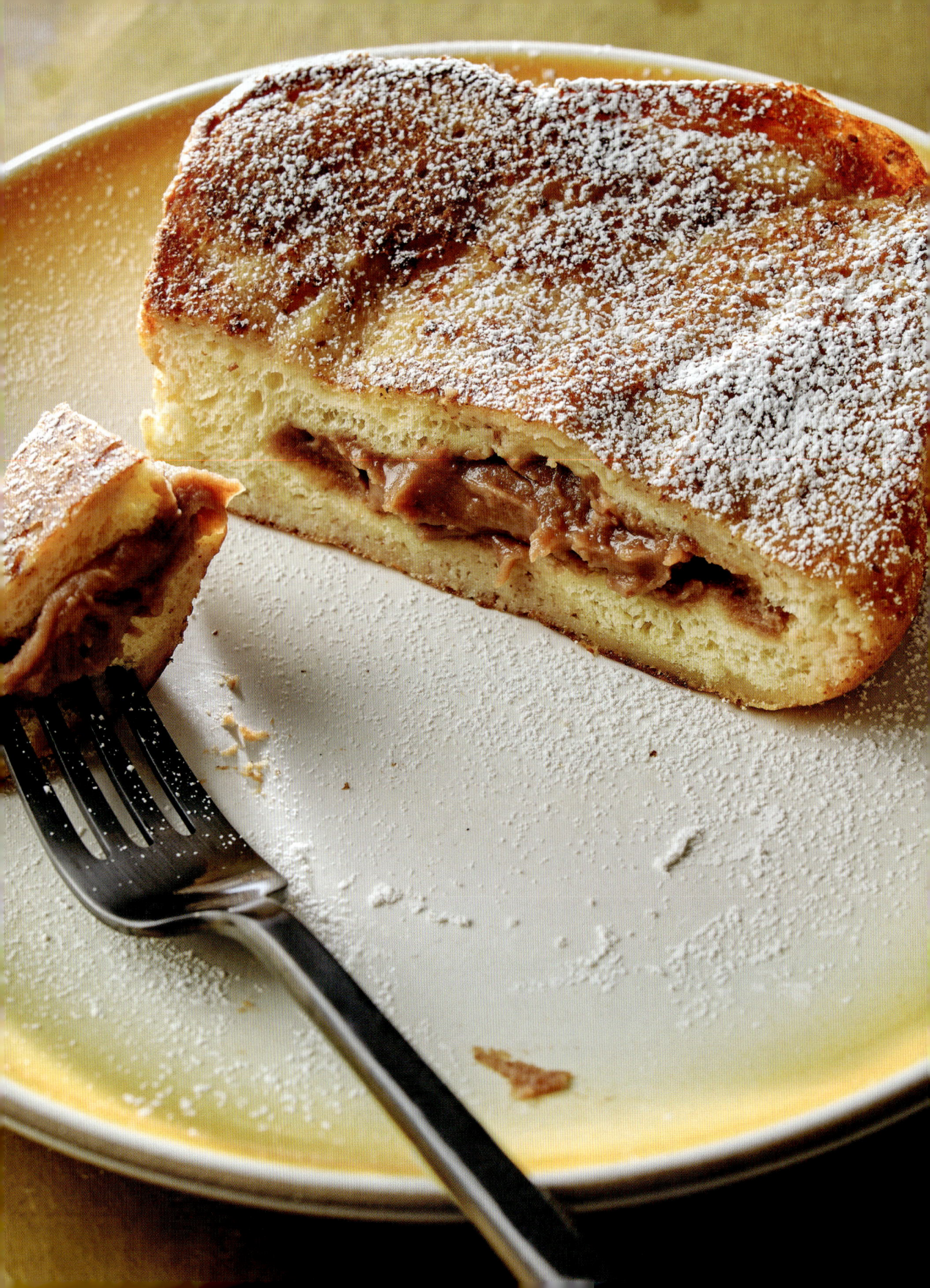

This is the kind of breakfast that makes you feel like you're at a fancy brunch spot — even if you're just in your pajamas at home. I got the idea from anko, a Japanese sweet bean paste traditionally made from adzuki beans and used in desserts like mochi and sweet buns. You can buy a can of anko at Asian grocery stores or online and scoop it straight from the can to stuff the French toast. Here, I go for a similar sweet bean paste using red kidney beans and coconut sugar. Either way, it's a great way to add lots of protein to your breakfast! And while you could add syrup, taste it first and ask yourself: Do I really need it?

SERVES 4

SWEET BEAN-STUFFED FRENCH TOAST

In a blender or food processor, blend the kidney beans with the liquid from the can and the coconut sugar on medium until smooth. Pour into a medium skillet and set over medium heat. Let the mixture come to a simmer, stirring often, and bubble into a thick paste, about 10 minutes. Transfer to a bowl. Let cool for about 15 minutes to allow the paste to set. Wash and dry the skillet.

Meanwhile, in a large shallow bowl, whisk together the soy milk, cornstarch, flaxseed, cinnamon, and vanilla. Set aside to thicken.

Using a serrated knife, cut a large slit in the bottom of each slice of bread to make a cavity, stopping before reaching the edges or cutting through to the other end. Pinch the sides of each slice of bread to open the cavity and use a butter knife to spread about a fourth of the kidney bean mixture inside.

Return the skillet to medium heat and melt 1 tablespoon of the vegan butter. Dip one of the stuffed bread slices in the thickened milk mixture, letting each side soak for about 10 seconds. Fry the slice in the skillet until browned, about 4 minutes per side. Repeat with the remaining slices, adding 1 more tablespoon of butter halfway.

Serve the stuffed French toast warm with a dusting of powdered sugar.

- 1 (15.5-ounce) can red kidney beans
- ¼ cup coconut sugar
- 1 cup unsweetened soy milk or other plant-based milk
- ¼ cup cornstarch
- 1 tablespoon ground flaxseed
- 1 teaspoon ground cinnamon
- 1 teaspoon pure vanilla extract
- 4 thick slices Bread of Champions (page 215) or store-bought brioche
- 2 tablespoons vegan butter
- Powdered sugar, for serving

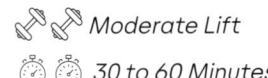 *Moderate Lift*

30 to 60 Minutes

Per serving
Calories: 572
Fat: 15g
Carbs: 84g
Fiber: 13g
Protein: 28g

Instead of using a store-bought egg substitute to make this frittata, I build a homemade blend using tofu, chickpeas, flaxseed, and cornstarch to create a texture that's creamy, tender, and rich, just like a traditional frittata, but with even better fuel — and almost twice the protein of an egg frittata. It's also loaded with veggies and topped with a gorgeous swirl of vibrant nut-free pesto (made with nutritional yeast instead of cheese) that takes it over the top.

SERVES 8 (MAKES 1 CUP OF PESTO)

VEGGIE & PESTO FRITTATA

Preheat the oven to 400°F.

Make the pesto: In a blender, combine the basil, nutritional yeast, lemon juice, olive oil, pepper, salt, and ¼ cup cold water. Blend on medium into a smooth, pourable pesto, about 30 seconds. If the pesto is a little thick, add 1 tablespoon of cold water and blend again. Pour into a bowl and wash out the blender.

Make the frittata: In a 12-inch cast-iron skillet, combine the tempeh and enough water to cover. Set over high heat and boil for about 10 minutes. (This removes the bitter flavor from the tempeh.) Drain the tempeh and set aside to cool on a plate; wipe the skillet dry.

Meanwhile, drain the tofu and add to a clean blender with the soy milk, chickpeas, nutritional yeast, cornstarch, flaxseed, 1½ teaspoons salt, ½ teaspoon pepper, onion powder, and turmeric together on high until completely smooth.

Heat the avocado oil over medium heat in the skillet you used for the tempeh. Once shimmering, add the leek, bell pepper, mushrooms, and a pinch of salt. Add the tempeh and cook, stirring often, until the vegetables soften, about 6 minutes.

Quick Pesto

2 cups packed basil leaves
¼ cup nutritional yeast
Juice of 1 lemon
2 tablespoons extra-virgin olive oil
1 teaspoon freshly ground black pepper
½ teaspoon salt

Frittata

8 ounces tempeh, cubed
16 ounces extra-firm tofu
1 cup unsweetened soy milk or other plant-based milk
1 (15.5-ounce) can chickpeas, rinsed
½ cup nutritional yeast
¼ cup cornstarch
2 tablespoons ground flaxseed
Kosher salt and black pepper
½ teaspoon onion powder
½ teaspoon ground turmeric
2 tablespoons avocado oil

Per serving — Calories: 444 | Fat: 20g | Carbs: 51g | Fiber: 11g | Protein: 23g

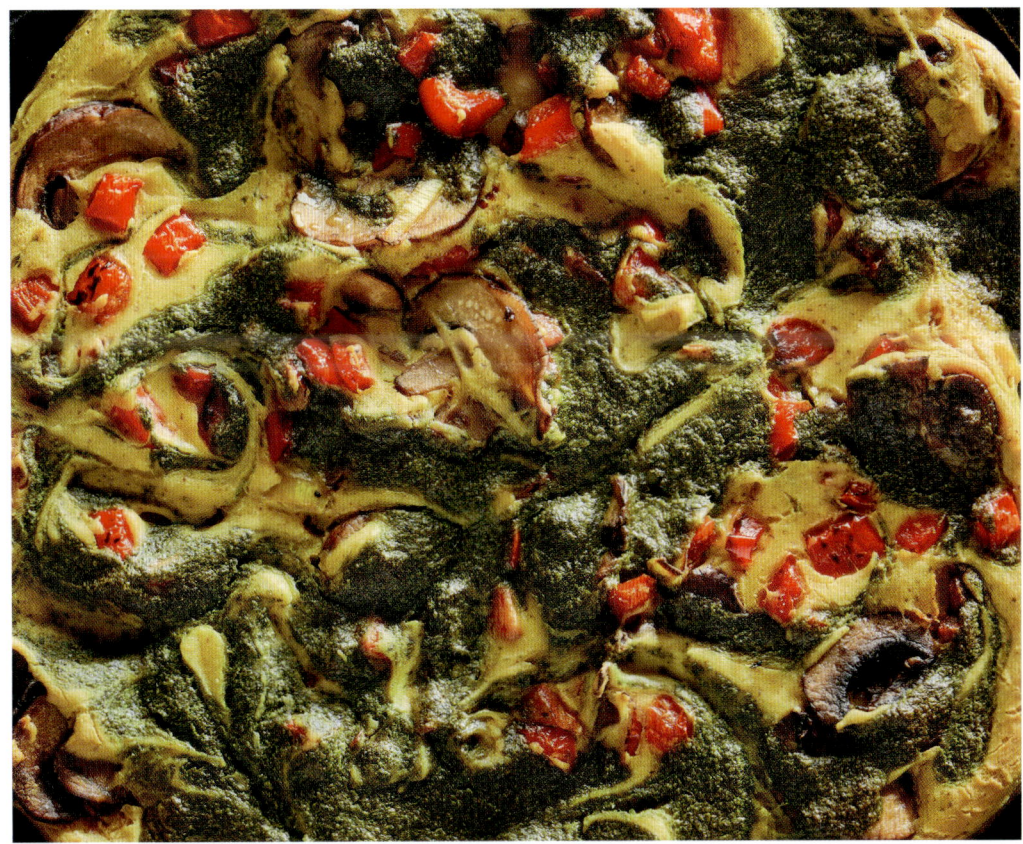

Remove the skillet from the heat. Pour the tofu mixture from the blender evenly around the skillet and stir to mix in the vegetables. Give the skillet a couple of firm shakes to evenly distribute. Spoon the pesto over the surface of the frittata, then use a chopstick or a butter knife to lightly swirl it into the mixture. Transfer to the oven and bake until the center of the frittata feels firm when you lightly press on it, 35 to 40 minutes.

Remove from the oven and let set for 10 minutes before slicing and serving.

Note: Double the pesto and refrigerate the extra in an airtight container for up to 5 days (or freeze for up to 1 month). I love having it around to dress up roasted vegetables, pastas, or grain bowls.

- 1 leek, tough green tops discarded, halved, cleaned well, and thinly sliced crosswise
- 1 red bell pepper, halved, seeded, and diced
- 8 ounces Baby Bella mushrooms, stems removed and caps thinly sliced

Moderate Lift

30 to 60 Minutes

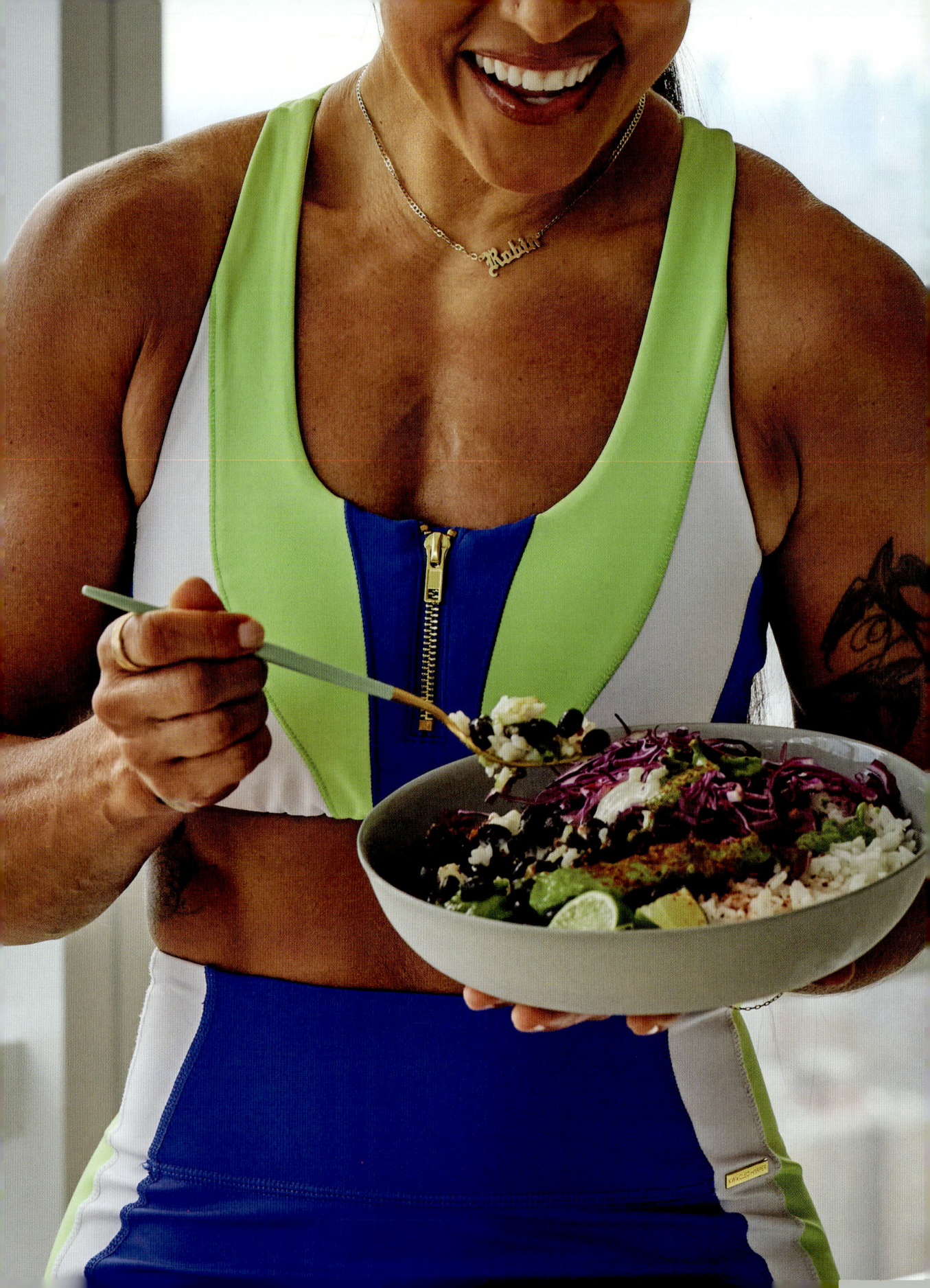

SKIP THE LUNCH SALAD

Hot take alert: If you think I'm a lunch salad girlie, well, think again. (You'll find my favorite *dinner* salads on pages 120 to 124!) Lunch should be a power move, not a pit stop. It's the meal that fuels the rest of your day, so why waste it on a bowl of leaves that'll leave you hungry an hour later? I load up on carbs when I need them most — midday, when my hustle is in full force and my body is craving fuel. The recipes in this chapter are stacked with the real secret weapons — protein, carbs, and fiber — to make sure you stay full, your energy stays steady, and your focus stays sharp. No crashes, no regrets — just meals that hit hard and keep you moving.

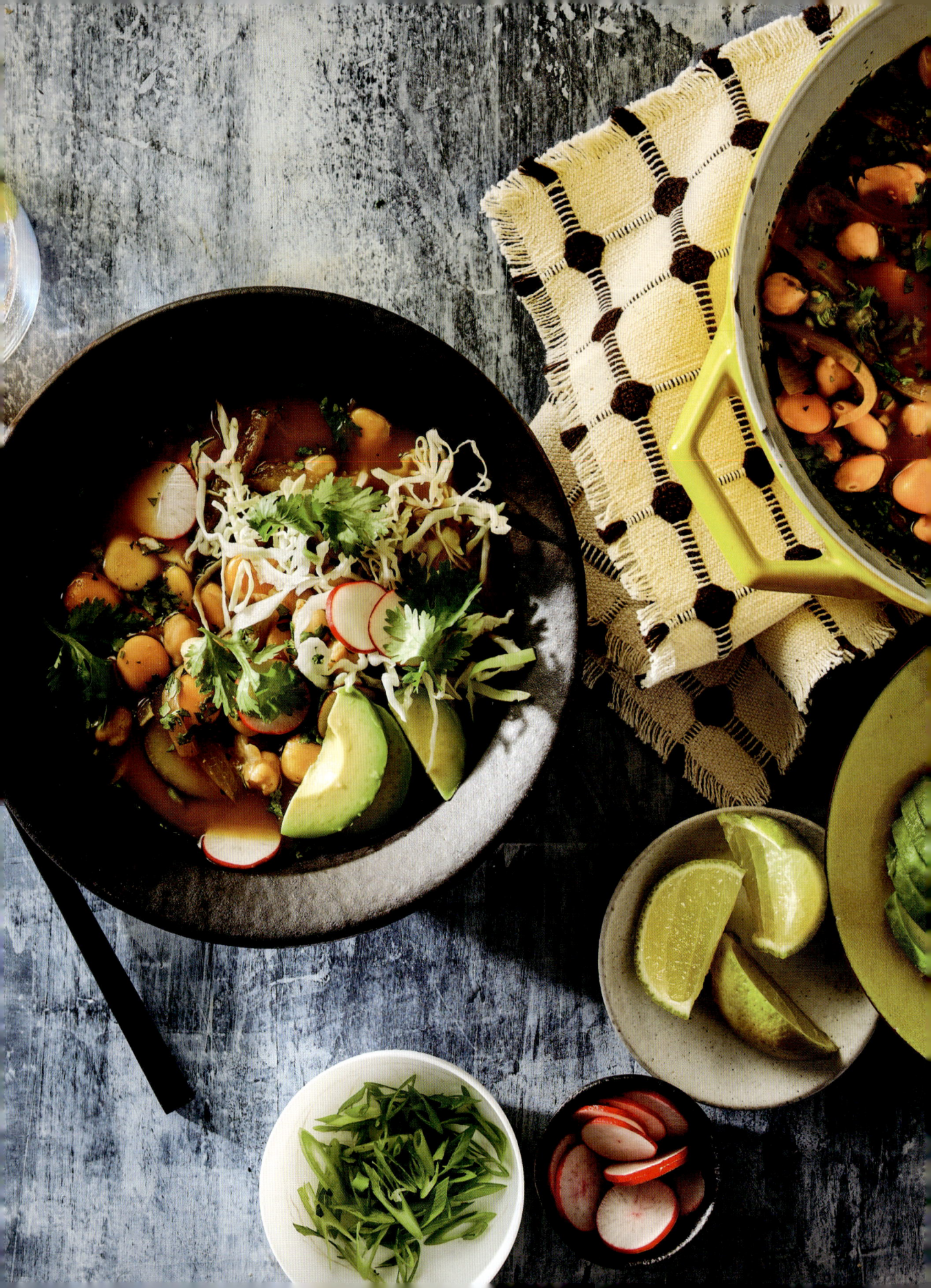

This soup doesn't just warm you up — it *restores* you. Think of it as an edible reset button, the perfect cure for sick days, stressful weeks, or those moments when you just need a little extra TLC in a bowl. Chickpeas step in for the traditional hominy, while lupini beans add an extra punch of protein to keep your energy high. Make a big batch, stash some in the freezer, and future you will be very grateful when life inevitably gets chaotic.

SERVES 4

CHICKPEA POZOLE

In a large Dutch oven, combine the vegetable stock, chickpeas, lupini beans, squash, onion, garlic, cilantro, chile powder, cumin, oregano, salt, and pepper. Set over high heat and bring to a boil, stirring often. Cover and reduce the heat to low. Simmer until the chickpeas are very tender, about 15 minutes.

Ladle the pozole into bowls and serve with your choice of toppings.

- 4 cups vegetable stock or Liquid Gold (page 235)
- 1 (15.5-ounce) can chickpeas, drained and rinsed
- 1 (8-ounce) jar lupini beans, drained and rinsed
- 1 large yellow squash or zucchini, cut into ½-inch pieces
- 1 medium white onion, halved and thinly sliced
- 2 garlic cloves, minced
- ½ cup chopped fresh cilantro
- 2 teaspoons ancho or chipotle chile powder
- 2 teaspoons ground cumin
- 1 teaspoon dried oregano
- 1 teaspoon kosher salt
- ½ teaspoon freshly ground black pepper
- Shredded cabbage, thinly sliced radishes, sliced avocado, thinly sliced scallions, fresh cilantro leaves, and lime wedges, for serving

 Easy Lift

 Under 30 Minutes

Per serving | **Calories: 272** | **Fat: 6g** | **Carbs: 40g** | **Fiber: 10g** | **Protein: 20g**

When possible, I prefer to make my own plant-based "meats" because I can control exactly what is in them. This Chipotle-inspired burrito bowl has a smoky and spicy, homemade, plant-based chorizo that's shockingly easy to throw together. Tajín adds a perfect citrusy kick, the black beans bring the fiber, and a creamy avocado salsa ties it all together.

SERVES 4 (MAKES 1 CUP SALSA)

CHORIZO BURRITO BOWL

Per serving
Protein: 42g
Calories: 586
Fat: 15g
Carbs: 78g
Fiber: 23g

Make the avocado salsa: In a blender, combine the tomatillos, avocado, cilantro, serrano, garlic, lime juice, salt, and 2 tablespoons of cold water. Blend on high to make a smooth sauce, about 1 minute. Refrigerate until ready to use, or up to 4 days.

Make the chorizo: In a medium bowl, combine the TVP, chili powder, paprika, cayenne, and vinegar. Taste for seasoning and add up to 1 tablespoon tamari if needed.

In a large nonstick skillet, heat the avocado oil over medium heat. When the oil is shimmering, add the TVP mixture in an even layer. Cook undisturbed until nicely browned, 4 to 5 minutes. Stir and cook for 2 more minutes to warm through. Remove to a bowl.

Make the bowls: In the same skillet (no need to wipe it out), add the black beans and ¼ cup water. Set over medium heat, stirring constantly, until the water boils off and the beans are warmed through, about 4 minutes. Remove from the heat.

Scoop ½ cup of the rice into each bowl. Add chorizo, black beans, avocado salsa, cabbage, sour cream, and a sprinkle of Tajín.

Dalina Says...
White and brown rice differ by only 1 to 2 grams of fiber per cooked cup so make whichever you prefer. Add black beans and you've got a power couple with all the essential amino acids for a complete protein. And Robin's homemade TVP chorizo brings extra flavor, protein, and fiber—without the processed additives in store-bought brands.

Avocado Salsa
2 tomatillos, husks removed, rinsed and halved
1 avocado, halved, and pitted
¼ cup packed cilantro leaves
1 serrano pepper, halved and seeded for less heat
2 garlic cloves
Juice of 1 lime
1 teaspoon kosher salt

Homemade Chorizo
½ pound hydrated TVP MVP (page 224) or ¾ cup dry TVP (follow package instructions to hydrate)
1 tablespoon chili powder
1 tablespoon smoked paprika
¼ teaspoon cayenne pepper
1 tablespoon cider vinegar
Tamari (optional) or soy sauce (optional)
2 tablespoons avocado oil

Bowls
1 (15.5-ounce) can black beans, rinsed
2 cups cooked white rice
Shredded purple cabbage, vegan sour cream (page 146), and Tajín, for serving

Moderate Lift
Under 30 Minutes

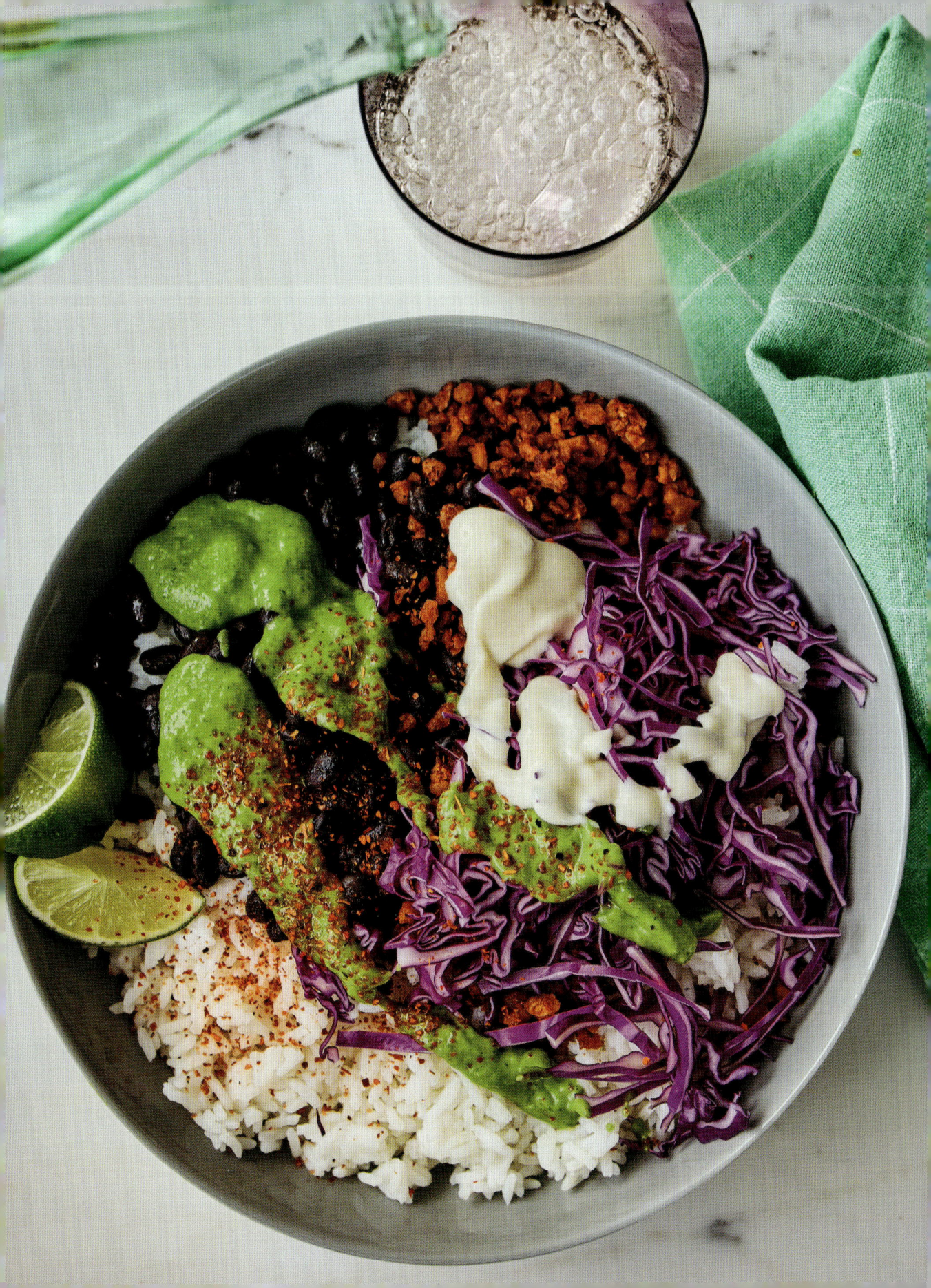

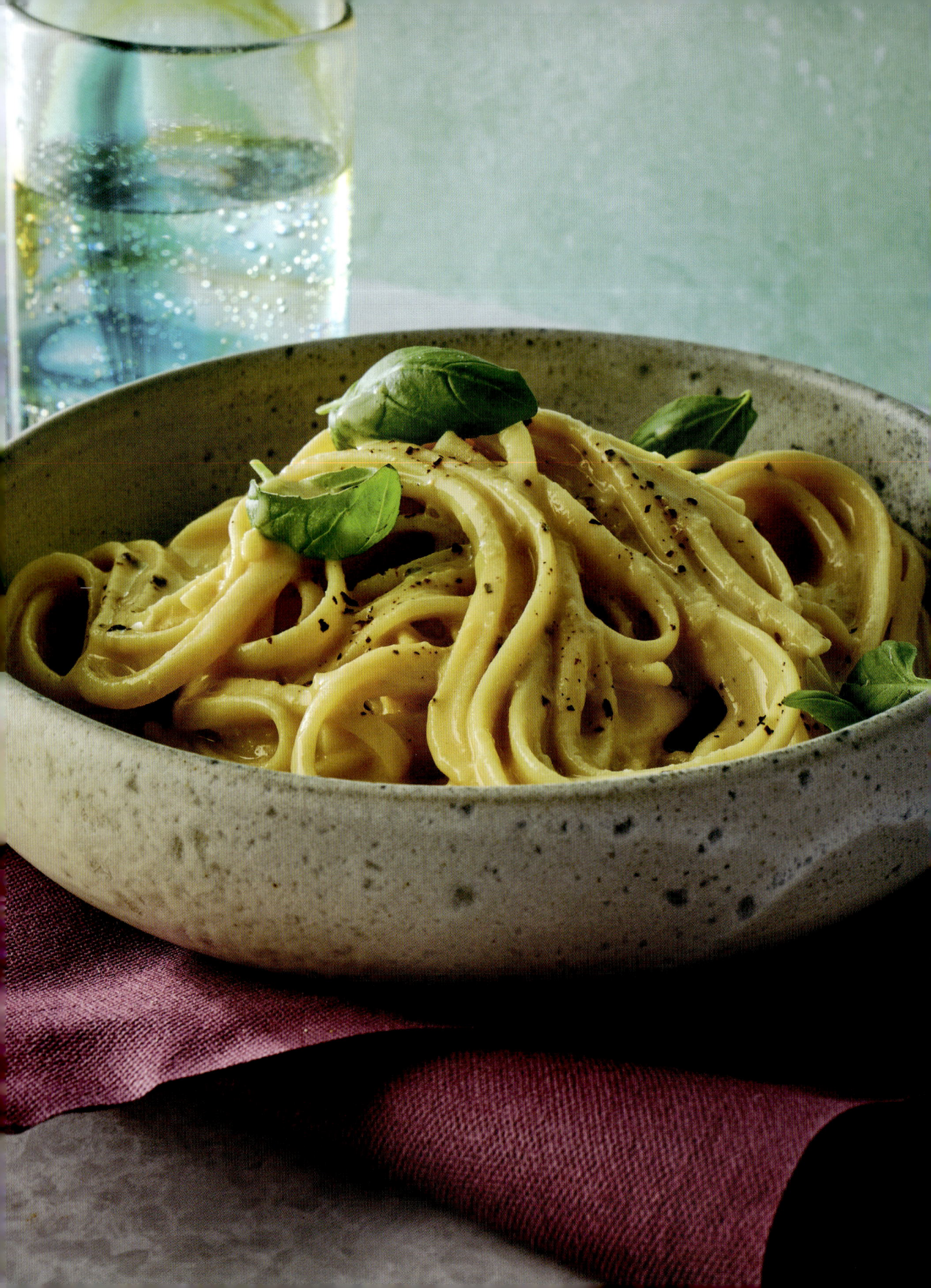

Everyone's out here trying to avoid carbs, but if you want real, lasting energy, nothing beats a lunch built on complex carbs! This is your new lunch hero — fast, filling, and with a protein-and-carb boost to power you through the rest of the day. Italians may send me hate mail for this one, but it's giving serious Olive-Garden-on-your-lunch-break vibes, with a creamy sauce powered with silken tofu and fiber-rich cannellini beans. It's for those moments when hunger strikes and you needed lunch like fifteen minutes ago. Nonna might side-eye it, but she'd still clean her plate.

SERVES 4

CREAMY ALFREDO PASTA

In a large pot, combine 4 quarts water and 1 tablespoon of the salt. Add the pasta and cook according to the package directions. Reserve 1 cup of the pasta cooking water before draining.

In a blender, combine the tofu, cannellini beans, garlic, nutritional yeast, pepper, the remaining 2 teaspoons salt, and the reserved pasta water. Blend on high until completely smooth, about 2 minutes. Taste for seasoning.

Return the pasta to the pot and add the alfredo sauce, stirring the two together. Set over medium heat and stir until the sauce warms through, about 3 minutes. Serve with a sprinkle of fresh basil.

Note: This is best eaten straight away — the sauce will firm up and be absorbed by the pasta as it cools. To heat up leftovers, add the pasta to a skillet with a splash of water, set over medium heat, and toss until warmed through.

- 1 tablespoon plus 2 teaspoons kosher salt
- 1 (8-ounce) box high-protein linguine
- 6 ounces silken tofu, drained
- 1 (15.5-ounce) can cannellini beans, drained and rinsed
- 2 garlic cloves
- ½ cup nutritional yeast
- 1 teaspoon freshly ground black pepper
- Chopped fresh basil, for serving

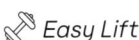 *Easy Lift*

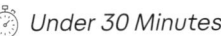 *Under 30 Minutes*

Per serving

Calories: 400

Fat: 6g

Carbs: 66g

Fiber: 14g

Protein: 29g

Per serving — Calories: 524 | Fat: 14g | Carbs: 78g | Fiber: 14g | Protein: 29g

Mac and cheese with peas is pure, wholesome nostalgia — but this version isn't just a throwback, it's a smart update. Red lentils bring sneaky protein and natural creaminess to the sauce, while white miso adds that deep, cheesy umami that keeps you going back for another bite. I turn up the heat with jalapeños (because spice training starts young in my family!), but if spice isn't your thing, you can leave them out and still get all the flavor. Either way, this dish is a potluck MVP, a perfect lunchtime make-ahead, and proof that comfort food can be just as nourishing as it is delicious. And the best part is no one will ever suspect it's secretly packed with protein. (Shhh, our little secret!)

SERVES 4

CREAMY MAC AND CHEESE

Set a colander in a large pot of water. Bring the water to a boil over high heat. Add the onion, carrot, cashews, and lentils to the colander and boil until the carrot is fork tender, about 15 minutes. Lift the colander to drain the water, then add the contents to a blender along with the soy milk, nutritional yeast, cornstarch, miso paste, lemon juice, Dijon, salt, garlic powder, onion powder, and turmeric. Blend on high to make a smooth "cheese" sauce, about 2 minutes.

Add more water to the pot if needed and heavily salt it. Add the pasta and cook according to the package directions. About 1 minute before the pasta is done, stir in the frozen peas, then drain.

Return the drained pasta and peas to the pot and add the sauce and jalapeños, if using. Set over medium heat and stir until the sauce thickens slightly, about 2 minutes. Serve immediately.

Note: The sauce will firm up as it cools. To heat leftovers, add the pasta to a skillet with a splash of water, set over medium heat, and toss until warmed through.

- 1 medium yellow onion, roughly chopped
- 1 medium carrot, roughly chopped
- ½ cup raw cashews
- ½ cup dry red lentils, rinsed and drained
- 1 cup unsweetened soy milk or other plant-based milk
- ½ cup nutritional yeast
- 1 tablespoon cornstarch
- 1 tablespoon white miso paste
- 1 tablespoon fresh lemon juice
- 1 tablespoon Dijon mustard
- 1 teaspoon kosher salt, plus more for the pasta
- 1 teaspoon garlic powder
- 1 teaspoon onion powder
- 1 teaspoon ground turmeric
- 1 (8-ounce) box high-protein pasta shells
- 1 cup frozen peas
- 4 jalapeños, diced (optional)

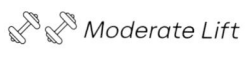 Moderate Lift

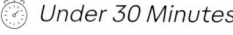 Under 30 Minutes

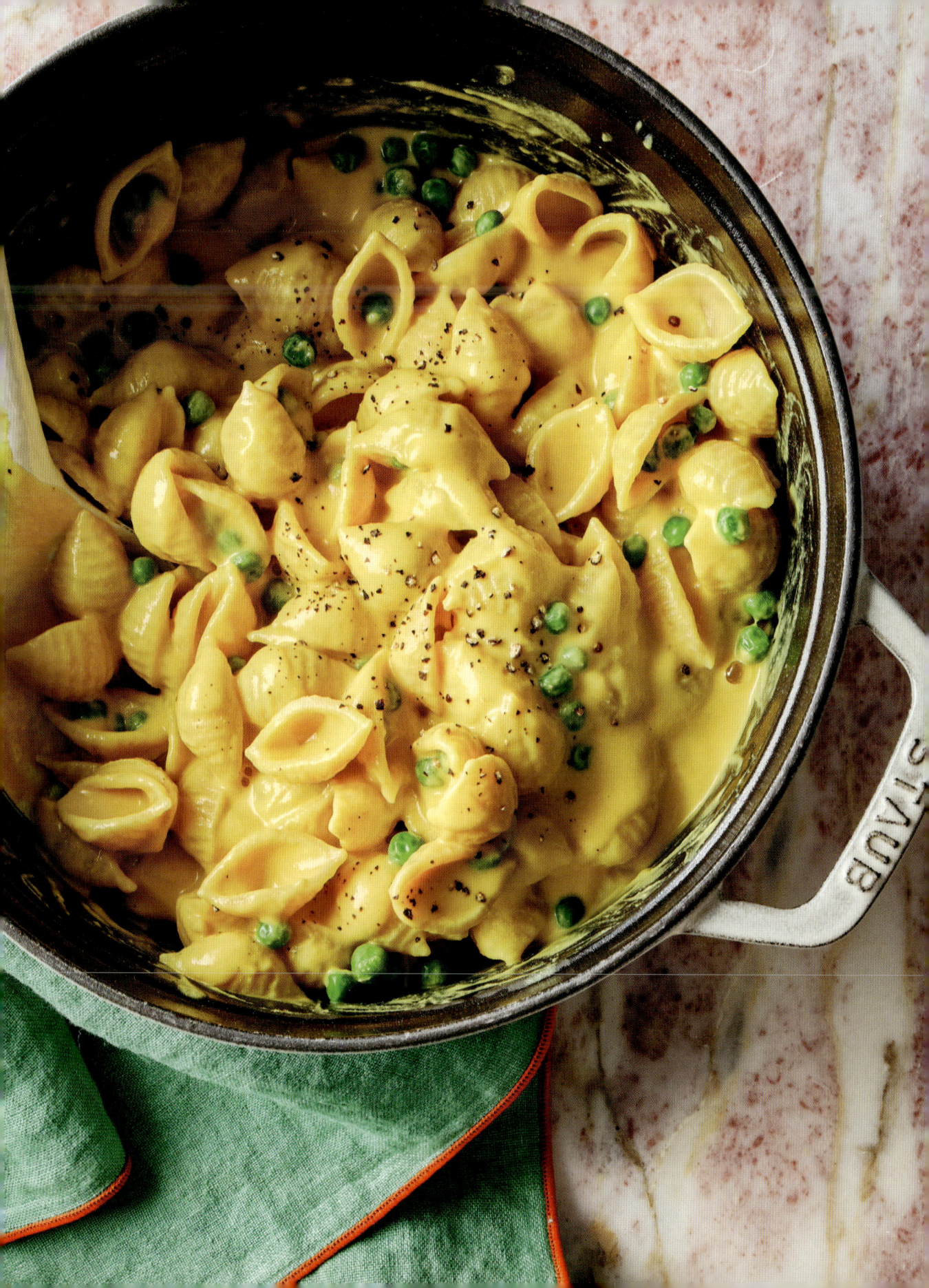

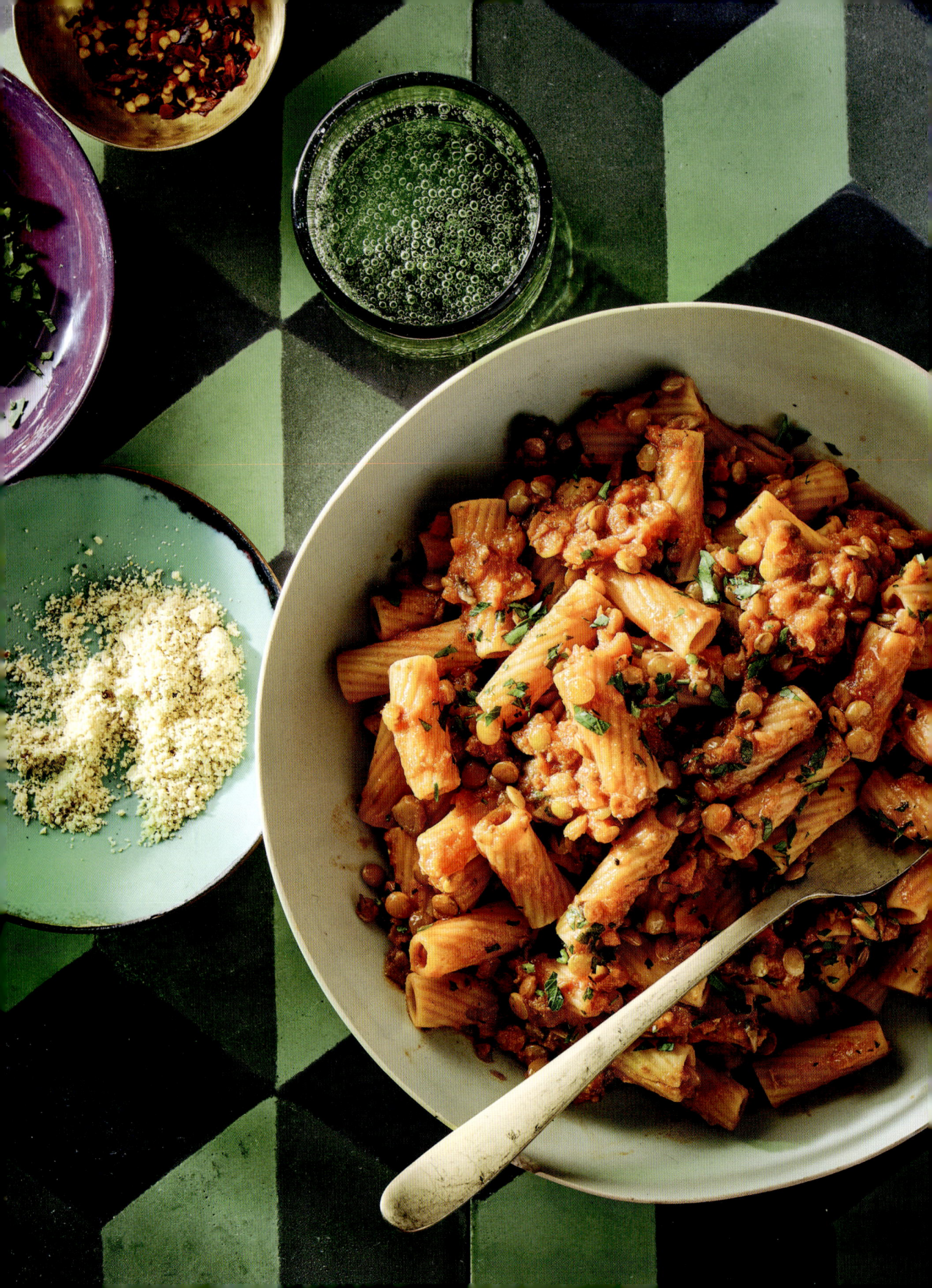

This dish is like a warm hug. It takes me right back to my days living near Little Italy in Manhattan, where the smell of red sauce practically followed me home. My version keeps all the I-need-a-second-bowl satisfaction, but is made in a fraction of the time (I chop everything up together in the food processor to get to the stove faster). For protein, I add lentils, and toss in mushrooms for their hearty, meaty texture. Fennel seeds and smoked paprika lend a deeply savory flavor. Oh, and the cashew parm should be sprinkled aggressively!

SERVES 8

MUSHROOM & LENTIL BOLOGNESE

In a food processor, combine the mushrooms, carrot, celery, onion, garlic, fennel seeds, oregano, cumin, and paprika. Process, scraping down the sides as needed, until the veggies are broken down into mostly small pieces, about 1 minute.

In a large Dutch oven or saucepan, heat the olive oil over medium-high heat. When the oil is shimmering, add the veggie mixture and season generously with salt, black pepper, and a pinch of red pepper flakes, if using. Stir occasionally, until the vegetables release moisture and soften, about 10 minutes.

Add the lentils, stock, tomato puree, and a good pinch of salt. Cover, reduce the heat to medium-low, and simmer until the lentils are cooked through, about 15 minutes. Stir in the soy milk and simmer until the sauce is thick, about another 5 minutes.

While the sauce is simmering, bring a large pot of salted water to a boil over high heat. Add the pasta and cook according to the package directions, then drain.

Add the pasta to the sauce and toss to coat completely. Serve the pasta hot with plenty of chopped parsley and cashew parm.

- 8 ounces sliced Baby Bella mushrooms
- 1 medium carrot, chopped
- 1 celery stalk, chopped
- 1 medium white onion, roughly chopped
- 2 garlic cloves
- 1 teaspoon fennel seeds
- 1 teaspoon dried oregano
- 1 teaspoon ground cumin
- 1 teaspoon smoked paprika
- 3 tablespoons extra-virgin olive oil
- Kosher salt and freshly ground black pepper
- Red pepper flakes (optional)
- 1 cup dry green lentils, rinsed and drained
- 1 cup vegetable stock or Liquid Gold (page 235)
- 1 (28-ounce) can tomato puree
- ½ cup unsweetened soy milk or other plant-based milk
- 2 (8-ounce) boxes high-protein rigatoni
- Chopped parsley and Cashew Parm (page 220)

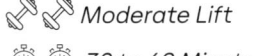 *Moderate Lift*

30 to 60 Minutes

Per serving

Calories: 446

Fat: 9g

Carbs: 75g

Fiber: 11g

Protein: 23g

Lentils used to intimidate me but they're one of the easiest, most versatile, most nutrient-packed foods out there (see page 233 for more). This curry uses quick-cooking red lentils, which effortlessly break down into creamy goodness. The silky element comes from a blended silken tofu mixture, but that's my twist — coconut milk would do the job just as well. Sometimes I serve this over rice, and sometimes I just eat it like stew — however you make it, you're getting a bowl full of fiber, protein, and pure comfort.

SERVES 4

RED LENTIL CURRY

In a blender, combine the silken tofu and ¼ cup water. Blend on high until completely smooth, about 1 minute.

In a large saucepan, heat the coconut oil over medium heat. When the oil is shimmering, add the garlic, ginger, and serrano. Cook, stirring often, until everything is very fragrant, about 1 minute. Stir in the curry powder, cumin, garam masala, turmeric, coriander, 2 teaspoons salt, and pepper until fragrant, about 30 seconds. Immediately add the stock and stir to scrape up any browned bits.

Stir in the lentils and tomatoes, then gently fold in the tofu cubes. Once the mixture comes to a simmer, cover and reduce the heat to low. Simmer until the lentils are very tender and the tofu is warmed through, about 15 minutes.

Pour in the silken tofu mixture and stir to combine. Simmer to warm through, about 1 minute more. Remove from the heat, stir in the lemon juice, and taste for seasoning.

Scoop ½ cup of the rice in each bowl, if using. Spoon the curry over the top and finish with a sprinkle of cilantro to serve.

- 6 ounces silken tofu, drained
- 1 tablespoon refined coconut oil
- 4 garlic cloves, grated
- 2-inch piece fresh ginger, peeled and grated
- 1 serrano pepper, minced (seeded for less heat)
- 1 tablespoon curry powder
- 2 teaspoons ground cumin
- 2 teaspoons garam masala
- 2 teaspoons ground turmeric
- 2 teaspoons ground coriander
- Kosher salt
- 1 teaspoon freshly ground black pepper
- 2 cups vegetable stock or Liquid Gold (page 257)
- 1 cup dry red lentils, rinsed
- 1 (14-ounce) can crushed tomatoes
- 1 (16-ounce) package extra-firm tofu, drained and cut into 1-inch cubes
- Juice of 1 lemon
- 2 cups cooked white rice (page 231; optional) and chopped fresh cilantro, for serving

Moderate Lift

Under 30 Minutes

Per serving (without rice) — Calories: 390 | Fat: 12g | Carbs: 45g | Fiber: 10g | Protein: 27g

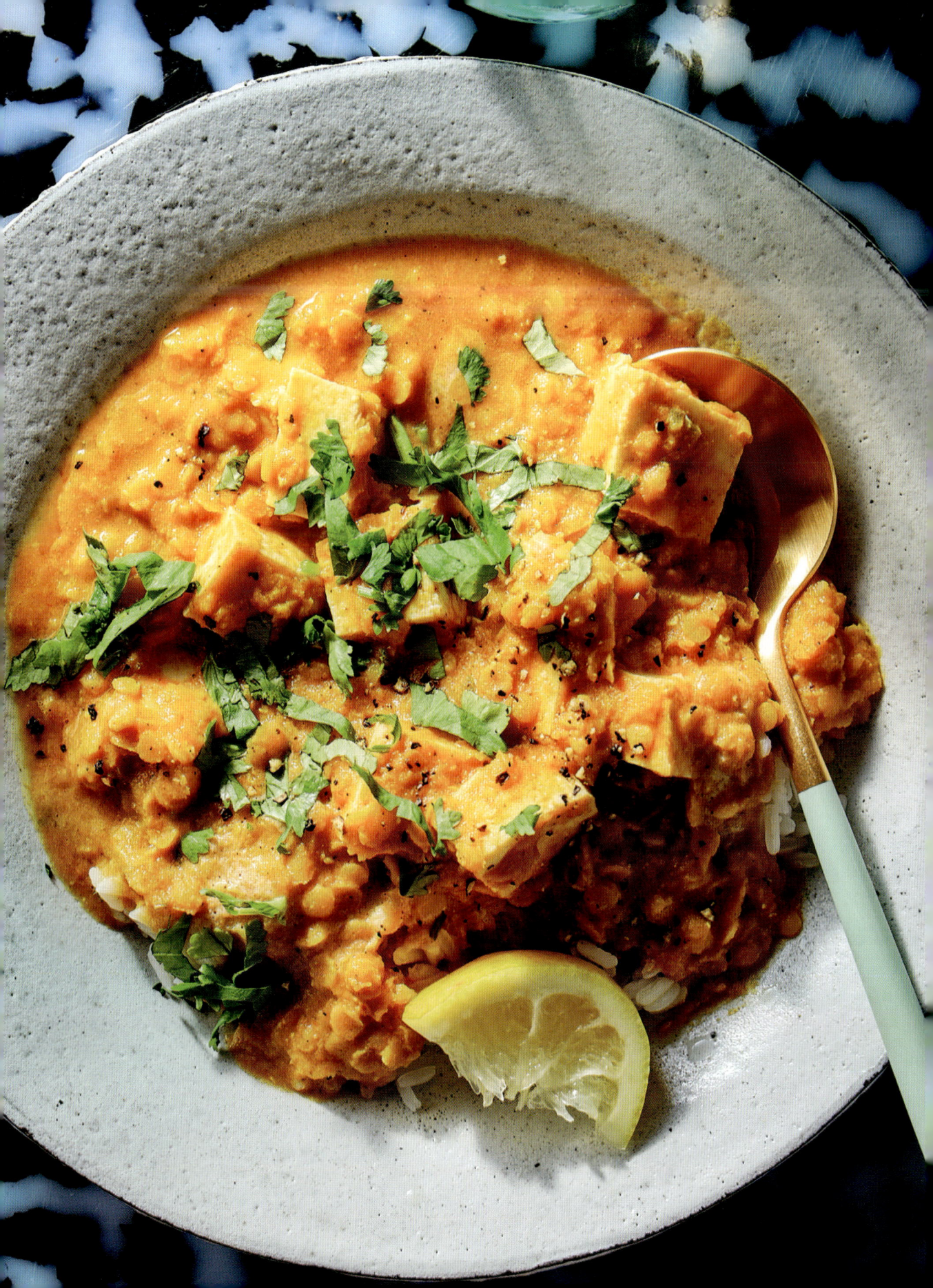

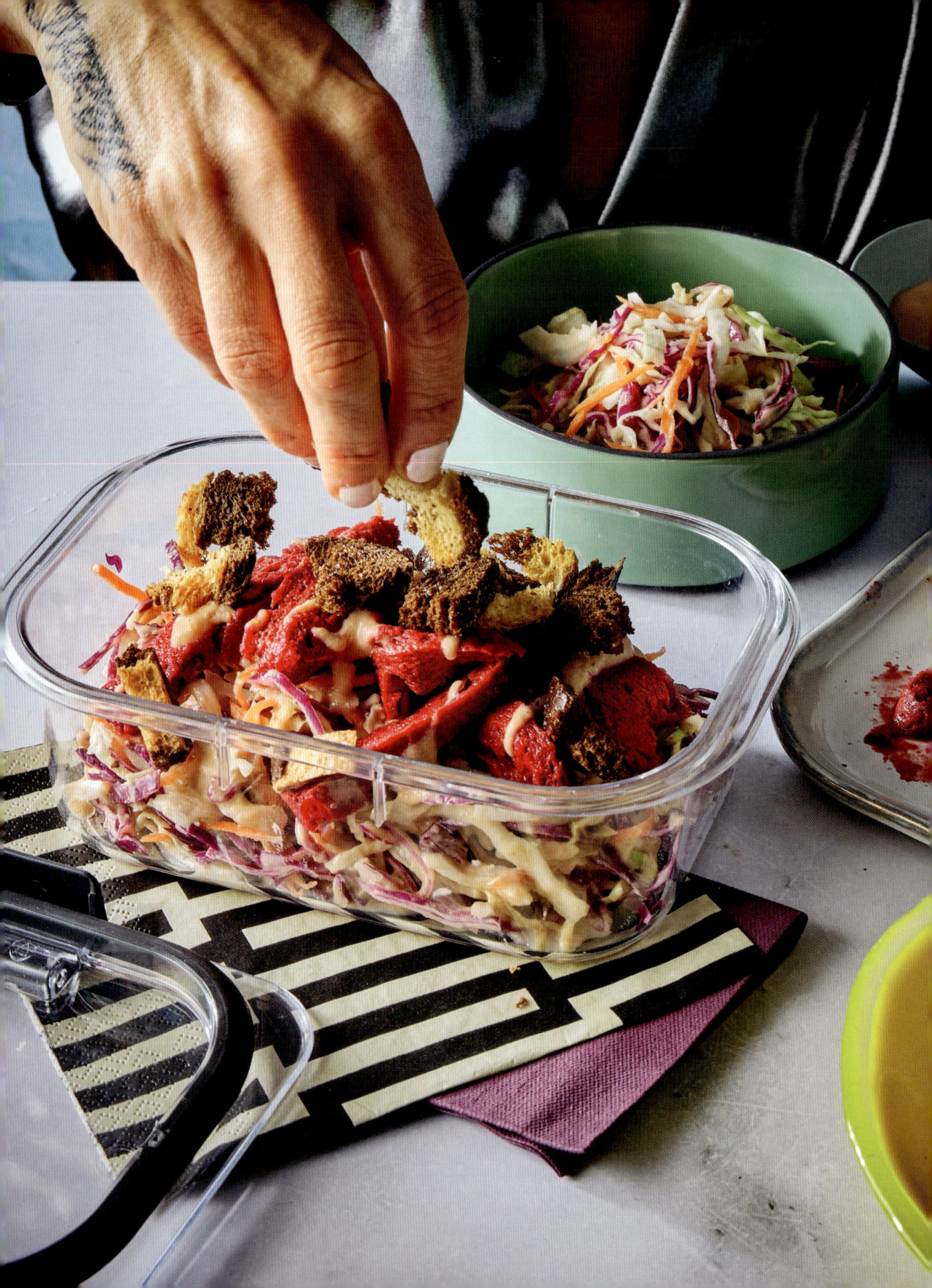

This is the ultimate Reuben meal-prep remix, a bowl piled high with all the classic flavors: pickle-and-beet-brined seitan (for that classic corned beef color and taste — and so good prepared with my homemade seitan), creamy Thousand Island dressing (made from tofu), and crispy rye croutons. Seitan has 31 grams of protein in 4 ounces — that's more than a similar portion of beef or chicken! You do have to brine the seitan at least 4 hours before you plan on serving this bowl — but since each bite is Meg Ryan–level *When Harry Met Sally* perfection, I think you'll agree it's worth the time.

SERVES 4 (MAKES 1 CUP DRESSING)

SEITAN REUBEN BOWL

Pickle the seitan: Thinly slice the seitan into long strips and arrange in a zip-top bag. Add the pickle brine, beet juice, pickling spice, garlic powder, and onion powder. Seal the bag and shake to combine. Refrigerate for at least 4 hours or overnight.

Make the Thousand Island dressing: In a blender, combine the tofu, ketchup, pickles, salt, and pepper. Blend on high to make a smooth dressing, about 1 minute. Transfer to an airtight container and refrigerate until ready to use, or up to 3 days.

Make the bowl: Preheat the oven to 400°F. Cut the bread slices into 1-inch pieces and arrange evenly on a rimmed baking sheet. Bake until toasted, about 10 minutes. (The croutons can be stored in an airtight container at room temperature for up to 3 days.)

To assemble each bowl, toss a fourth of the slaw with 2 tablespoons of the dressing to lightly coat. Arrange the slaw at the bottom of a serving bowl, then lay a few pieces of the seitan on top. Spoon over a little more dressing and sprinkle a few of the croutons on top. Serve immediately.

Seitan
1 pound seitan, homemade (page 222) or store-bought strips
½ cup dill pickle brine
¼ cup beet juice
1 teaspoon pickling spice
1 teaspoon garlic powder
1 teaspoon onion powder

Thousand Island Dressing
6 ounces silken tofu, drained
¼ cup sugar-free ketchup
8 dill pickle slices
1 teaspoon kosher salt
1 teaspoon freshly ground black pepper

Bowl
4 slices marble rye bread
1 (10-ounce) bag vegetable slaw mix

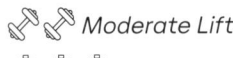 *Moderate Lift*
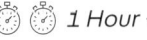 1 Hour +

Per serving
Calories: 420
Fat: 3g
Carbs: 37g
Fiber: 6g
Protein: 30g

Protein: 24g | Fiber: 27g | Carbs: 80g | Fat: 6g | Calories: 453
Per serving, without quinoa

When I went vegan, I zeroed in on recipes that felt familiar, easy, and totally satisfying to help ease into my new way of eating. This is exactly that kind of recipe, packed with three types of hearty beans, smoky spices, and a touch of cocoa powder to deepen the flavor and give it that rich, slow-cooked taste — no hours of simmering required. It'll quickly become your go-to for a repeatable, customizable meal. For even more protein and fiber, I'll serve the chili over quinoa — sometimes, especially after an intense workout, I just need to eat something deeply fortifying to help my body recover. If you really want to level up, spoon this chili over the Stacked Nacho Fries (page 173) or pair it with Tempeh Buffalo Dip (page 174) for a full-on game day spread — no actual game required.

SERVES 4

THREE-BEAN CHILI

In a large Dutch oven, heat the avocado oil over medium heat. When the oil is shimmering, add the onion, garlic, and jalapeños. Cook, stirring often, until the onion softens, about 4 minutes. Add the chili powder, cocoa powder, and paprika, and cook, stirring often, until fragrant, about 30 seconds. Immediately add the stock and stir to scrape up any browned bits.

Stir in the black beans, kidney beans, pinto beans, tomatoes, salt, and pepper. Once the mixture comes to a simmer, cover and reduce the heat to low. Simmer until the beans are very tender, about 15 minutes. Remove from the heat, stir in the lime juice, and taste for seasoning.

Scoop ½ cup of the quinoa into each bowl, if using. Spoon the chili over the top and finish with a dollop of sour cream and a sprinkle of scallions before serving.

1 tablespoon avocado oil
1 medium red onion, diced
3 garlic cloves, minced
2 jalapeños, diced (seeded for less heat)
3 tablespoons chili powder
1 tablespoon cocoa powder
2 teaspoons smoked paprika
2 cups vegetable stock or Liquid Gold (page 235)
1 (15.5-ounce) can black beans, drained and rinsed
1 (15.5-ounce) can kidney beans, drained and rinsed
1 (15.5-ounce) can pinto beans, drained and rinsed
1 (28-ounce) can diced tomatoes
1 teaspoon kosher salt, plus more as needed
½ teaspoon freshly ground black pepper
Juice of 1 lime
2 cups cooked quinoa (page 231; optional), store-bought or homemade vegan sour cream (page 146), and thinly sliced scallions, for serving

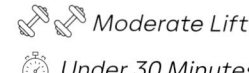
Moderate Lift
Under 30 Minutes

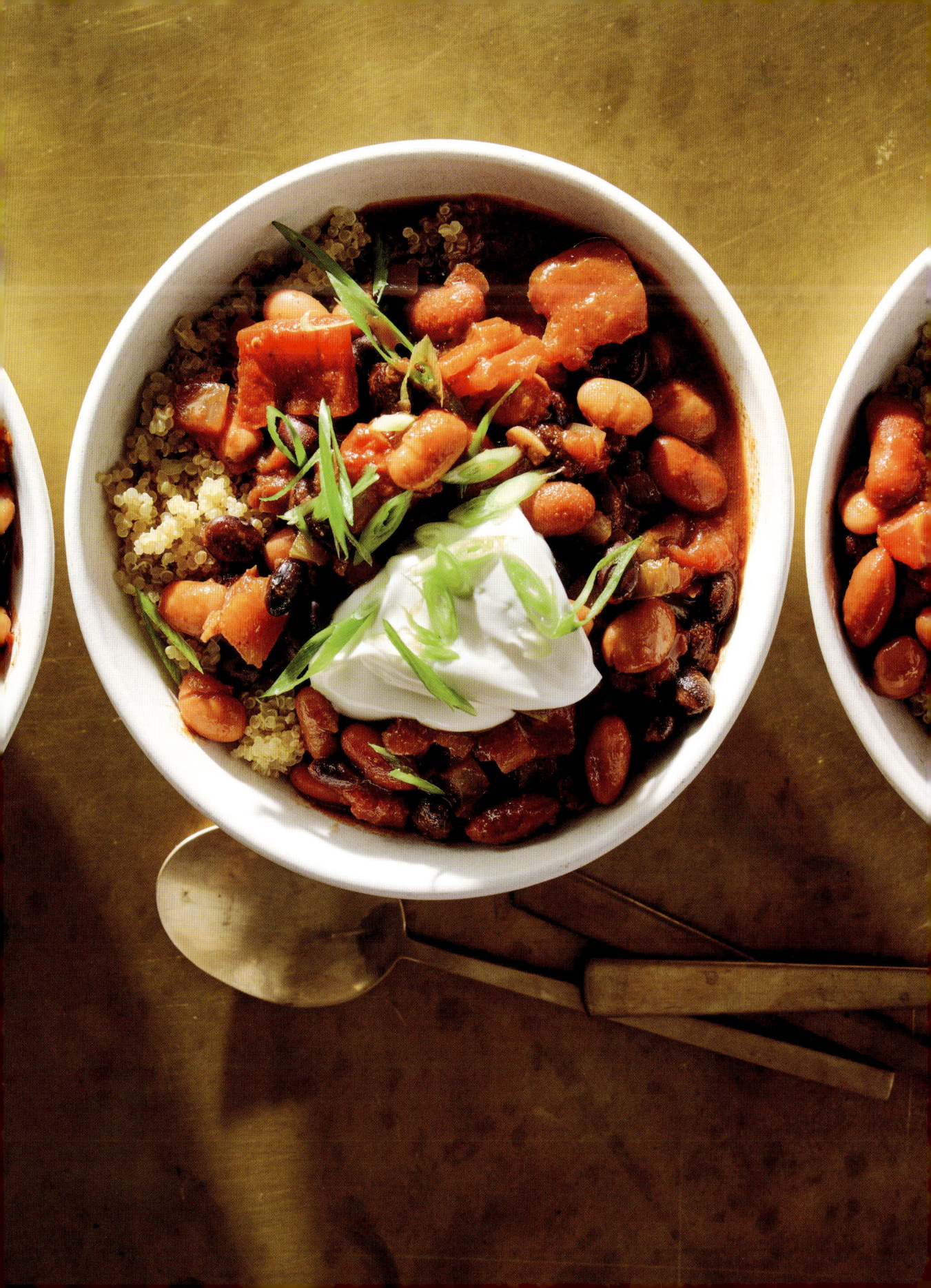

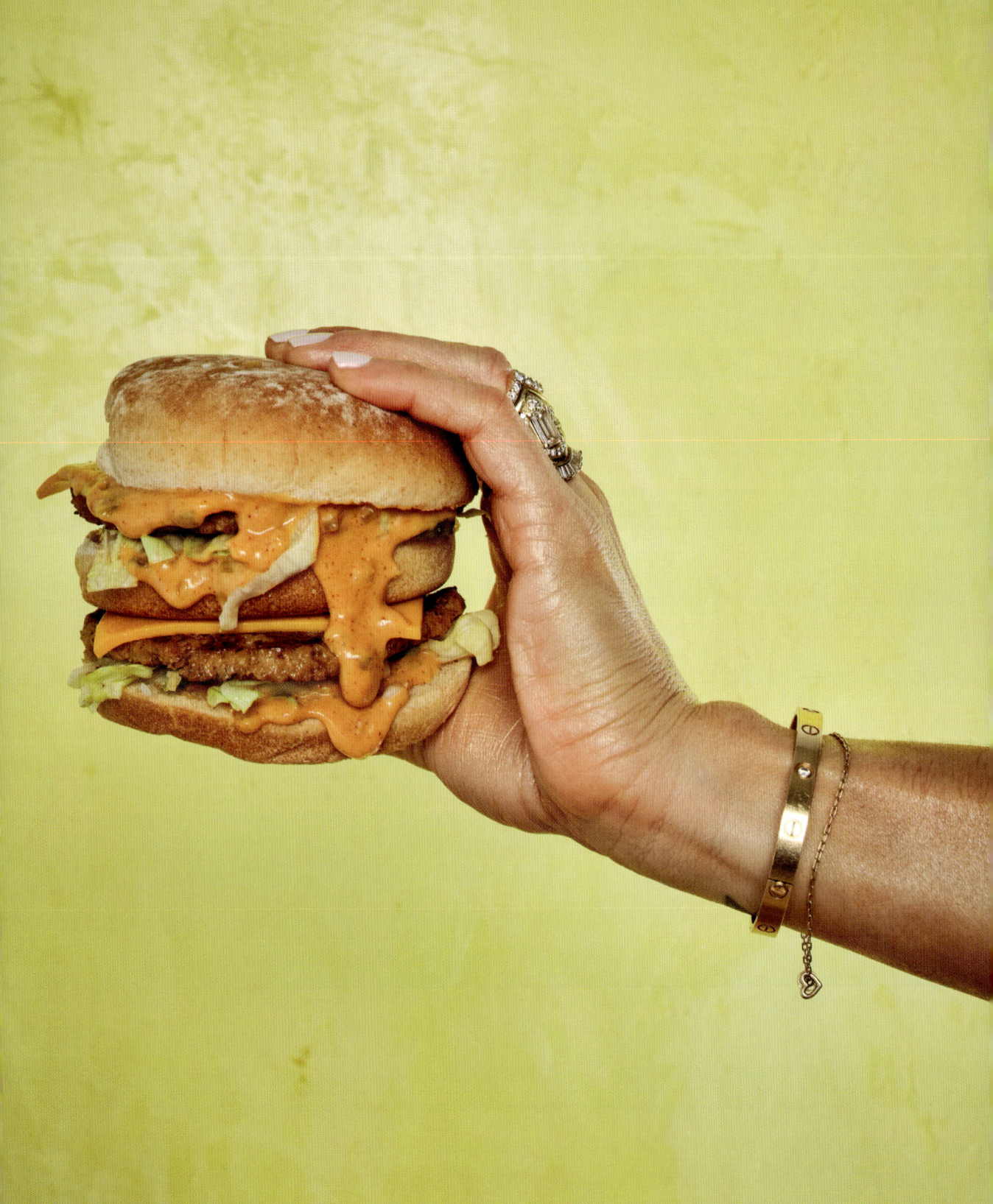

I ♥ SANDWICHES

This chapter is basically my love letter to road trip food made healthier — inspired by fast-food classics, gas station gems, and deli counter staples I thought I'd never get to eat again after going vegan. My versions hit just as hard, especially because they're loaded with plant-based protein, so your body enjoys them just as much as you do. So, if you thought sandwiches were out of the question because you're eating more plants, training hard, or trying to fuel your macros, think again. When you need something quick to make, easy to take on the go, satisfying, and endlessly adaptable, a sandwich always delivers. These sandwiches bring the flavor, the nostalgia, and the fuel to keep you going.

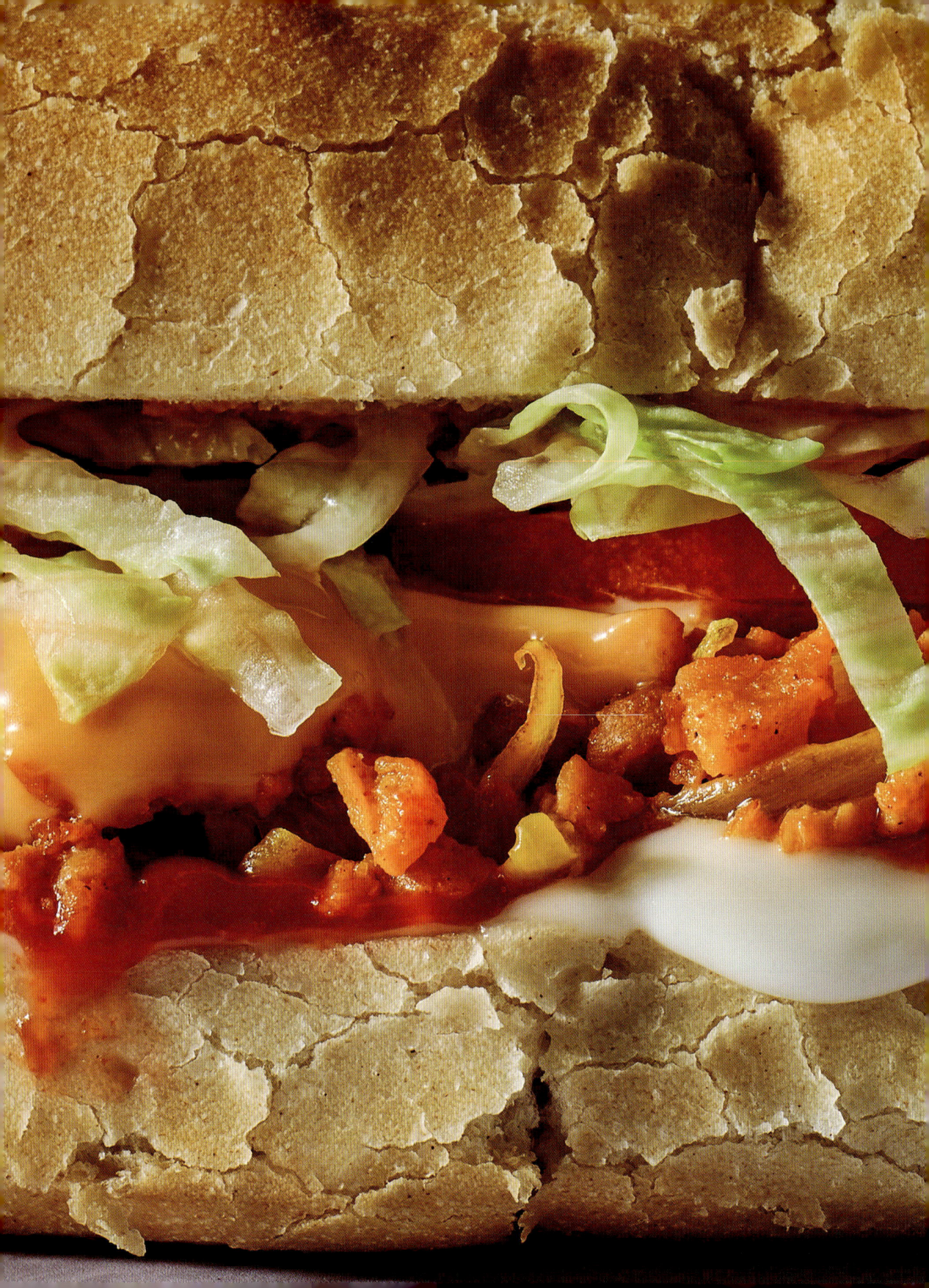

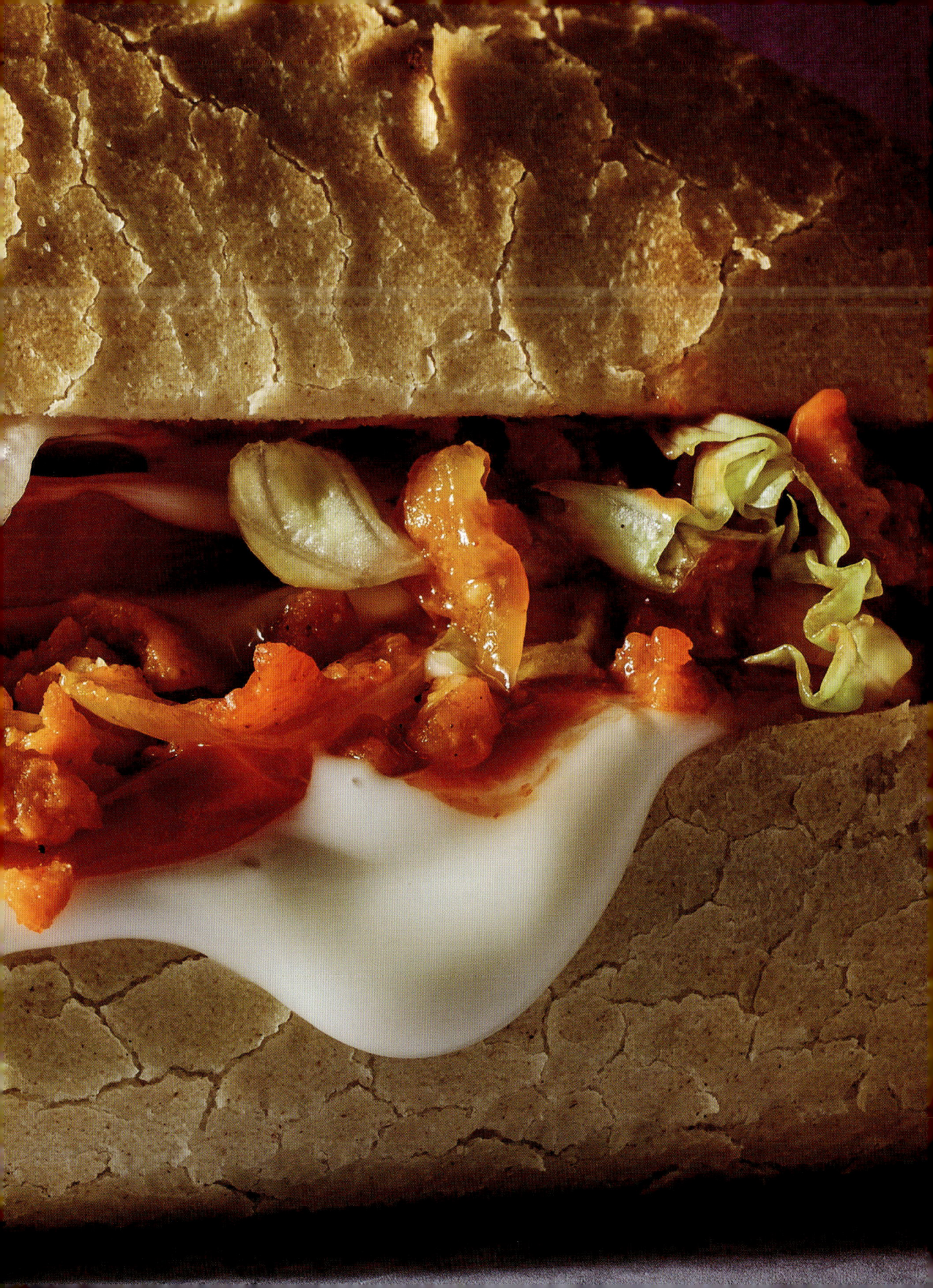

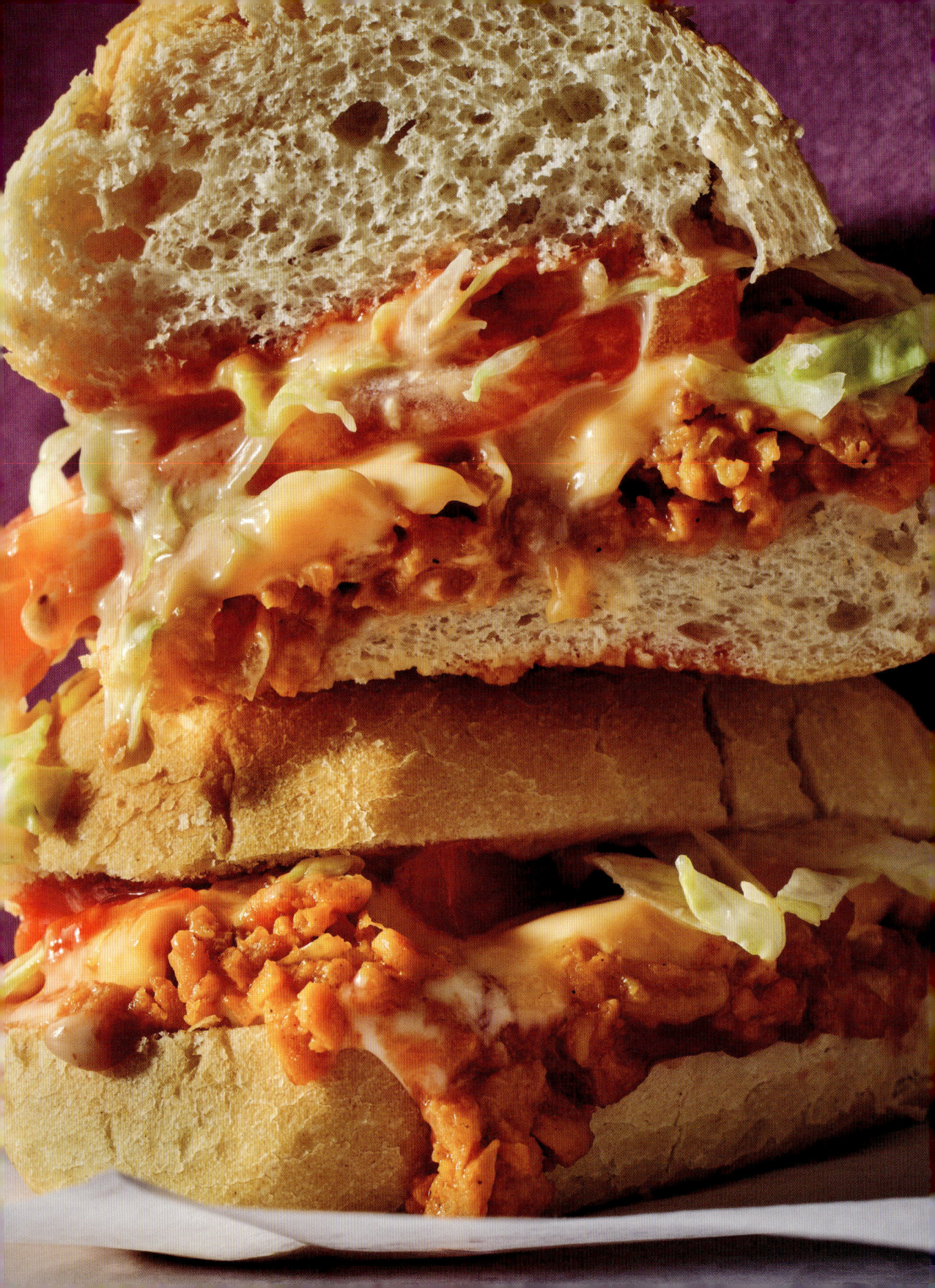

New Yorkers know: the bodega chopped cheese is iconic. Essentially, it's ground beef, chopped up right on the griddle, topped with melted cheese, then stuffed into a hero roll with lettuce, tomato, and all the classic condiments. It's the late-night, post-everything, grab-it-on-the-go sandwich that never misses. When I lived in my downtown NoLita apartment, I'd go out on my fire escape, yell my order across the street (the owner always seemed to be outside on a smoke break), and my sandwich would be waiting for me by the time I hit the sidewalk. This version keeps that energy alive — savory, melty, messy in the best ways. The TVP-based "meat" in this version brings all the texture, the seasoning is on point, and the combo of ketchup, mayo, and shredded lettuce is nonnegotiable. You don't need a bodega cat staring you down to enjoy this one — just a big appetite.

MAKES 2 SANDWICHES

BODEGA CHOPPED CHEESE

Make the TVP meat: In a medium bowl, mix the hydrated TVP, nutritional yeast, liquid smoke, onion powder, garlic powder, and ¼ teaspoon pepper.

Make the chopped cheese: In a large cast-iron skillet, heat the avocado oil over medium. When it is just barely smoking, add the meat mixture with the onion. Season with a good sprinkle each of Sazón and adobo, then use a flat spatula to toss with the meat-and-onion mixture. Cook, tossing occasionally, until the onion is soft, about 6 minutes.

Use the spatula to divide the mixture into two portions. Drape two slices of cheese over each portion. Add a splash of water to the skillet and cover to melt the cheese, about 1 minute. Remove from the heat.

Spread open the hoagie rolls and give each a coat of ketchup and mayo. Use the spatula to transfer the two portions of meat onto the rolls (it's ok if the cheese gets mixed in at this point). Layer on some tomato slices and 1 cup of shredded lettuce. Press the roll shut and wrap in a sheet of parchment paper for the real bodega feeling. Slice each sandwich in half before serving.

TVP Meat
- ¼ pound hydrated TVP MVP (page 224) or 6 tablespoons rehydrated TVP
- 1 tablespoon nutritional yeast
- ½ teaspoon liquid smoke
- ¼ teaspoon onion powder
- ¼ teaspoon garlic powder
- Freshly ground black pepper

Chopped Cheese
- 1 tablespoon avocado oil
- ½ large white onion, halved and thinly sliced
- Sazón and adobo seasonings
- 4 slices vegan American cheese
- 2 hoagie rolls, split
- Sugar-free ketchup
- Vegan mayo
- 1 beefsteak tomato, thinly sliced
- 2 cups shredded lettuce

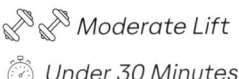 *Moderate Lift*

Under 30 Minutes

Per sandwich
Calories: 620
Fat: 24g
Carbs: 84g
Fiber: 9g
Protein: 30g

This is my ultimate meal prep flex — saving me minutes (and sanity) all week long. I make this salad with soy curls (dried soy strips made from whole soybeans that get rehydrated for an easy meat substitute) in a big batch to last in the fridge all week. Whether tucked into a lettuce cup, a high-protein wrap, or high-protein bread (or frankly, just snacked on with a spoon!), it brings a perfect herby-crunchy-tangy-meaty bite. Yogurt keeps things light and protein packed, and I always add whatever farmers' market pickles I'm obsessing over that week. Post-workout, pre-Zoom, or smack in the middle of midday life, I can grab a quick bite and keep it moving.

MAKES 8 SANDWICHES, WRAPS, OR STUFFED LETTUCE CUPS (6 CUPS CH*CKEN SALAD)

CLASSIC CHI*KEN SALAD

In a large bowl, combine the soy curls with enough hot tap water to cover. Let hydrate for 10 minutes, then drain thoroughly.

Wipe the large bowl dry, then whisk together the yogurt, nutritional yeast, mustard, salt, pepper, garlic powder, and onion powder. Add the drained soy curls, celery, scallions, pickles, lemon juice, and dill. Fold to mix all the ingredients evenly, then cover the bowl with plastic wrap and refrigerate for at least 30 minutes or overnight to let the flavors meld. The salad lasts for up to 5 days in the fridge.

Pile on bread, roll in a wrap, or spoon into lettuce cups.

Note: While some grocery stores are starting to stock soy curls, they're often easier to find online. Or, if you don't want to wait for a delivery (or hunt them down), two drained cans of chickpeas, lightly smashed, are a great substitute!

8 ounces dehydrated soy curls (see Note)
1 cup plain vegan Greek yogurt
2 tablespoons nutritional yeast
2 tablespoons grainy mustard
2 teaspoons kosher salt, plus more as needed
1 teaspoon freshly ground black pepper
1 teaspoon garlic powder
1 teaspoon onion powder
2 celery stalks, diced
2 scallions, thinly sliced
½ cup finely chopped pickles of your choice
Juice of 1 lemon
2 tablespoons roughly chopped fresh dill
16 slices high-protein bread, such as Hero, or 8 high-protein wraps, or 8 butter lettuce cups

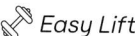 *Easy Lift*

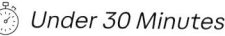 *Under 30 Minutes*

Per sandwich — Calories: 250 | Fat: 10g | Carbs: 33g | Fiber: 29g | Protein: 25g

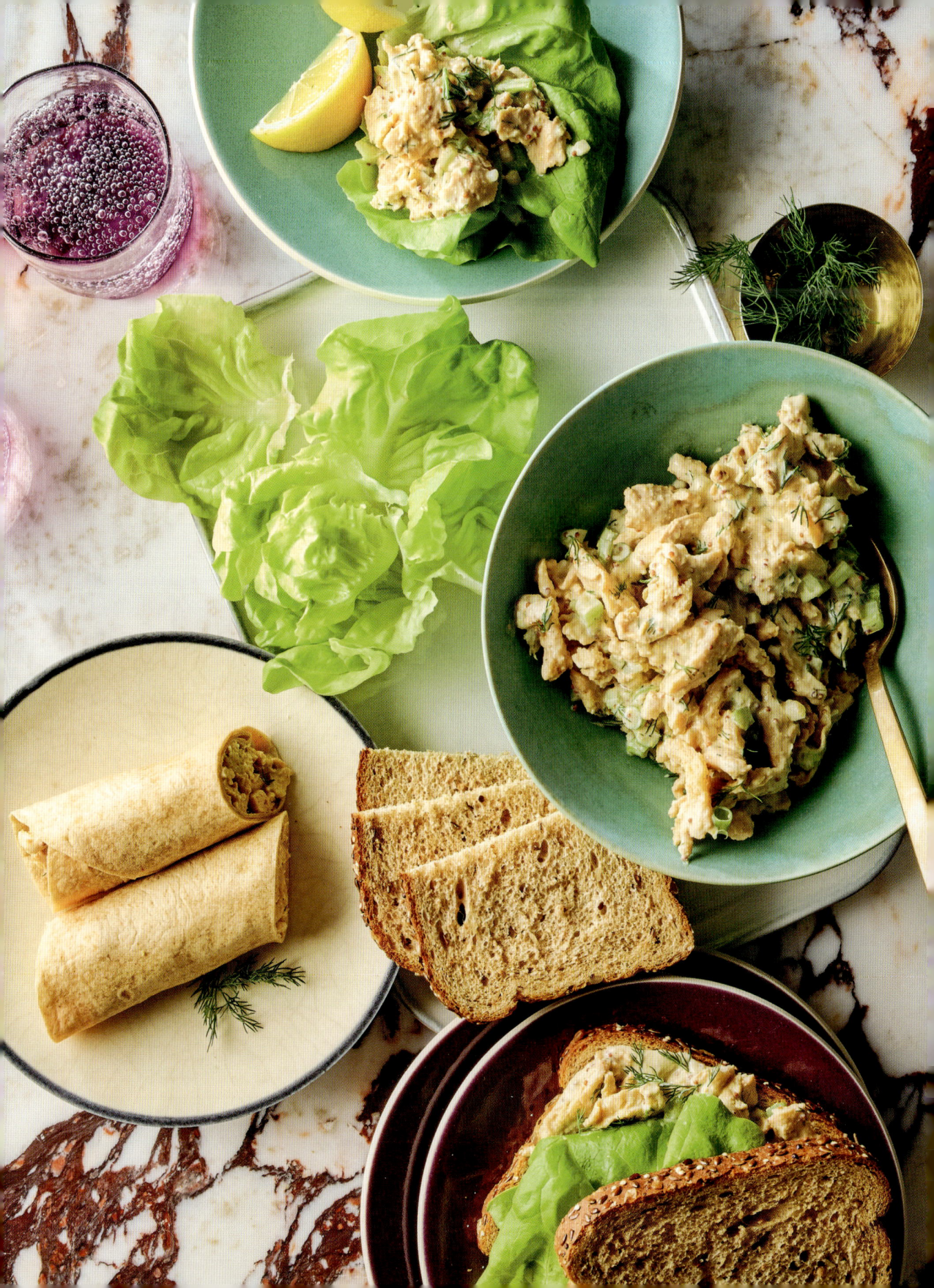

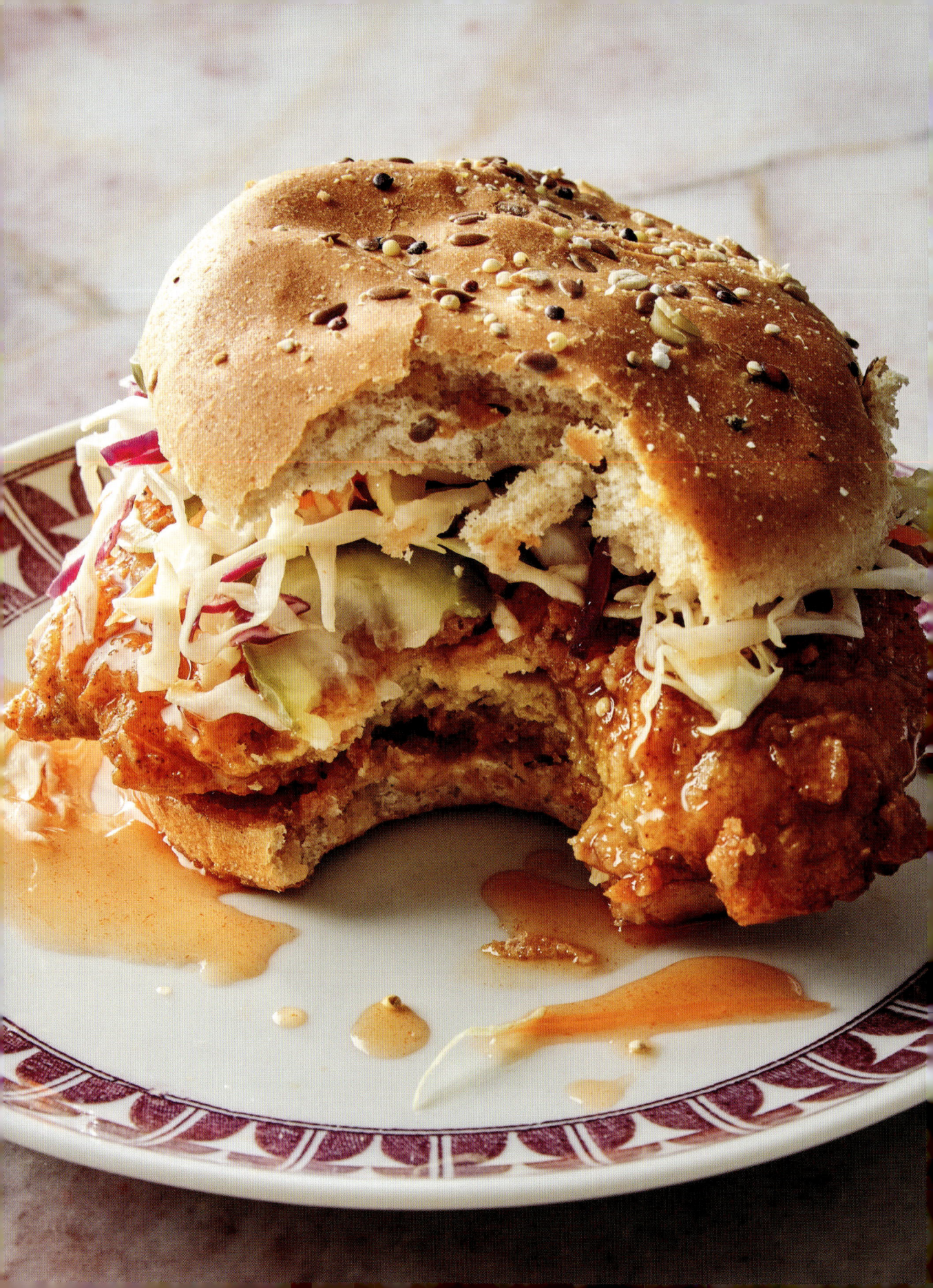

This is the crispy, crunchy, spicy-sweet-drizzled-to-perfection sandwich to end all others. Ok, so it's not an everyday thing, but when you're craving something fried that goes all in, this is it. It takes me straight back to being a kid — after the dentist, my mom would let me pick whatever fast food I wanted as a reward. It was usually a sandwich like this. This is my grown-up, plant-powered version that hits all the same notes — crispy, fried, stacked high with a crunchy slaw — but actually fuels me for whatever's next. Give that seitan the time it deserves — at least 4 hours to marinate — because you can't rush greatness.

MAKES 4 SANDWICHES

FRIED NO-CHICK DELUXE

Cut the seitan into 4 equal pieces. In a zip-top bag, combine the soy milk, 2 tablespoons of the hot sauce, the pickle brine, vinegar, onion powder, and garlic powder. Add the seitan, seal the bag, and shake to mix the marinade and coat the seitan. Refrigerate for at least 4 hours, but ideally overnight.

Remove the seitan pieces to a plate and pour the marinade into a shallow bowl. Whisk 2 tablespoons of the flour into the marinade to thicken. In another shallow bowl, whisk the remaining 1 cup flour with the cornstarch, baking powder, and Cajun seasoning. Working with one piece at a time, dip the seitan in the marinade, letting the excess drip off, then toss in the flour mixture to coat evenly. Dip back in the marinade and dredge in the flour a second time. Transfer to a wire rack to rest while dredging the rest of the seitan.

In a large saucepan, heat the vegetable oil over medium heat until it registers 375°F on a thermometer. While the oil is heating, whisk the agave and remaining ¼ cup hot sauce together in a medium bowl and keep nearby.

When the oil is ready, carefully lower two pieces of the seitan into the saucepan. Fry until deep brown all over, flipping halfway, 3 to 4 minutes. Transfer to the wire rack to drain while frying the remaining two pieces. While the seitan is still hot, carefully toss it in the agave mixture to coat, then return to the wire rack to set.

To assemble the sandwiches, set the fried seitan on the bottom buns. Pile some slaw on top and spoon some of the remaining spicy agave on top. Layer on a few pickle slices and press on the top buns. Serve hot.

½ pound DIY Seitan (page 222)
2 cups unsweetened soy milk or other plant-based milk
¼ cup plus 2 tablespoons hot sauce
2 tablespoons dill pickle brine
2 tablespoons apple cider vinegar
1 tablespoon onion powder
1 tablespoon garlic powder
1 cup plus 2 tablespoons all-purpose flour
1 cup cornstarch
2 tablespoons baking powder
2 tablespoons Cajun seasoning
2 quarts vegetable oil
½ cup agave syrup
4 high-protein burger buns, such as Hero
Cabbage slaw and dill pickle slices, for serving

Heavy Lift
1 Hour +

Per sandwich
Calories: 666
Fat: 36g
Carbs: 67g
Fiber: 27g
Protein: 31g

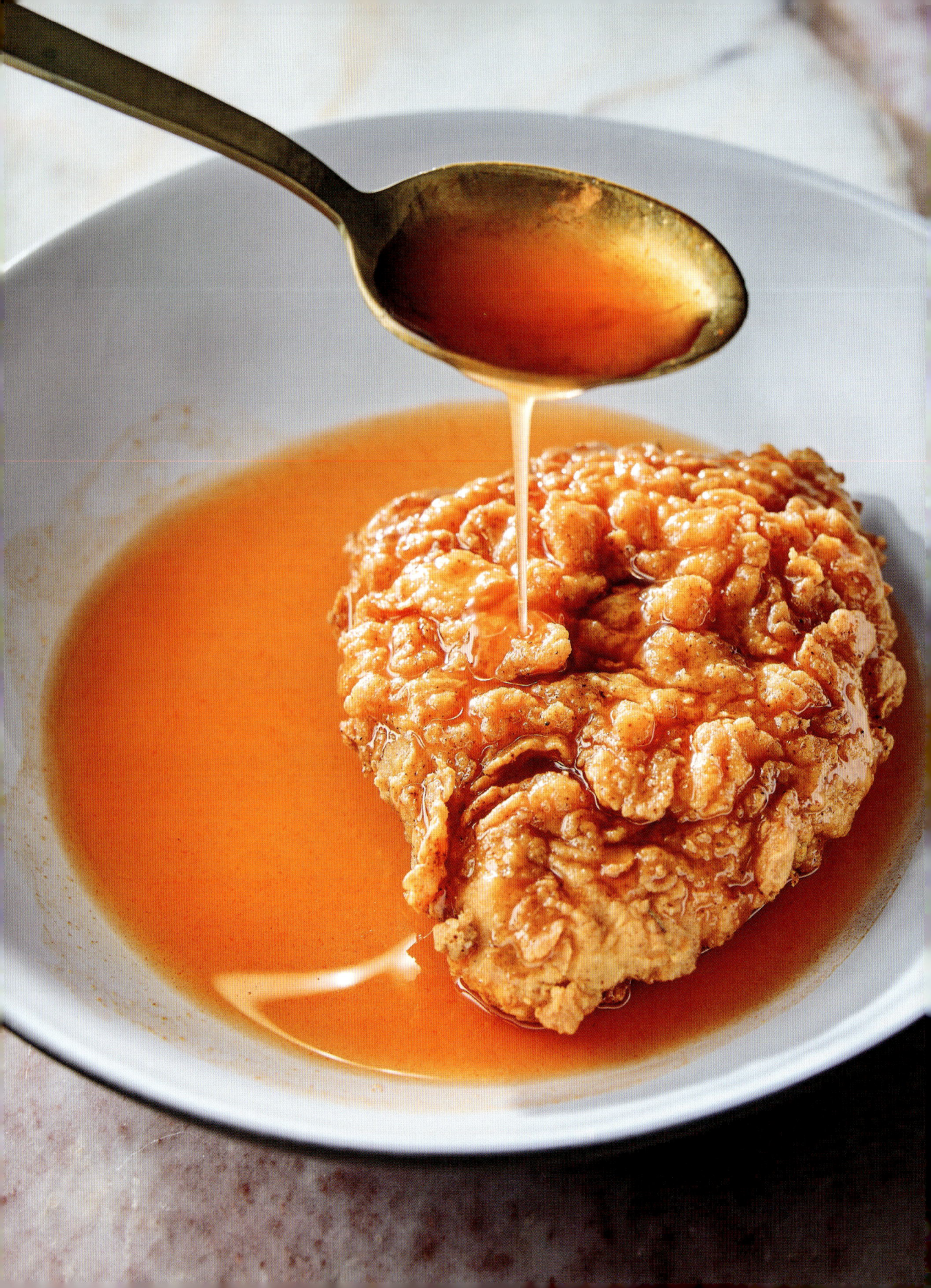

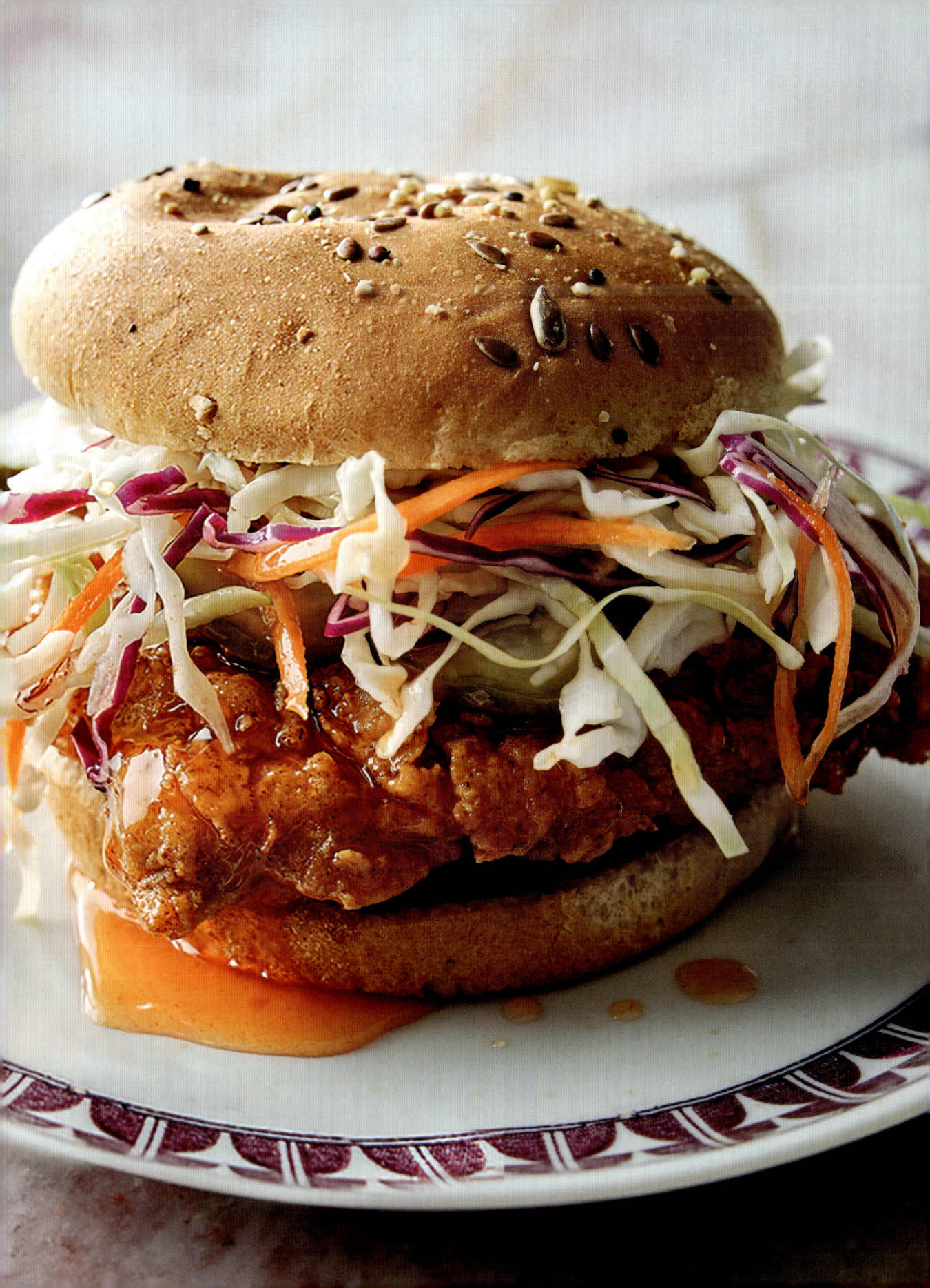

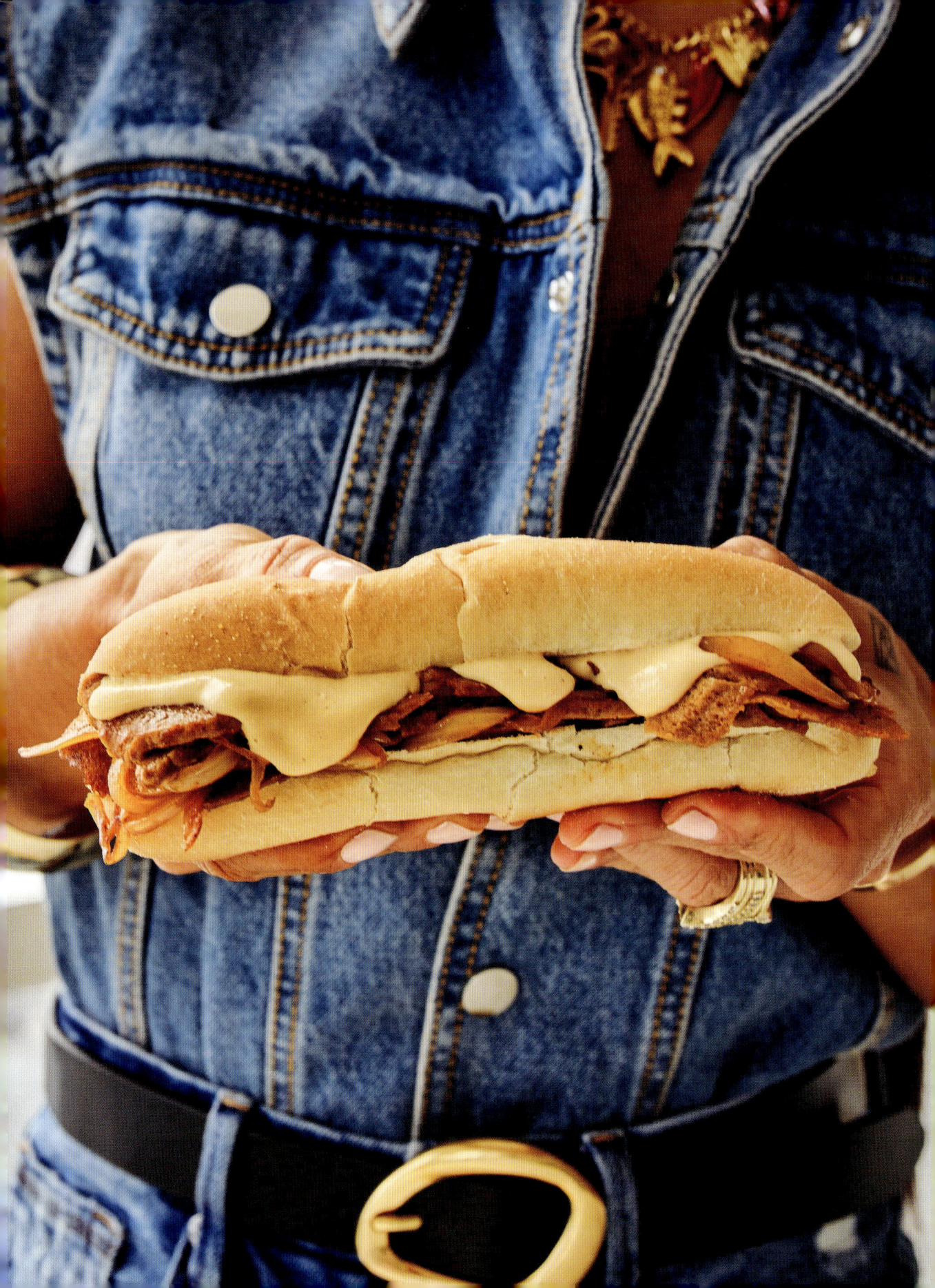

I might be a New Yorker now, but at my core I'm a Philly girl forever. And Philly takes its cheesesteaks very seriously. The city's vegan scene is thriving, so I know I have to bring my A-game with this one. When I went plant based, I thought I was saying goodbye to cheesesteaks forever, which was devastating. But this version has all the essentials: thinly sliced seitan that soaks up every bit of smoky, savory flavor and a silky, bright orange plant-based turn on Cheez Whiz (because if your whiz isn't neon, it's not right). And yes, we're doing it "wit" — which means "with onions" for those new to the lingo. Philly, I hope this "jawn" did you proud!

MAKES 4 SANDWICHES

I'M FROM PHILLY CHEESESTEAK

Make the vegan steak: Thinly slice the seitan to make long strips. In a large nonstick skillet, evenly spread out the seitan, then pour over the Worcestershire sauce, soy sauce, avocado oil, paprika, garlic powder, and liquid smoke. Use tongs to toss and coat evenly. Let rest for 5 minutes to marinate.

Add the onion and set the skillet over medium heat. Cook, undisturbed, as the seitan slowly steams off liquid and the onion softens, about 10 minutes. Once the liquid has evaporated, season with a pinch of salt and pepper. Stir occasionally until the onion and seitan are brown all over, about 5 minutes. Remove from the heat.

Vegan Steak

- 1 pound seitan, homemade (page 224) or store-bought strips
- 2 tablespoons vegan Worcestershire sauce
- 2 tablespoons soy sauce or tamari
- 1 tablespoon avocado oil
- 1 teaspoon smoked paprika
- 1 teaspoon garlic powder
- 1 teaspoon liquid smoke
- 1 large white onion, thinly sliced
- Kosher salt and freshly ground black pepper

Per sandwich

Calories: 670

Fat: 17g

Carbs: 65g

Fiber: 4g

Protein: 35g

Recipe continues...

I ♥ Sandwiches 95

While the seitan cooks, make the whiz: In a small saucepan, bring 1 cup water to a boil over high heat. Remove from the heat and add the cashews. Soak until soft, about 10 minutes, then drain and return to the same saucepan. Add the soy milk, hot sauce, onion powder, and garlic powder. Set over medium heat and bring to a simmer. Immediately (but carefully) pour the mixture into a blender and add the vegan cheese. Blend on medium speed until smooth, about 1 minute. Taste for seasoning, adding salt if needed. Cover the blender to keep the sauce warm.

Split each hoagie roll, pile on some seitan and onions using tongs, then pour over a healthy amount of whiz. Press together and serve immediately.

Whiz

¼ cup raw cashews
½ cup unsweetened soy milk or other plant-based milk
1 teaspoon hot sauce
¼ teaspoon onion powder
¼ teaspoon garlic powder
4 ounces vegan cheddar cheese, shredded
Kosher salt

4 hoagie rolls, split

Moderate Lift

Under 30 Minutes

```
┌─────────────────────────────────────────────┐
│  Dalina Says...                             │
│  Robin's plant-based cheesesteak offers satisfac-
│  tion and nutrition, which is always the goal. The
│  sautéed onions add fiber and antioxidants, while
│  the plant-based protein (seitan) and cashew-based
│  whiz keep you full while giving lots of flavor.
└─────────────────────────────────────────────┘
```

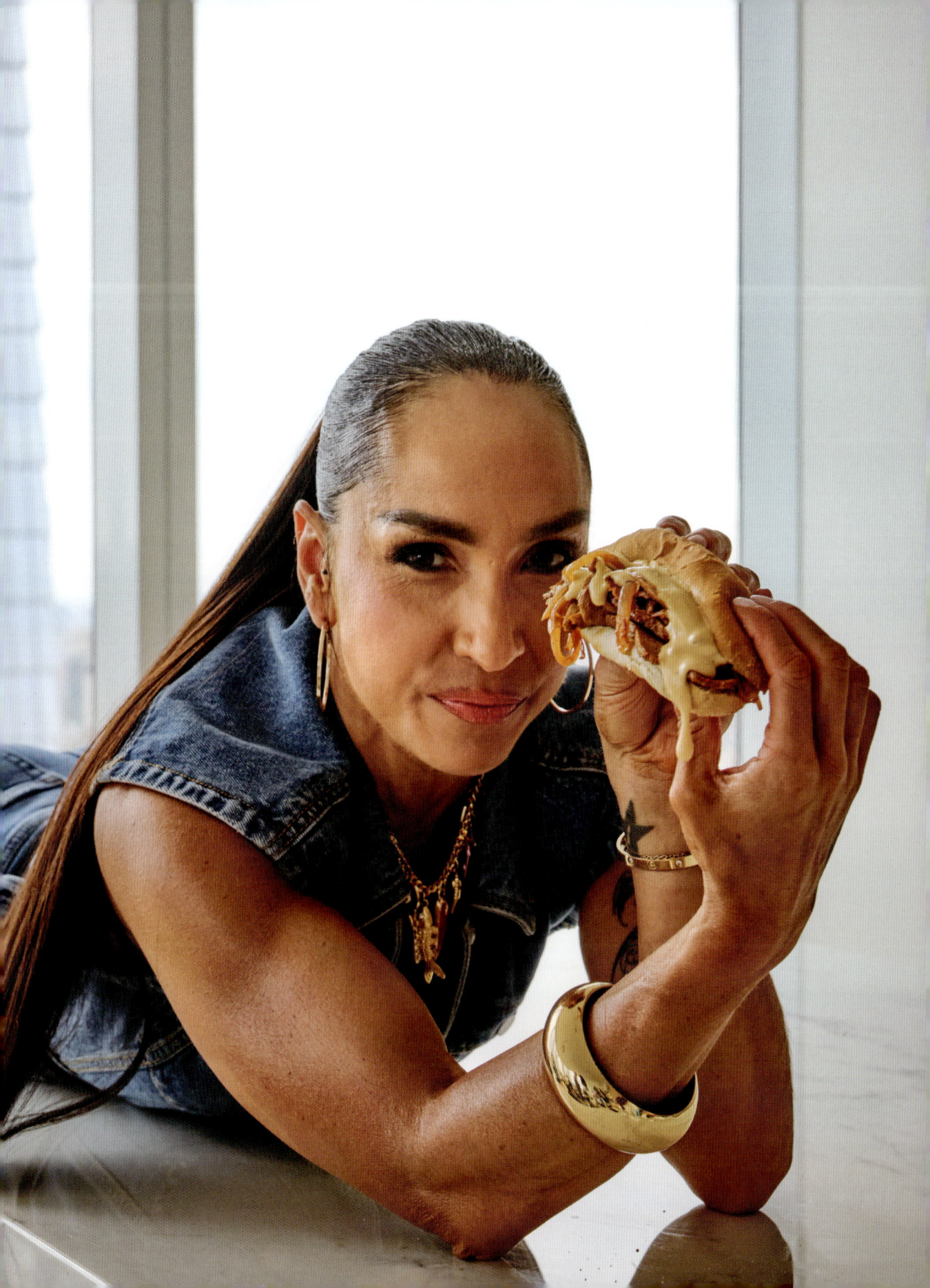

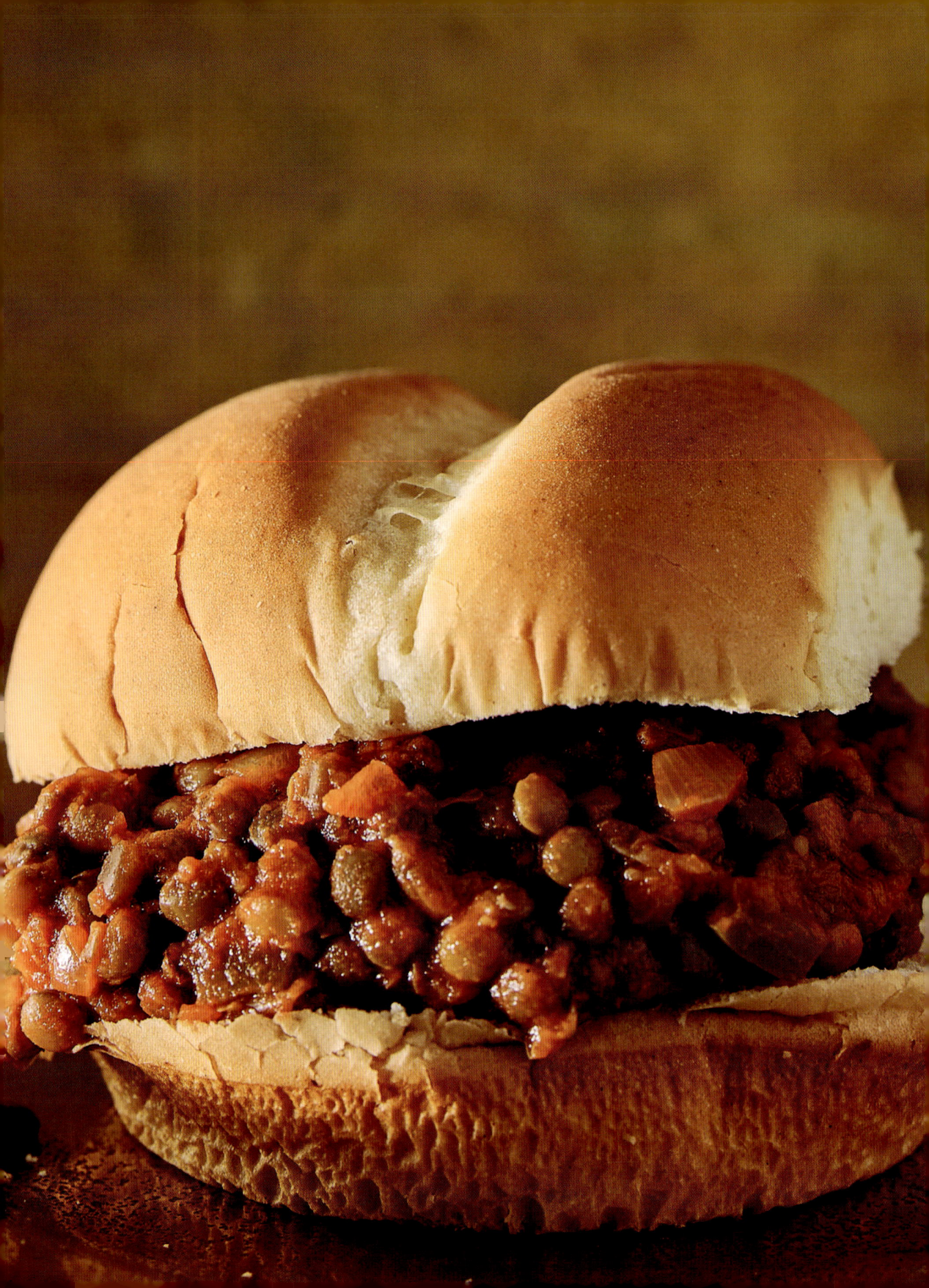

Traditional sloppy Joes are way too sweet and ketchupy for my taste. I like to think my version is a little more refined — still hearty and meaty from the lentils, with a smoky, savory sauce that's just the right amount of tangy. Serve the hearty filling on high-protein buns and watch them disappear. Napkins definitely required.

MAKES 4 SANDWICHES

LENTIL SLOPPY JOES

Preheat the oven to 200°F. In a large skillet, heat the avocado oil over medium heat. When the oil is shimmering, add the onion, bell pepper, and garlic. Cook, stirring often, until the pepper is soft, about 4 minutes.

Stir in the tomato sauce, coconut sugar, Worcestershire sauce, chili powder, salt, paprika, red pepper, and black pepper. Let the mixture come to a simmer, then stir in the lentils to coat. Simmer until the lentils are warmed through and the sauce is thickened, about 5 minutes.

While the lentils are simmering, split the burger buns and arrange on the oven rack to toast. Divide the sloppy Joe mixture among the toasted buns and serve immediately.

- 2 tablespoons avocado oil
- ½ medium white onion, diced
- ½ green bell pepper, seeded and diced
- 2 garlic cloves, minced
- 1 (15-ounce) can tomato sauce
- 2 tablespoons coconut sugar
- 2 tablespoons vegan Worcestershire sauce or coconut aminos
- 1 tablespoon chili powder
- 1 teaspoon kosher salt
- 1 teaspoon smoked paprika
- ½ teaspoon red pepper flakes
- ½ teaspoon freshly ground black pepper
- 2 cups cooked lentils (page 233)
- 4 high-protein burger buns, such as Hero

 Easy Lift

 Under 30 Minutes

Per sandwich

Calories: 400

Fat: 13g

Carbs: 69g

Fiber: 34g

Protein: 22g

Fast, filling, and easy to eat with one hand, this burrito has smoky beans, a killer vegan queso, and just enough heat to keep things interesting. Plus, it's just as good at room temperature, so go ahead and toss one in your bag as a purse snack for later. You'll thank me when hunger strikes!

MAKES 4 BURRITOS

PLANT-POWERED BEAN & CHILE BURRITOS

Make the vegan queso: In a large saucepan, heat the avocado oil over medium heat. When the oil is shimmering, add the onion and cook, stirring occasionally, until translucent, about 4 minutes. Stir in the garlic and continue to cook until fragrant, about 2 minutes. Add the potato, carrot, cashews, and 2 cups water. Increase the heat to high and bring to a boil. Reduce the heat to medium and simmer until the potato and carrot are very soft and the cashews are swollen, 10 to 15 minutes. Remove from the heat and let cool for 10 minutes.

Carefully pour the vegetables and liquid into a blender. Add the nutritional yeast, miso, salt, mustard, and turmeric. Blend on high until the mixture is smooth, 1 to 2 minutes. Pour into a bowl and taste for seasoning. Use immediately or let cool completely and refrigerate in an airtight container for up to 5 days. (See sidebar.)

Vegan Queso

1 tablespoon avocado oil
½ small white onion, diced
1 garlic clove, thinly sliced
1 small russet potato, peeled and cut into ½-inch cubes
1 small carrot, cut into ¼-inch rounds
¼ cup raw cashews
¼ cup nutritional yeast
1 tablespoon white miso
1 teaspoon kosher salt, plus more as needed
1 teaspoon yellow mustard
½ teaspoon ground turmeric

```
Queso on Repeat

This queso makes plenty for leftovers and can
be drizzled over Seitan Fajitas (page 145) or
Stacked Nacho Fries (page 173), used as a dip
for Crispy Air-Fried Tofu Nuggets (page 169) or
Pizza Bites (page 170), or served with chips and
salsa for an easy snack. Reheat the queso in the
microwave or in a saucepan over low heat,
stirring frequently.
```

Recipe continues...

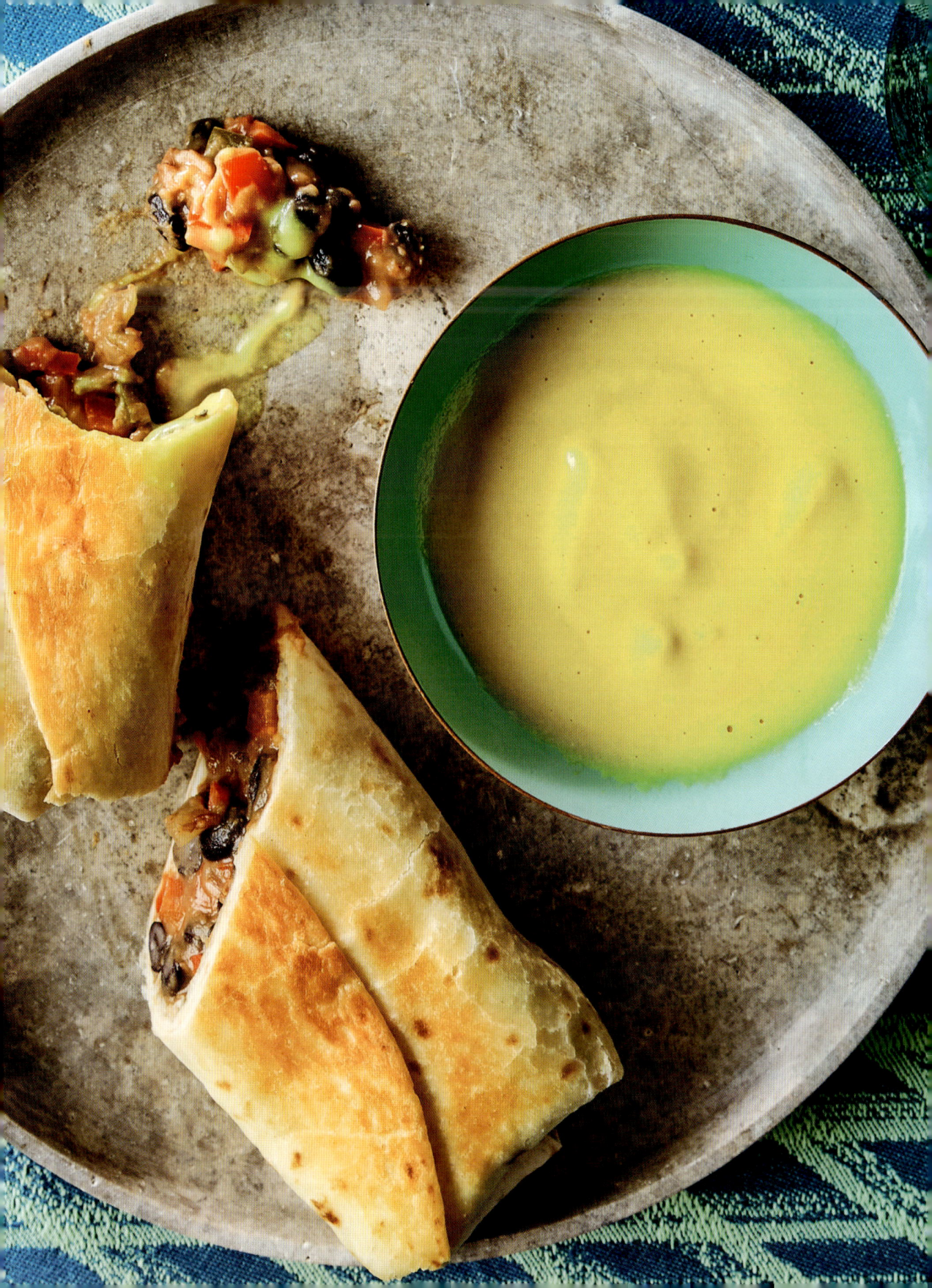

Make the burritos: In a large nonstick skillet, heat 1 tablespoon of the avocado oil over medium heat. When the oil is shimmering, add the onion and bell pepper. Cook, stirring occasionally, until the onion is translucent, about 4 minutes. Add the refried beans, black beans, jalapeños, salt, cumin, and paprika. Cook until warmed through, about 4 minutes, then transfer to a bowl to cool slightly.

Wipe out the skillet. Set over high heat and warm the tortillas for about 10 seconds on each side until soft. Lay the tortillas out on a clean work surface. Scoop the bean filling evenly in the center of each tortilla, leaving space around the edges. Fold in the sides first, then tuck the bottom edge over the filling and roll up tightly while keeping everything snug.

In the same skillet, heat the remaining 1 tablespoon avocado oil over medium heat. When the oil is shimmering, arrange the burritos, seam side down, evenly around the skillet. Cook until the bottoms are browned, about 2 minutes, then flip and cook to brown the other side, another 2 minutes. I like serving the hot burritos with the warm queso in a bowl on the side for dunking.

Burritos

2 tablespoons avocado oil
½ small white onion, diced
1 red bell pepper, seeded and diced
1 (15.5-ounce) can vegan refried beans
1 (15.5-ounce) can black beans, drained and rinsed
¼ cup drained pickled jalapeños, diced
1 teaspoon kosher salt
1 teaspoon ground cumin
½ teaspoon smoked paprika
4 (12-inch) high-protein tortillas, such Hero

 Moderate Lift

 30 to 60 Minutes

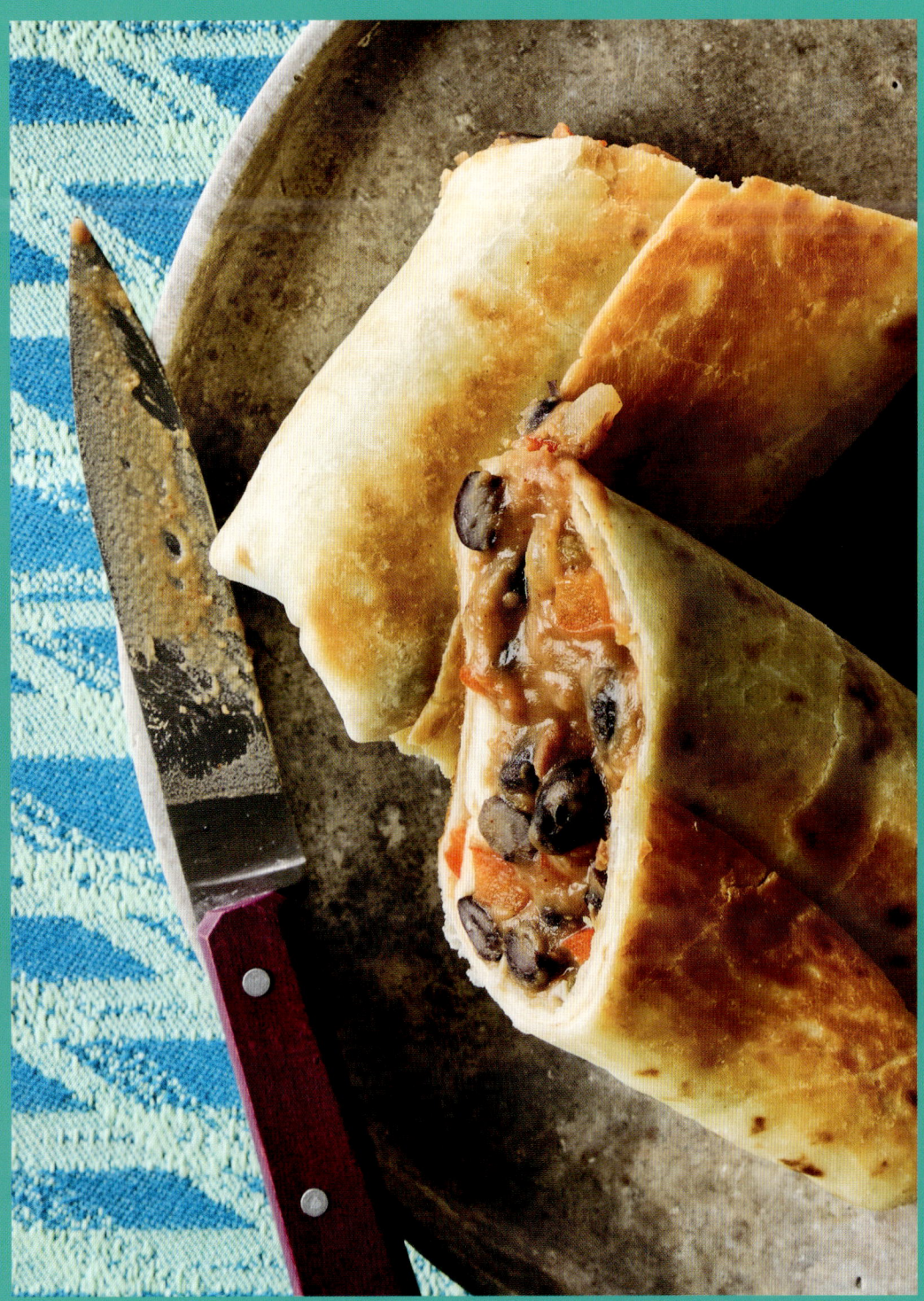

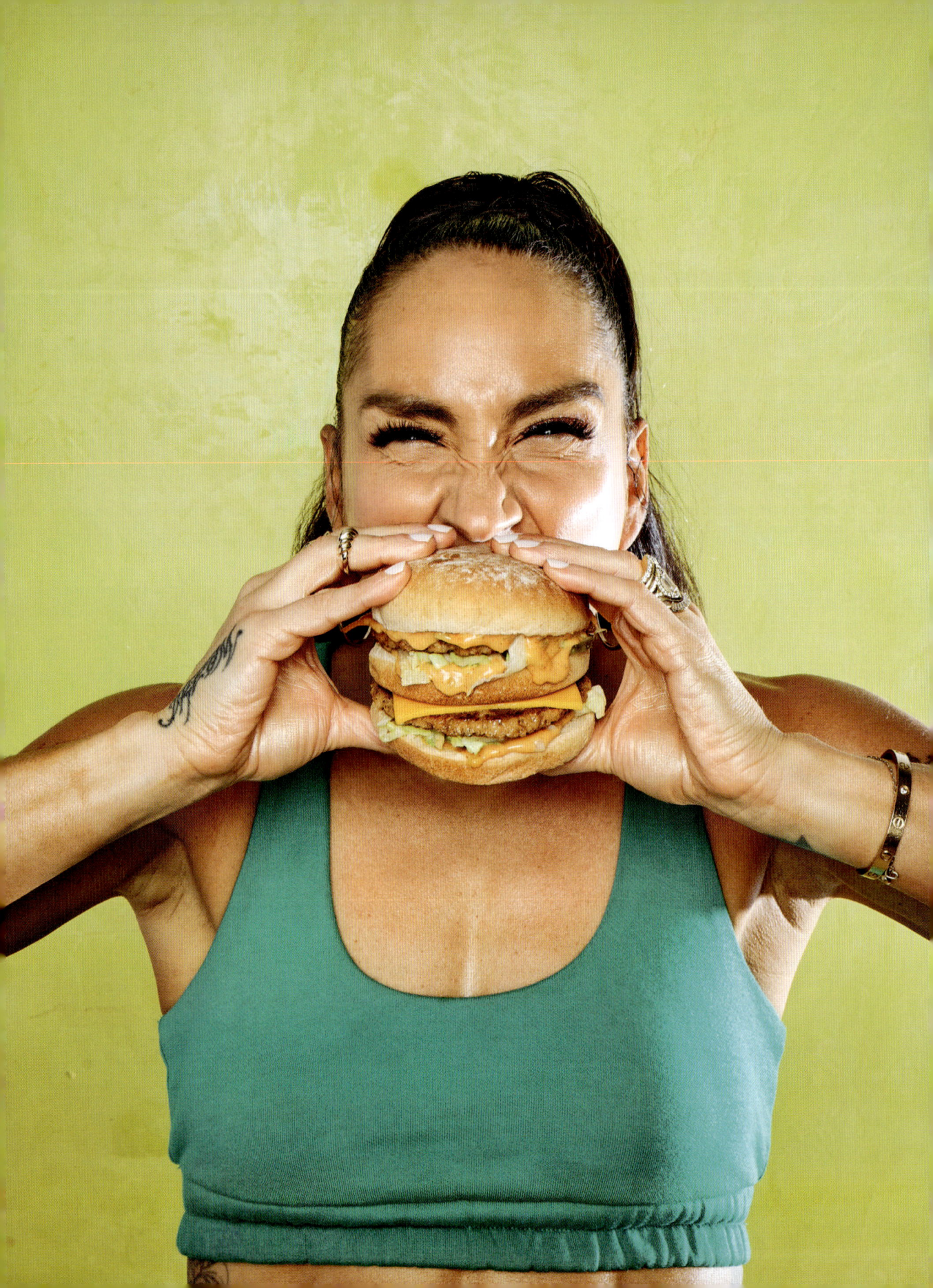

This might just be my all-time favorite recipe in the book. The flavors hit exactly like the real deal — savory, smoky, tangy, and perfectly stacked between three layers of soft, squishy buns. The special sauce is spot-on, the homemade patties are juicy, and the whole thing delivers. If you're in a time crunch, no shame in grabbing your favorite plant-based burger and building it up with all the fixings. But these burgers are packed with big, bold flavor and are easy to prep ahead of time for a burger on command. Yeah, the macros are up there, but let's be real — some things are worth it. This is the kind of meal you make when you're really having a Mac attack but want it plant-based and packed with protein. I'm convinced even the most die-hard carnivore won't be able to resist.

MAKES 4 BURGERS

VEGAN BIG STACK

Per burger

Calories: 757

Fat: 28g

Carbs: 94g

Fiber: 25g

Protein: 38g

Make the sauce: In a medium bowl, whisk together the mayonnaise, ketchup, mustard, relish, vinegar, onion powder, garlic powder, and paprika. Transfer to an airtight container and refrigerate until ready to use or up to 5 days.

Make the patties: In a large bowl, whisk together the mayonnaise, flaxseed, nutritional yeast, miso, soy sauce, Worcestershire sauce, onion powder, garlic powder, paprika, liquid smoke, and black pepper. Add the TVP and stir to coat. Add the breadcrumbs and flour and stir until it forms a solid mixture.

Lay a piece of parchment or wax paper on a clean work surface and coat with nonstick spray. Divide the burger mix into 8 equal portions (about 2 ounces each) and roll into balls. Evenly space the balls across the parchment. Coat another piece of parchment with nonstick spray and place it on top of the balls. Use a drinking glass to press each ball into a ¼-inch-thick patty. Cut the parchment into squares around each patty and stack the patties on a plate. (The plate can be wrapped and refrigerated for up to 3 days if you want to make these ahead — or freeze in a zip-top freezer bag for up to 1 month.)

Recipe continues...

Sauce
- ½ cup vegan mayonnaise
- 2 tablespoons sugar-free ketchup
- 1 tablespoon yellow mustard
- 1 tablespoon sweet relish
- 1 teaspoon rice wine vinegar
- ½ teaspoon onion powder
- ½ teaspoon garlic powder
- ½ teaspoon smoked paprika

Patties
- ¼ cup vegan mayonnaise
- 2 tablespoons ground flaxseed
- 2 tablespoons nutritional yeast
- 1 tablespoon white miso paste
- 1 tablespoon soy sauce
- 1 tablespoon vegan Worcestershire sauce
- 1 teaspoon onion powder
- 1 teaspoon garlic powder
- 1 teaspoon smoked paprika
- 1 teaspoon liquid smoke
- ½ teaspoon freshly ground black pepper
- 1 pound hydrated TVP MVP (page 224) or 1½ cups dry TVP (follow package instructions to hydrate)

I ♥ Sandwiches

Make the burgers: Separate all the buns. We're going to use all 8 of the bottom buns and 4 of the top buns. (Reserve those other tops for your own extra delicious top bun–only sandwiches.) Each burger will get a base, center, and top bun; I like to organize them cut side up in vertical lines so I can do a quick burger assembly line.

On all of the top, bottom, and center buns, spread 1 tablespoon of sauce. On all of the bottom buns, layer some onion and lettuce. On all of the center buns, layer onion, lettuce, and pickles. Keep the buns at the ready for the burgers.

In a large nonstick skillet, heat the avocado oil over medium heat. When the oil is shimmering, peel the top parchment off two patties. Set them, burger side down, in the skillet, then peel the other parchment off. Sear for about 3 minutes, then flip. Lay a slice of cheese on each burger and add a splash of water to the skillet (to help melt the cheese faster). Cover and cook until the cheese is melted and the burgers are nicely browned, about another 3 minutes. Transfer one patty to the bottom bun. Stack the center bun on top, then lay on the second patty. Press on the top bun.

Continue searing and assembling the remaining burgers, adding more oil to the skillet as needed. Serve hot.

½ cup plain breadcrumbs
¼ cup all-purpose flour
Nonstick cooking spray

Burgers
8 high-protein burger buns, such as Hero
Finely diced white onion
Shredded iceberg lettuce
Dill pickle slices
1 tablespoon avocado oil, plus more as needed
8 slices vegan American cheese

Heavy Lift

30 to 60 Minutes

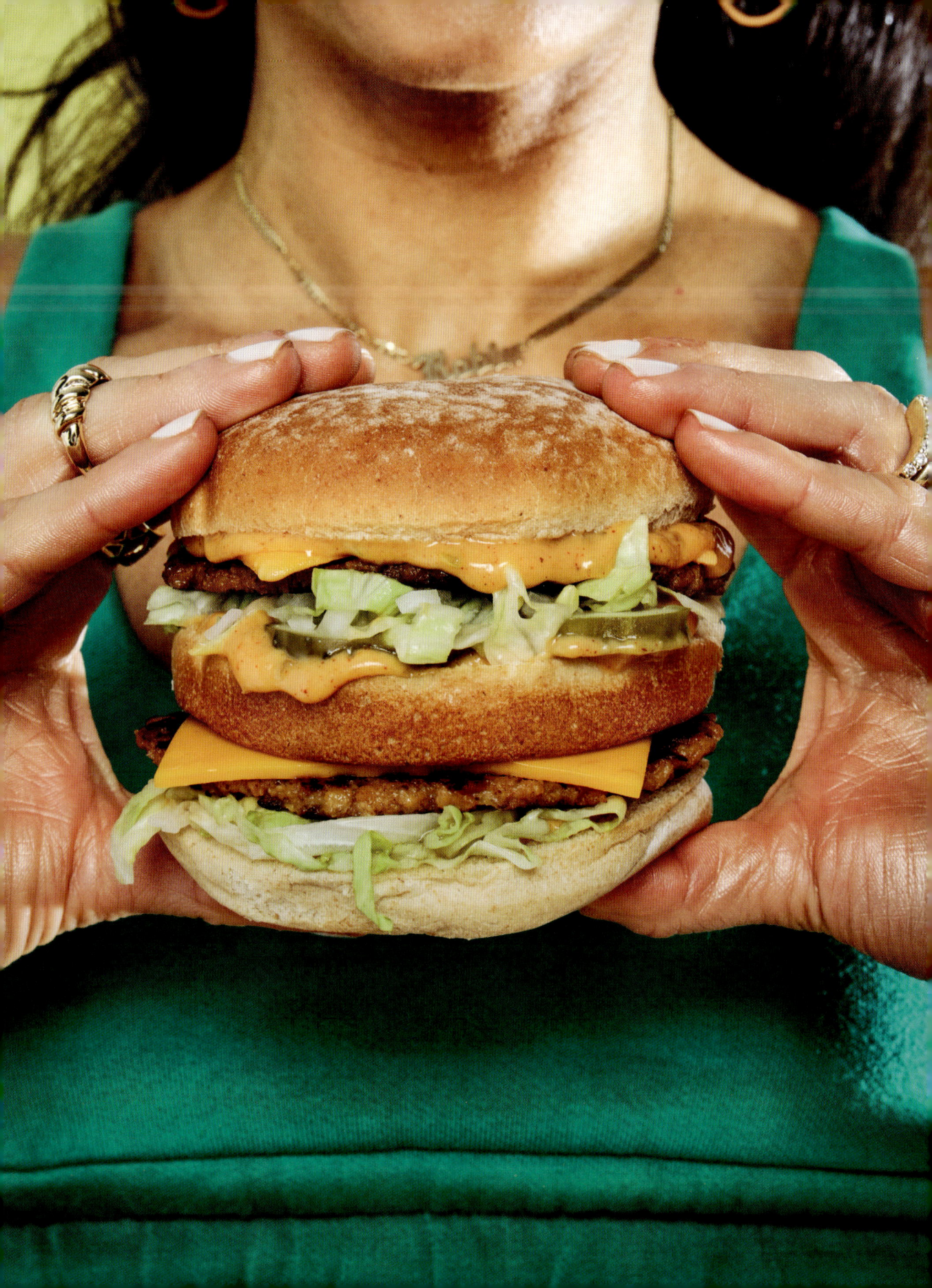

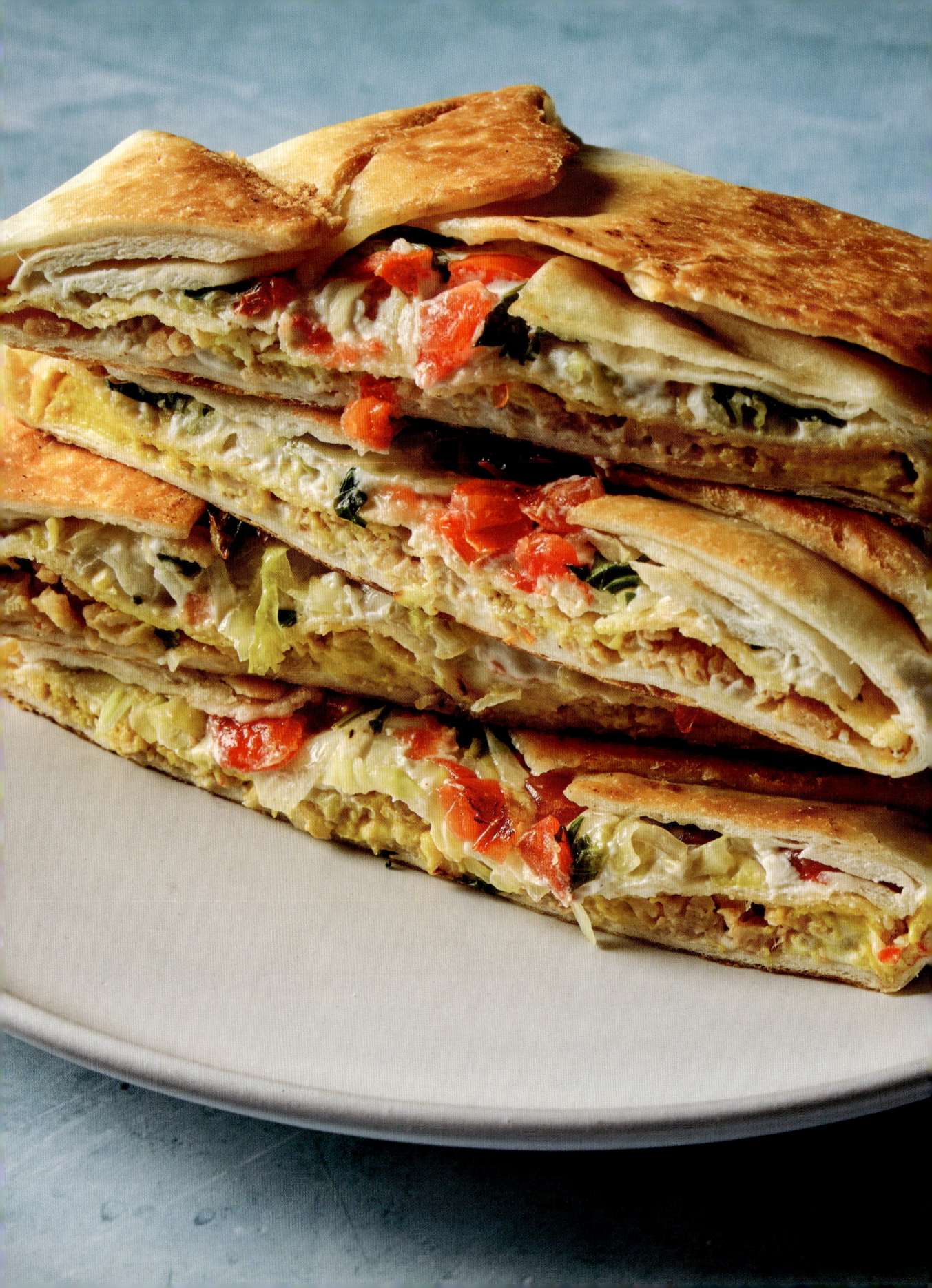

Listen, I have *strong* feelings about the crunchwrap. As a kid, I'd save my allowance for two things at the Willow Grove Mall in Pennsylvania: a trip to Spencer's Gifts (yes, I wanted that clear phone) and a stop at Taco Bell. This version gives you all the crunch, the nacho "cheese," and the pure joy of biting into the perfect wrap.

MAKES 4 WRAPS

FULLY LOADED CRUNCHY WRAP

Make the nacho cheese: In a small saucepan, combine the soy milk and cashews. Set over high heat and bring to a boil. Reduce the heat to low, cover, and simmer until the cashews are very soft, about 15 minutes.

Pour the mixture into a blender, along with the jalapeño brine, onion powder, garlic powder, and salt. Blend on high until smooth. Add the cheese and blend again for a creamy cheese sauce.

Make the wraps: In a large skillet, combine the hydrated TVP, lime juice, taco seasoning, and ½ cup water. Set over medium heat and stir often as the mixture comes to a simmer. Let the water boil off, about 5 minutes. Remove from the heat and let cool slightly.

In a large nonstick skillet over high heat, warm the tortillas for about 10 seconds on each side until soft. Lay the tortillas out on a clean work surface. Spread 1 tablespoon of the sour cream in the center of each tortilla. Scoop the TVP mixture evenly in the center of each tortilla, leaving space around the edges. Spoon about 2 tablespoons of the nacho cheese on top, then gently press the tostada in the center. Spread 1 more tablespoon of sour cream on each tostada, then make a small pile of lettuce, tomato, and cilantro.

Fold half of the tortilla into the center, then fold the corner up. Fold the next corner up, and continue creating pleats in a circular pattern, until it's fully closed. (A little sour cream will help it stick, if needed.)

In the same skillet, heat the avocado oil over medium heat. When the oil is shimmering, set a wrap, seam side down, in the center of the skillet. Cook until browned, about 2 minutes, on each side. Continue toasting the rest, adding a little more avocado oil as needed. Enjoy warm.

Nacho Cheese
- ½ cup unsweetened soy milk or other plant-based milk
- ¼ cup raw cashews
- 1 tablespoon pickled jalapeño brine
- ½ teaspoon onion powder
- ½ teaspoon garlic powder
- ¼ teaspoon kosher salt
- 4 ounces shredded vegan cheddar cheese

Wraps
- ½ pound hydrated TVP MVP (page 224) or ¾ cup dry TVP (follow package instructions to hydrate)
- Juice of 1 lime
- 3 tablespoons taco seasoning
- 4 (12-inch) high-protein tortillas, such Hero
- ½ cup vegan sour cream, (page 146), plus more as needed
- 4 hard tostadas
- Shredded iceberg lettuce
- Diced tomatoes
- Chopped fresh cilantro
- 1 tablespoon avocado oil, plus more as needed

Moderate Lift

Under 30 Minutes

Per wrap
Calories: 647
Fat: 32g
Carbs: 78g
Fiber: 27g
Protein: 40g

I ♥ Sandwiches

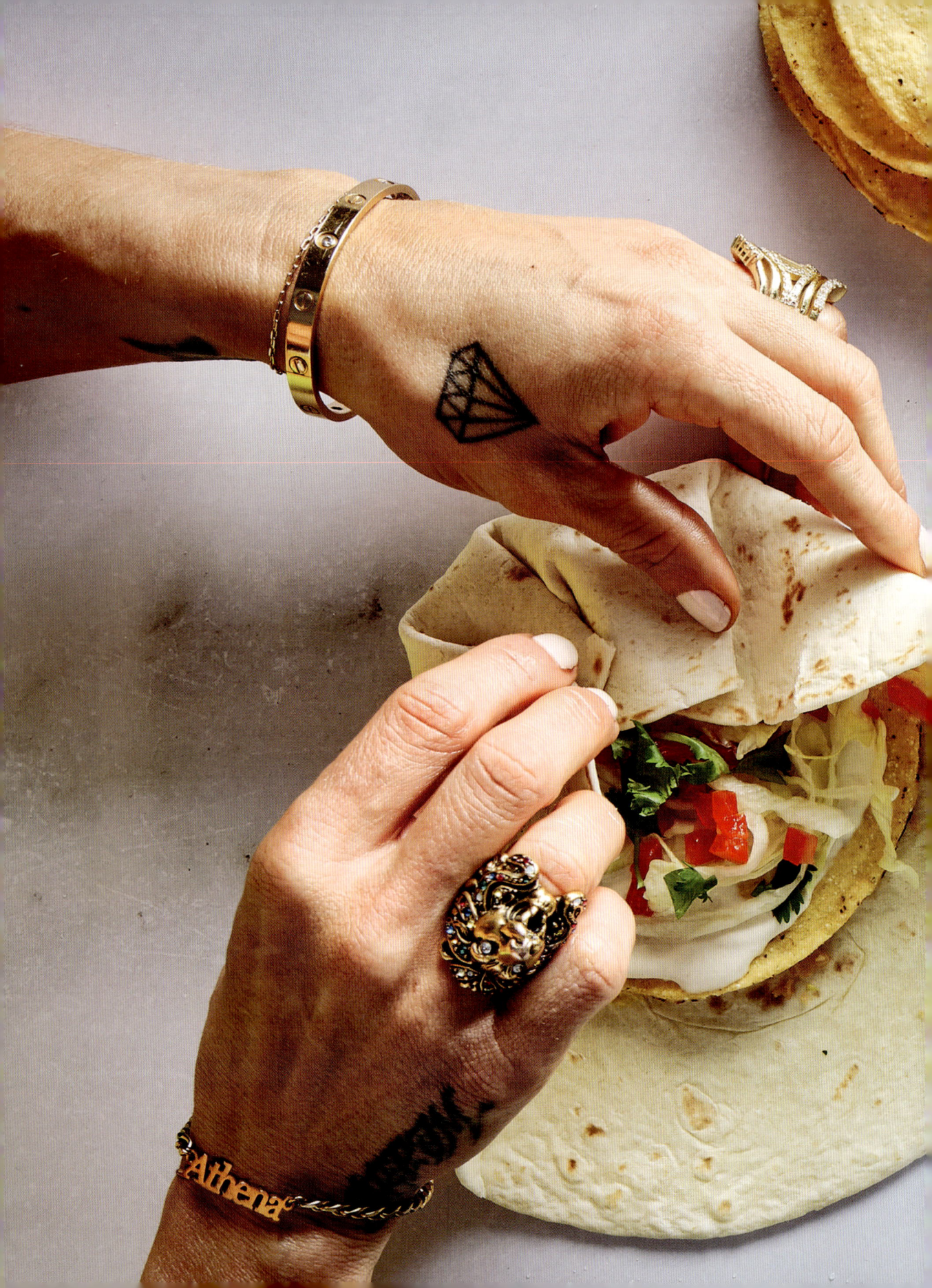

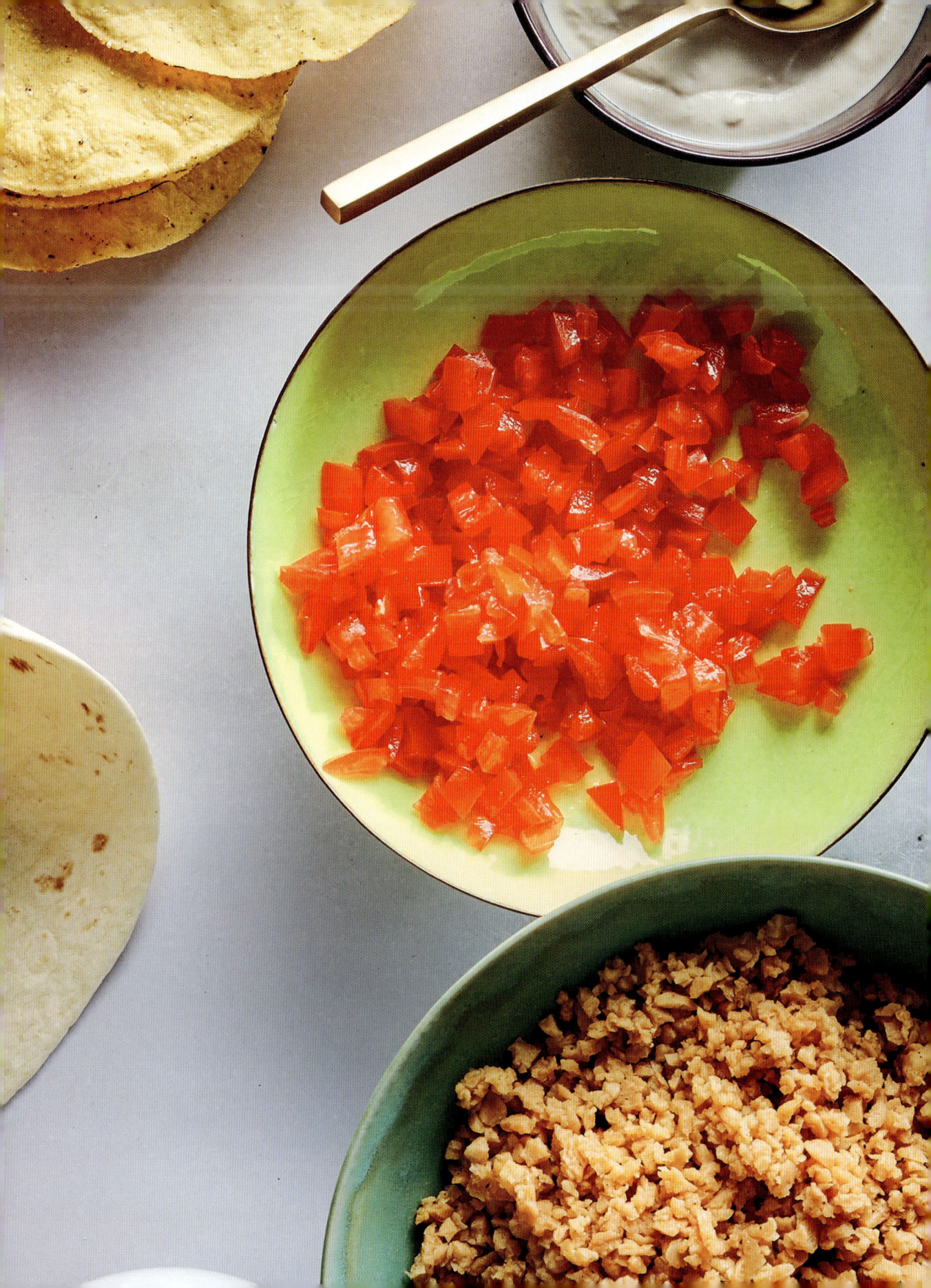

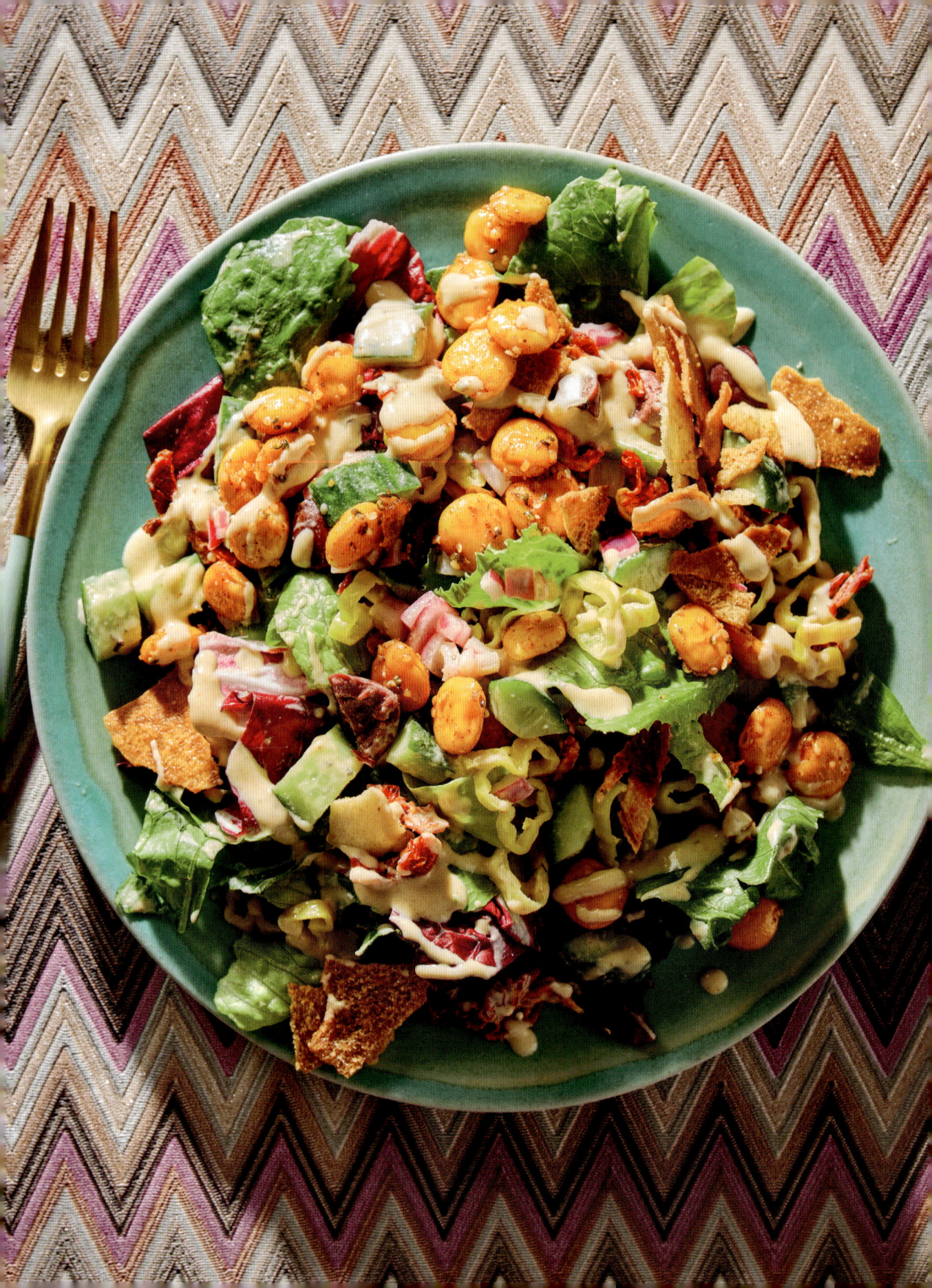

EAT YOUR VEGGIES

Hot take alert: I don't eat salads for lunch — no, I save them for the end of the day. Whether I'm training or chasing my kids or jumping from one meeting into another, when I'm hustling all day, raw veggies can be too much for my stomach to digest — this is why I'm not, and will never be, a lunch salad girlie (instead, I go hard on carbs when I need energy the most — I even wrote a whole chapter on it; see page 65). As the day winds down, though, I shift away from quick-burning calories and move to veggie-heavy salads and raw bowls for dinner. Raw vegetables take longer to digest and eating them later gives my body time to slow down, absorb the nutrients, and start the recovery process without competing with the high-energy demands of my daytime hustle. This chapter is packed with my favorites, from veg-loaded bowls to hearty salads (no bunny food here!) and maki rolls that are filling, flavorful, and exactly what you need to prepare your body for a restorative night's sleep without feeling weighed down.

Bold, bright, and absolutely bursting with flavor — this bowl is one of my all-time favorite meal preps to have on hand for the week. Marinated watermelon and tofu cubes bring the poke vibes, while crisp veggie ribbons and tangy kimchi add the perfect crunch. Use whatever's in season to build out your bowl (if watermelon isn't an option, just double up on the tofu). The real game changer is an edamame-ginger dressing that adds a rich, creamy texture with an unexpected punch (make a double batch to drizzle over everything — you won't regret it!). Fun fact: When Athena was born and I was breastfeeding, I ate this constantly — she smelled like ginger for the first year of her life. (Naturally, she loves it now.) Ginger is my ride-or-die ingredient, thanks to its anti-inflammatory superpowers and that zingy kick I can't get enough of.

SERVES 4

KIMCHI GINGER POKE BOWL

Make the poke: In an airtight container, whisk together the tamari, vinegar, sesame oil, mirin, lime juice, ginger, and red pepper flakes, if using. Add the tofu and watermelon. Cover and refrigerate for at least 2 hours or overnight.

Meanwhile, make the edamame and ginger dressing: In a blender, combine the edamame, tofu, ginger, garlic, vinegar, and salt. Blend on low to break up the ingredients, then blend on high to make a smooth, emulsified dressing, about 1 minute, stopping to scrape down the sides as needed. Use immediately or refrigerate in an airtight container for up to 1 week. (The dressing will thicken in the refrigerator, so whisk in 1 tablespoon warm water to bring it back to a runny, spoonable texture before using.)

Assemble the bowl: Add rice to a medium serving bowl, then arrange pieces of the marinated tofu and watermelon on top, with some kimchi tucked alongside. Finish with vegetable ribbons and a good drizzle of the dressing and garnish with scallions and sesame seeds. Serve immediately.

Poke
½ cup tamari or soy sauce
¼ cup rice wine vinegar
3 tablespoons toasted sesame oil
3 tablespoons mirin or agave syrup
Juice of 2 limes
2-inch piece fresh ginger, peeled and grated
1 teaspoon red pepper flakes (optional)
8 ounces extra-firm tofu, drained and cut into ¼-inch cubes
8 ounces seedless watermelon, cut into ¼-inch cubes

Recipe continues...

Per serving
Calories: 514
Fat: 11g
Carbs: 89g
Fiber: 4g
Protein: 21g

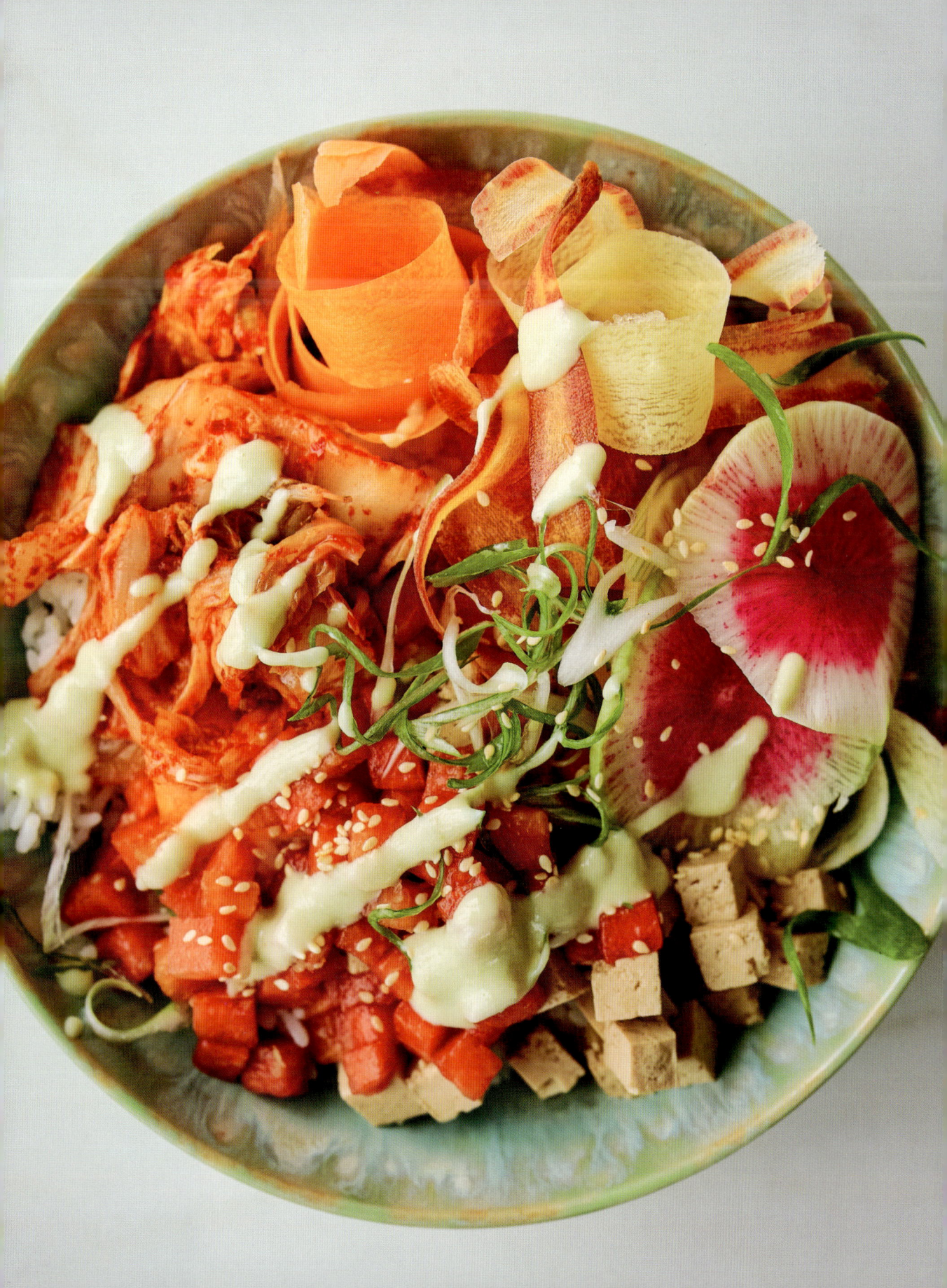

Pro Tip: Prep extra ingredients ahead of time and store them in the fridge so you'll be ready to plate up a masterpiece at a moment's notice. Precut your tofu and watermelon for the week, but don't add them to the marinade until the night before. The good news is one batch of marinade will get you through the week!

> ## How to Make Vegetable Ribbons
> Any firm vegetable, like rainbow carrots, English cucumber, watermelon radish, zucchini, or yellow squash, is ready to be a ribbon. Scrub and dry the vegetable, leaving the peel intact. Run a vegetable peeler down the length to create long, thin ribbons. I stack my ribbons in separate airtight containers and season with a good pinch of salt and enough rice wine vinegar to barely submerge them. Soak for at least 15 minutes or refrigerate for up to 2 weeks. The ribbons will get more pliable and tart the longer they sit. When you're ready to use them, drape, fold, or roll the ribbons to zhuzh up your grain bowl, sandwich, wrap, salad, or pizza.

Edamame and Ginger Dressing
½ cup shelled edamame, thawed if frozen
2 ounces extra-firm tofu, drained
1-inch piece fresh ginger, peeled and thinly sliced
1 garlic clove
2 tablespoons rice wine vinegar
1 teaspoon kosher salt

Bowl
1 cup cooked white rice (see Grains for Days, page 231)
½ cup kimchi, whole or roughly chopped
Vegetable ribbons (see sidebar)
Thinly sliced scallions and toasted sesame seeds, for serving

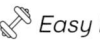 *Easy Lift*

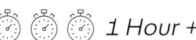 *1 Hour +*

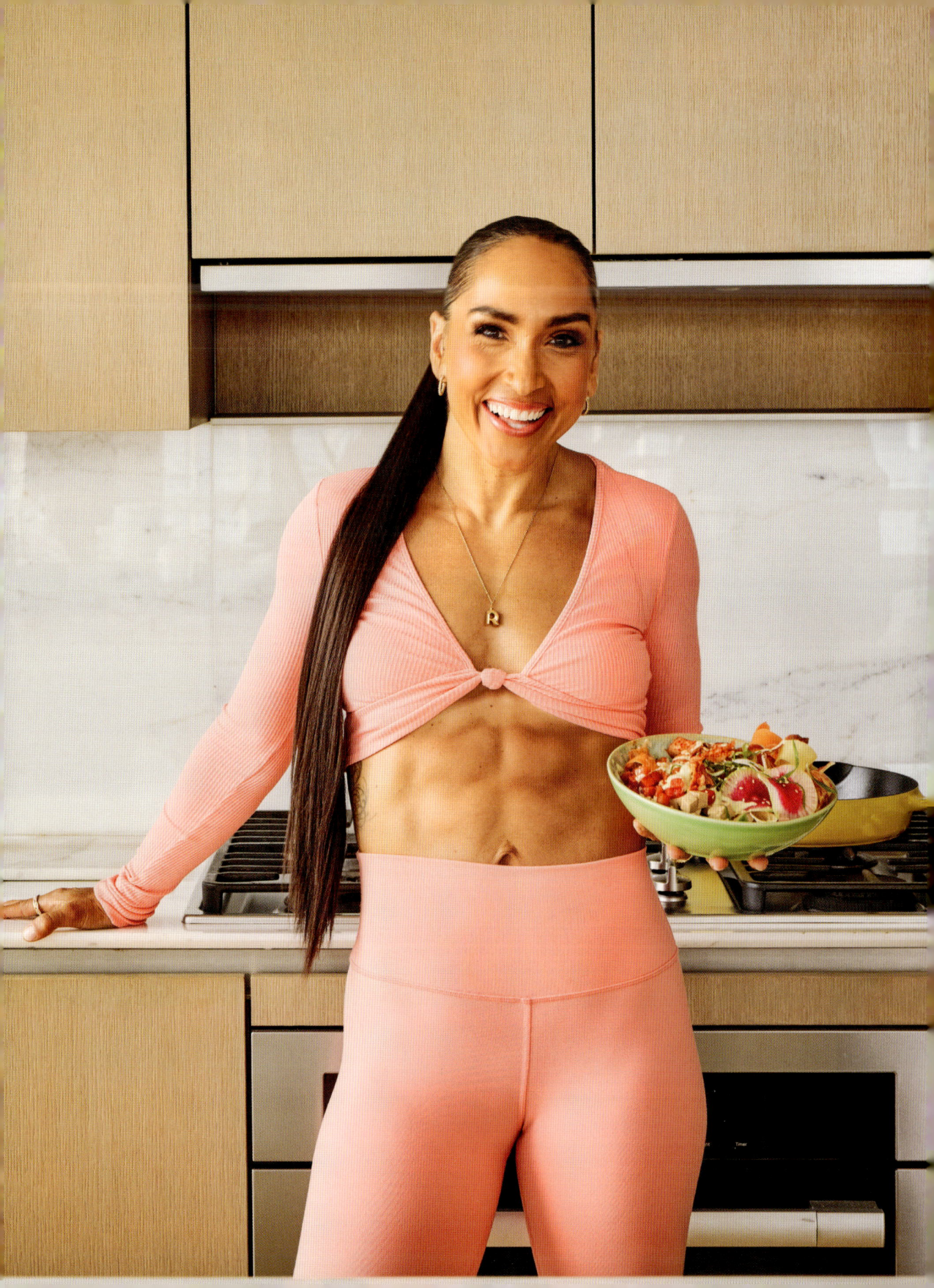

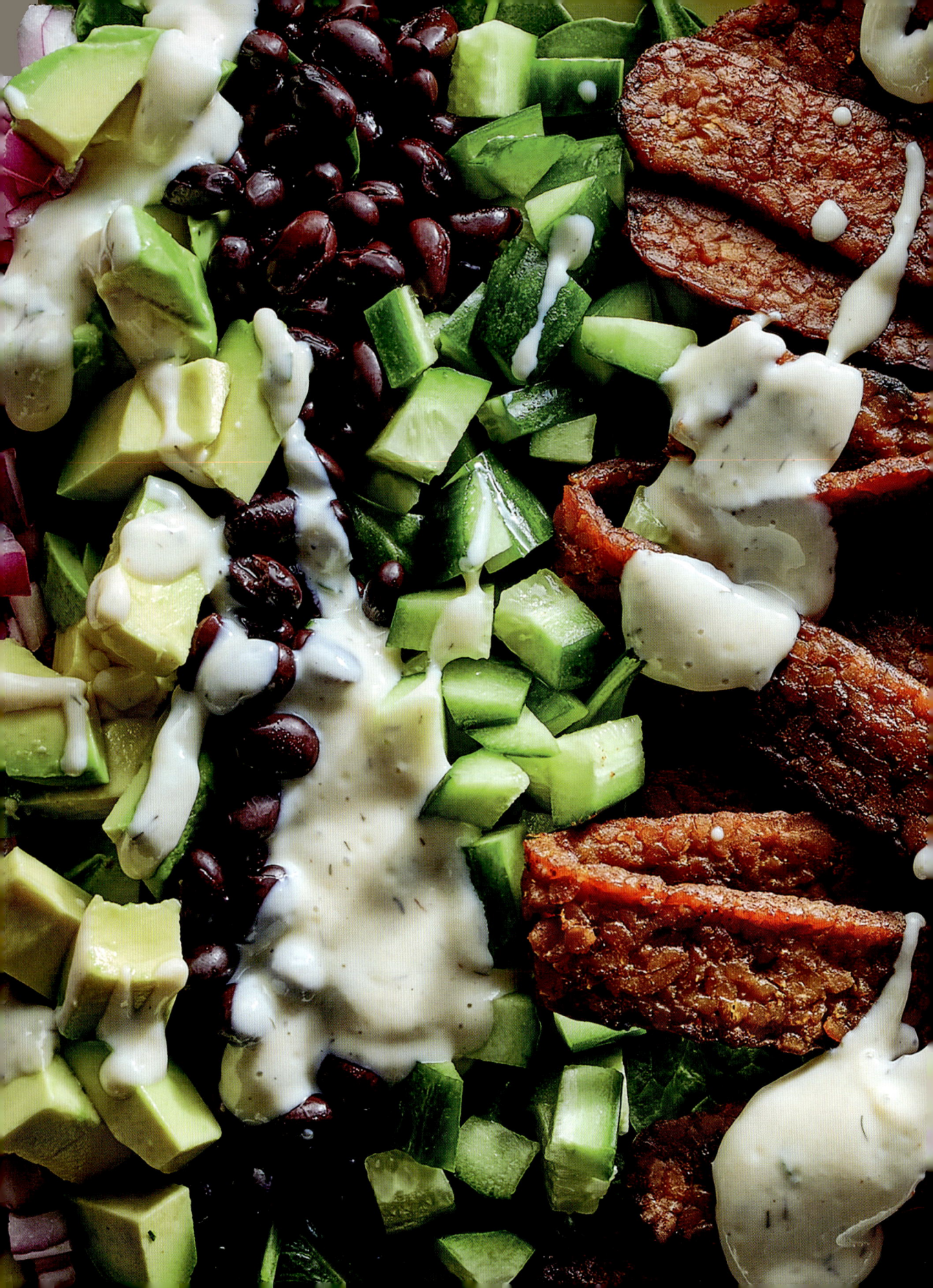

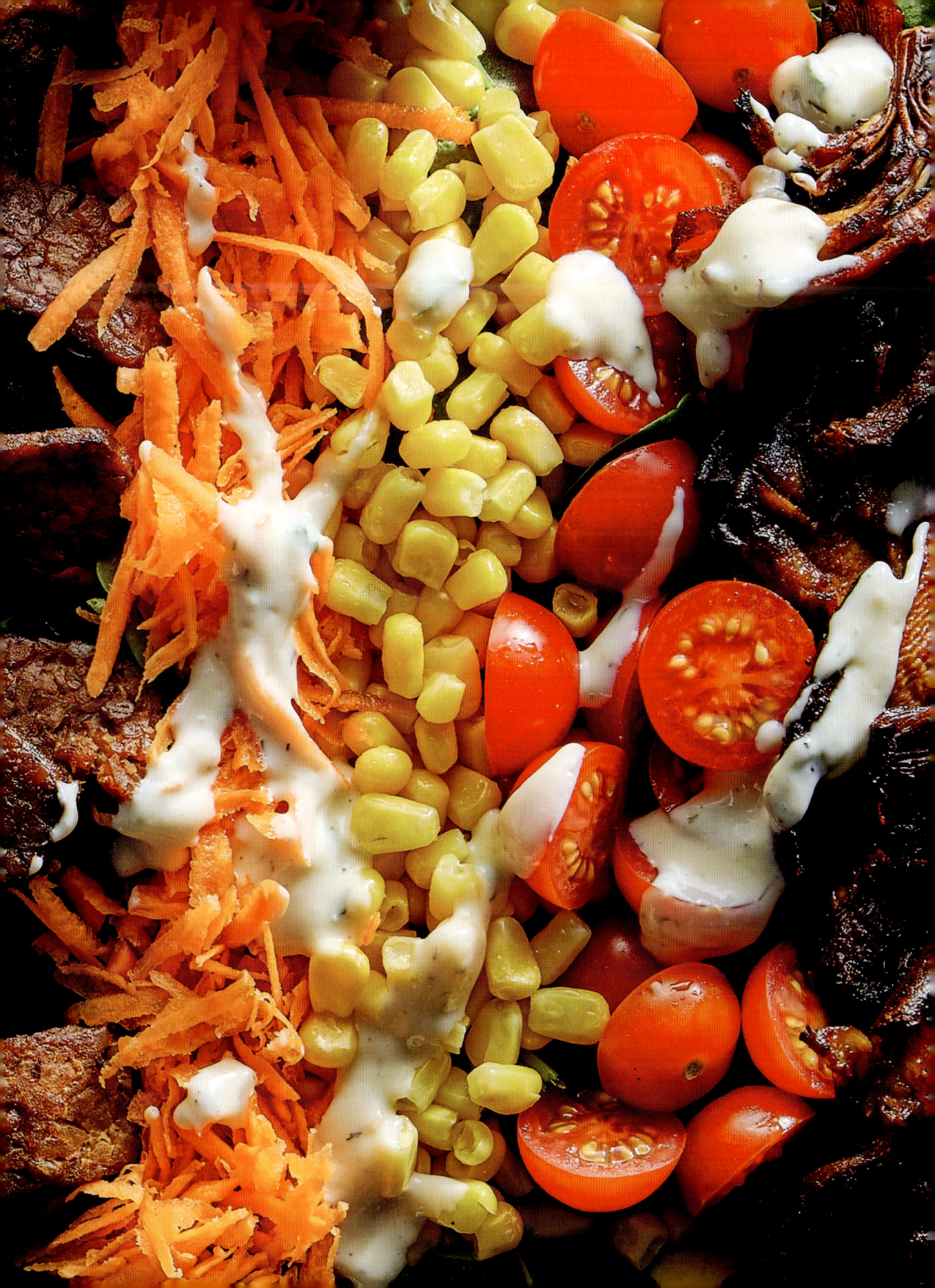

Per serving — Calories: 618 | Fat: 25g | Carbs: 77g | Fiber: 26g | Protein: 31g

When I went vegan, two of the things I missed most were bacon and cheese. Here, standing in for bacon we have crispy mushrooms and charred tempeh, delivering the savory bite I need, while avocado provides the fatty richness of cheese. And then there's the star of the show: tofu ranch dressing. Ranch is always a good idea, whether you're dipping chips, spreading it on a sandwich, or drizzling it over pizza. Unlike most vegan dressings that lean on coconut for creaminess, this one uses silken tofu to pack in protein while keeping the fat content light.

SERVES 4

LOADED COBB SALAD

Make the mushroom and tempeh: Preheat the oven to 450°F. Line a rimmed baking sheet with parchment paper. Arrange the tempeh and mushrooms on the prepared baking sheet. In a small bowl, whisk together the coconut aminos, vegetable oil, and liquid smoke, if using. Spoon the mixture evenly over the tempeh and mushrooms and toss to coat them. Bake until the mushrooms are crisp and browned and the tempeh is charred around the edges, 10 to 15 minutes, rotating the baking sheet halfway through the cooking time. Season with a light pinch of salt and a few good cracks of pepper. Use immediately or let cool completely on the baking sheet and refrigerate in an airtight container for up to 3 days. Recrisp in a 450°F oven for 5 to 10 minutes as needed.

Make the salad: To a large serving bowl, add a base layer of spinach. Top with neat piles of the black beans, tomatoes, corn, carrots, cucumbers, onion, avocados, mushrooms, and tempeh. Drizzle a healthy amount of the ranch dressing on top (I like to keep the rest on the side for backup). Serve immediately.

Mushrooms and Tempeh

8 ounces tempeh bacon, or regular tempeh cut in ¼-inch-thick slices
1 (3.5-ounce) container oyster mushrooms, ripped into shreds
3 tablespoons coconut aminos or tamari
2 tablespoons vegetable oil
½ teaspoon liquid smoke or smoked paprika (optional)
Kosher salt and freshly ground black pepper

Salad

4 cups baby spinach
1 (15.5-ounce) can black beans, drained and rinsed
2 cups grape tomatoes, quartered
2 cups corn kernels, fresh or thawed from frozen
2 cups shredded carrots
4 mini cucumbers, diced
1 small red onion, diced
2 ripe avocados, pitted, peeled, and diced
Tofu Ranch Dressing (recipe follows)

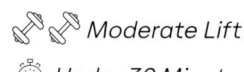 *Moderate Lift*

Under 30 Minutes

This dressing is a game changer — rich, creamy, and perfectly tangy. It makes plenty, but go ahead and double the recipe — you'll want to have some in the fridge for later.

MAKE 1½ CUPS

TOFU RANCH DRESSING

In a blender, combine the tofu, miso, onion powder, garlic powder, vinegar, and salt. Blend on low until smooth. Scrape the dressing into a small bowl and whisk in the dill, chives, and pepper. Taste for seasoning, adding more salt if needed.

Any leftover ranch, if such a thing even exists, can be refrigerated in an airtight container for up to 3 days. The vinegar will thicken the dressing as it sits, so whisk in 1 tablespoon warm water to loosen it up again before serving.

- 1 (12.3-ounce) package silken tofu, drained
- 2 tablespoons white miso
- 1 teaspoon onion powder
- 1 teaspoon garlic powder
- 1 teaspoon white wine vinegar
- ½ teaspoon kosher salt, plus more as needed
- 1 teaspoon dried dill
- 1 teaspoon dried chives
- 1 teaspoon freshly ground black pepper

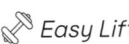 *Easy Lift*

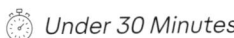 *Under 30 Minutes*

Per ¼ cup (6 servings)

Calories: 52 | Fat: 2g | Carbs: 4g | Fiber: 0g | Protein: 5g

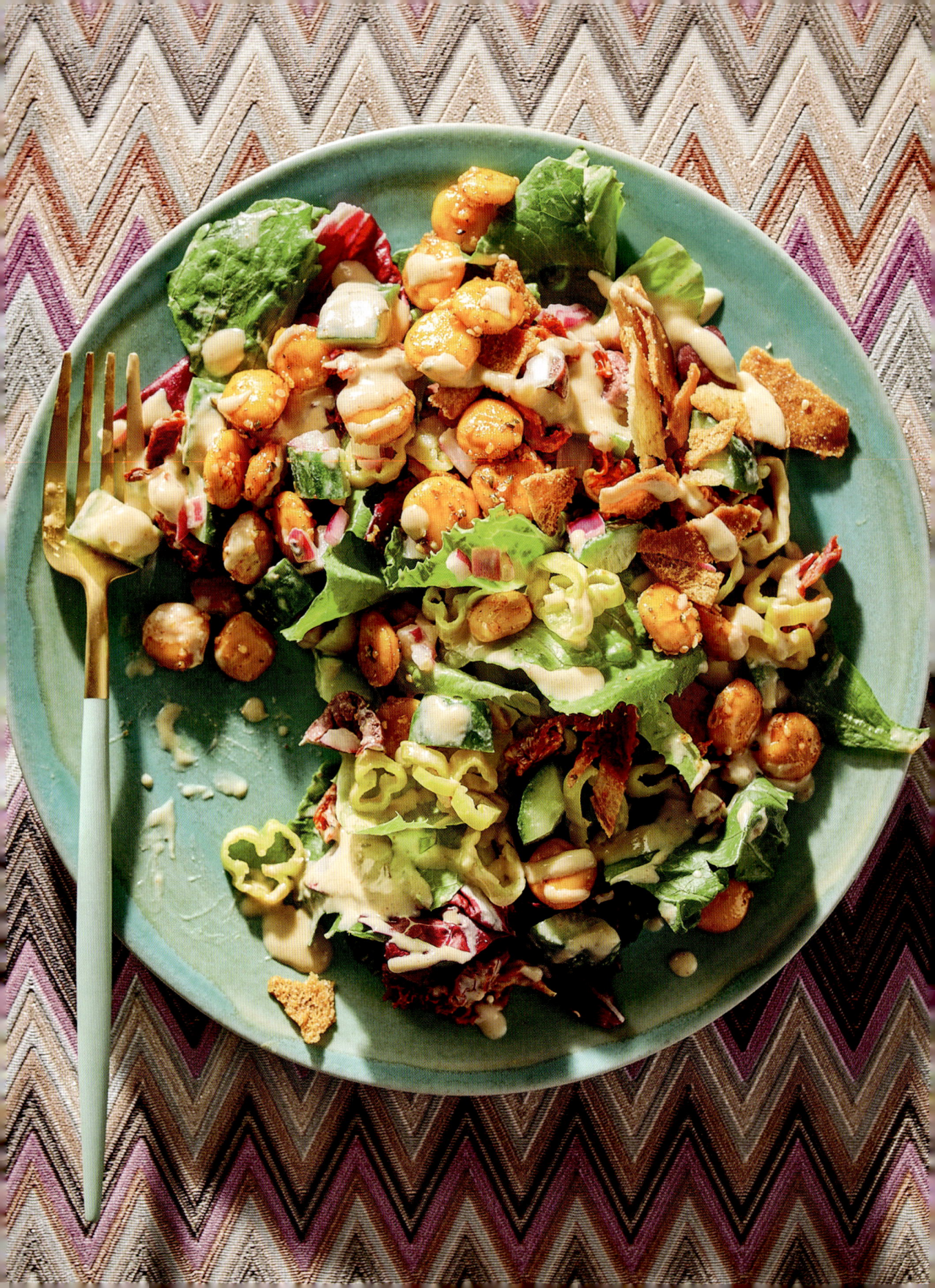

Atlas always signs "more" when I make this salad and, honestly, I can't blame him. It's fresh, crisp, and endlessly adaptable. One of those recipes that started in my rotation early and never left. Raid your fridge for stray veggies and half-used jars of olives or roasted red peppers, and let it all come together. The hummus-based dressing is creamy and protein-packed.

SERVES 4

MED CHOPPED SALAD

Per serving

Calories: 307 | Fat: 15g | Carbs: 38g | Fiber: 8g | Protein: 21g

Make the seasoned lupini beans: Preheat the oven to 250°F. Line a rimmed baking sheet with parchment paper. Drain and rinse the lupini beans, spread them out on paper towels and pat dry. Transfer the beans to the prepared baking sheet and toss with 1 tablespoon olive oil, hemp seeds, paprika, salt, and cayenne, if using. Bake until the beans are warmed through and fragrant, about 15 minutes. Set aside.

Meanwhile, make the hummus dressing: In a small bowl, whisk the hummus, yogurt, lemon juice, Dijon, 2 teaspoons salt, oregano, cumin, coriander, paprika, red pepper flakes (if you want a spicy kick), and 2 tablespoons warm water. Taste for seasoning, adding more salt if needed. Use immediately or refrigerate in an airtight container for up to 1 week. (The dressing will thicken in the fridge, so whisk in 1 tablespoon warm water to bring it back to a runny, spoonable texture before using.)

Make the salad: In a small bowl, stir together the onion, vinegar, and salt. Set aside to lightly pickle.

Add the lettuce and radicchio to a large bowl. Finely chop the pepperoncini and sun-dried tomatoes and add to the bowl with the cucumbers. Drain the onion and add to the bowl along with the hummus dressing. Toss to completely coat the salad.

Serve topped with the crispy lupini beans and crushed pita chips for crunch.

Lupini Beans
1 (8-ounce) jar lupini beans
Extra-virgin olive oil
1 tablespoon hemp seeds
1 teaspoon smoked paprika
½ teaspoon kosher salt
¼ teaspoon cayenne pepper (optional)

Hummus Dressing
½ cup hummus, any flavor
¼ cup plain vegan Greek yogurt
¼ cup fresh lemon juice
2 tablespoons Dijon mustard
Kosher salt
2 teaspoons dried oregano
1 teaspoon ground cumin
1 teaspoon ground coriander
1 teaspoon smoked paprika
½ teaspoon red pepper flakes (optional)

Salad
1 small red onion, diced
½ cup white wine vinegar
Kosher salt
1 head romaine, chopped
1 head radicchio, chopped
12 pepperoncini
12 sun-dried tomatoes
4 mini cucumbers, diced
Pita chips or protein chips

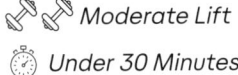 *Moderate Lift*

Under 30 Minutes

Per serving · Calories: 338 · Fat: 22g · Carbs: 23g · Fiber: 5g · Protein: 20g

I love kale, probably more than any other green. It's sturdy, reliable, and can handle whatever you throw at it — including a crispy, protein-packed topping that makes basic croutons look like amateurs. Think crunchy tempeh, nutty quinoa, and hearty lentils, all coming together for the ultimate salad upgrade. Add a silky tahini dressing, and you've got a salad that eats like a meal. If you've sworn off kale salad, it's probably because you met one that was tough and tragically un-massaged. I like my kale silky, tender, and easy on the digestive system — and yes, I've got massage tips below to help you show it some love. Bonus: This salad is perfect for meal prep — just store everything separately until you're ready to assemble. And when the meal-prepped kale is on its last legs? Toss it in a skillet for a quick sauté and use it as the base for a tofu scramble or stir-fry.

SERVES 4

THE BIG (KALE) SALAD WITH TEMPEH "CROUTONS"

Make the tempeh "croutons": Preheat the oven to 425°F. Line a rimmed baking sheet with parchment paper and add the tempeh crumbles, lentils, quinoa, olive oil, a generous pinch of salt, and a small pinch of cayenne, if using. Toss to coat and spread into a single layer. Bake, stirring every 5 minutes, until the lentils and quinoa are crisp and the tempeh is browned, 15 to 20 minutes. Remove from the oven and stir in the pumpkin seeds. Let cool on the baking sheet for at least 10 minutes, or cool completely. Use immediately or store in an airtight container at room temperature for up to 3 days.

Tempeh "Croutons"

4 ounces tempeh, crumbled

¼ cup rinsed canned lentils or cooled homemade lentils (page 233)

¼ cup cooled cooked quinoa (see Grains for Days, page 233)

2 tablespoons extra-virgin olive oil

Kosher salt

Cayenne pepper (optional)

¼ cup raw pumpkin seeds

Make the tahini dressing: In a small bowl, whisk together the tahini, nutritional yeast, lemon juice, maple syrup, salt, and ¼ cup warm water. The consistency should be slightly runny. Taste for seasoning, adding more salt if needed. Use immediately or refrigerate in an airtight container for up to 1 week. (The dressing will thicken in the refrigerator, so whisk in 1 tablespoon warm water to bring it back to a runny, spoonable texture.)

Make the salad: Strip the kale leaves from the stems (discard the stems) and tear into uneven pieces. Pile the leaves in a large bowl, coat with the lemon juice and a healthy pinch or two of salt, and massage well (see Pro Tip).

Spoon about ¼ cup of the tahini dressing over the kale and toss to coat. Sprinkle on the croutons, then spoon the remaining dressing over the top before serving.

Pro Tip: Give your kale the spa treatment it deserves. Massaging your kale with plenty of acid and salt helps break down its tough fibers for easier digestion and nutrient absorption. Simply add the acid and salt called for in the recipe and then crunch the leaves between your fingers until they're wilted and deep green. Really get in there and give them the full shiatsu, it's totally worth it. Do a taste test — I like my kale buttery soft, with just enough chew to remind you it's still a green goddess.

Tahini Dressing
⅓ cup tahini
2 tablespoons nutritional yeast
2 tablespoons fresh lemon juice
1 tablespoon pure maple syrup
1 teaspoon kosher salt, plus more as needed

Salad
2 bunches lacinato kale
Juice of 2 lemons
Kosher salt

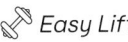 *Easy Lift*

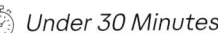 *Under 30 Minutes*

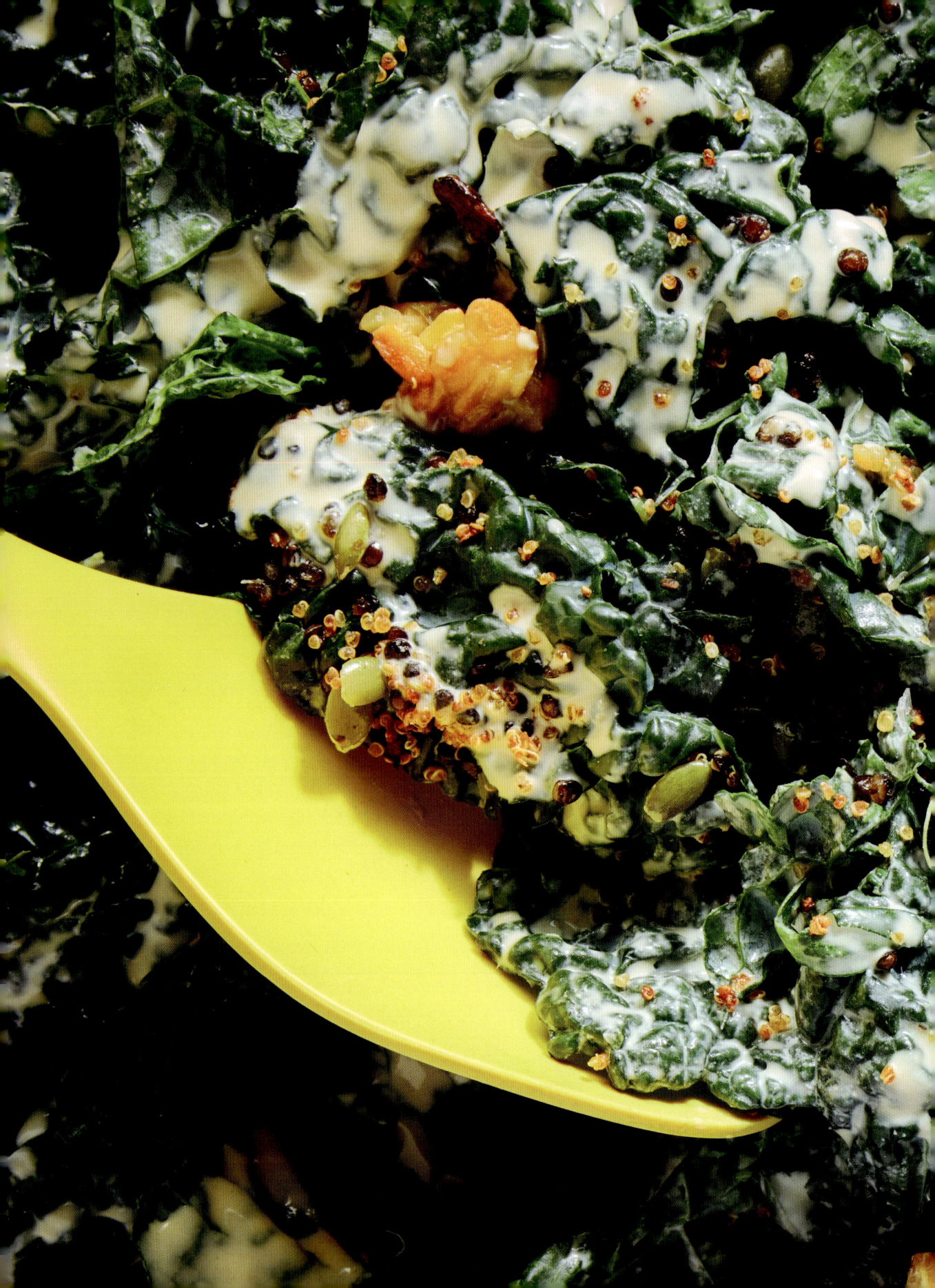

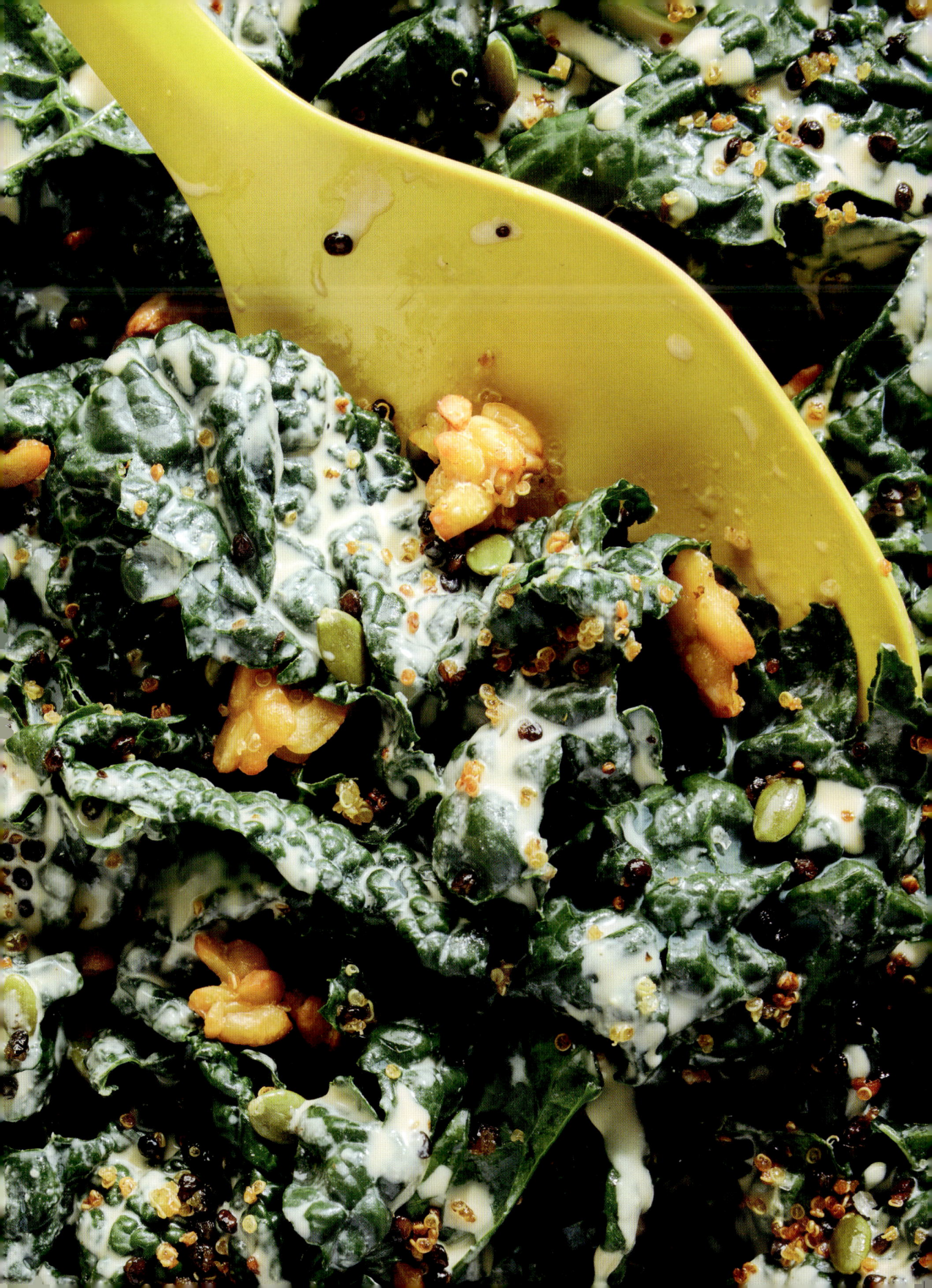

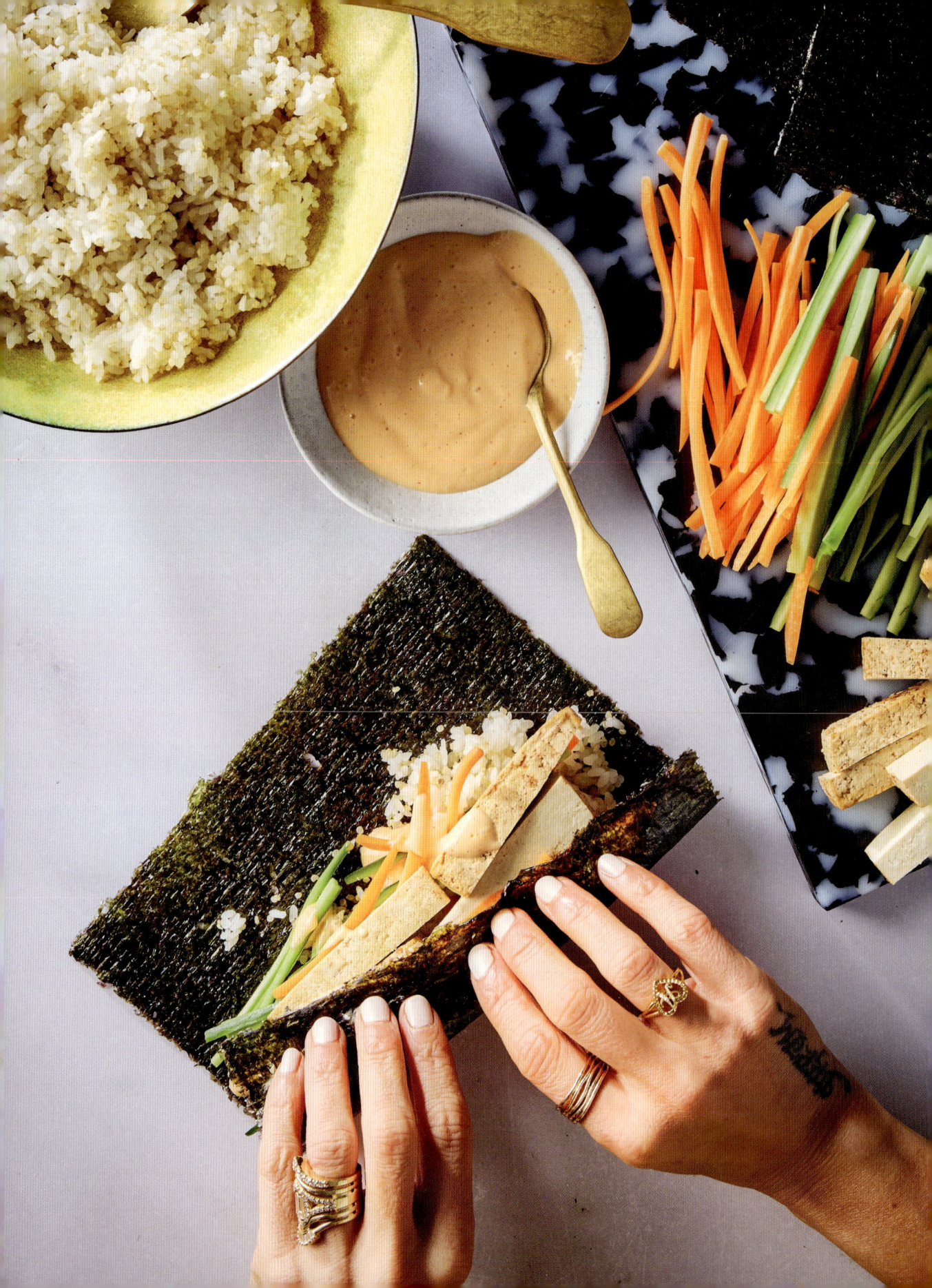

There's something so satisfying about eating with your hands, right? When I'm craving sushi, these hand rolls hit the spot. Quinoa mixed into the rice gives them a protein boost, making them extra filling and satisfying. And let's talk about the sriracha mayo — it's the kind of sauce that takes everything to the next level. This meal is just as fun to assemble as it is to eat, making it perfect for little kitchen helpers. Just a heads up: nori gets soggy if it sits too long, so prep everything ahead of time and roll as you go. The rice-quinoa mixture and fillings will keep in the fridge for up to 5 days, so you can have fresh hand rolls on demand all week.

MAKES 4 LARGE HAND ROLLS

VEGAN HAND ROLLS

In a small bowl, stir the rice, quinoa, and tamari together to fully combine. Let sit for 5 minutes so the rice can absorb any excess liquid. Cut the tofu lengthwise to make 4 equal strips and pat dry with paper towels.

Working with one sheet at a time, lay the nori on a clean work surface. Use wet hands to evenly press about ⅓ cup of the rice mixture across the bottom half of the sheet. Diagonally arrange a small bundle of cucumber and carrot sticks on top of the rice, then lay a piece of tofu on top. Finish with a generous tablespoon of sriracha mayo.

Starting on the rice side, lift the bottom corner of the nori over the ingredients, then continue rolling diagonally across the rest of the nori. Dip a finger in water and press to seal the nori shut. Serve immediately with more mayo on the side for dipping.

- 1 cup cooked and cooled white rice (see Grains for Days, page 231)
- ⅓ cup cooked and cooled quinoa (see Grains for Days, page 231)
- 1½ tablespoons tamari or coconut aminos
- 1 (7-ounce) block baked tofu
- 4 sheets nori
- 1 mini cucumber, cut into thin matchsticks
- 1 small carrot, cut into thin matchsticks
- Sriracha Mayo (recipe follows)

 Easy Lift

 Under 30 Minutes

Per serving (2 rolls) | Calories: 288 | Fat: 10g | Carbs: 29g | Fiber: 4g | Protein: 21g

This spicy, creamy sauce brings the flavor everywhere — hand rolls, grain bowls, sandwiches, you name it. It's the ultimate condiment to keep on hand when you want a little extra heat.

MAKES 1 CUP

SRIRACHA MAYO

In a blender, combine the tofu, sriracha, miso, and salt. Blend on low until smooth. Taste for seasoning. Scrape into an airtight container or squeeze bottle. Use immediately or refrigerate for up to 1 week. The mayo will be runny right out of the blender but will thicken into a mayo texture after a few hours in the fridge.

8 ounces silken tofu, drained
2 tablespoons sriracha
1 tablespoon white miso
¼ teaspoon kosher salt

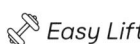 *Easy Lift*

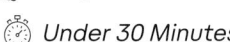 *Under 30 Minutes*

Per ¼ cup — Calories: 49 | Fat: 2g | Carbs: 4g | Fiber: 1g | Protein: 4g

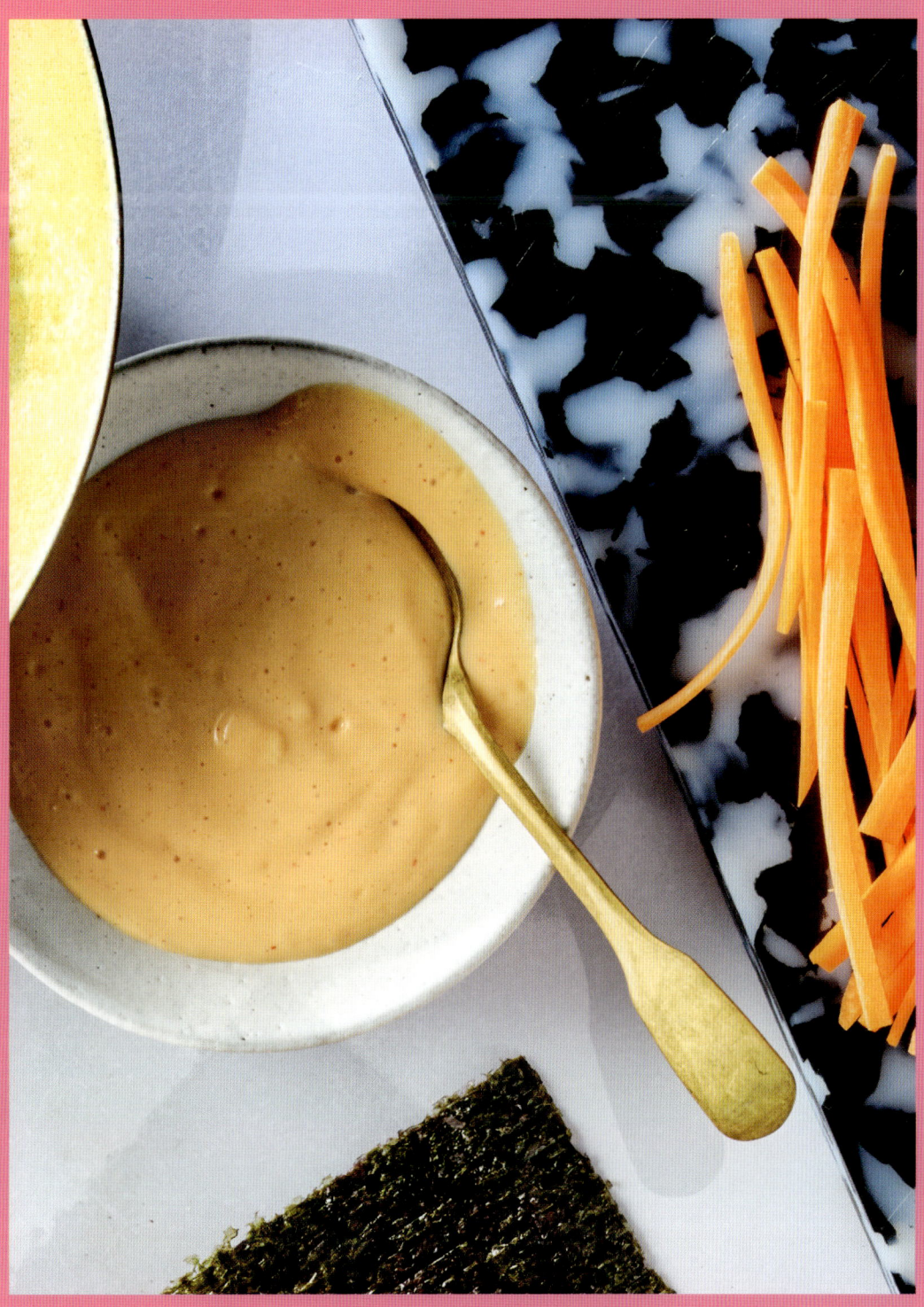

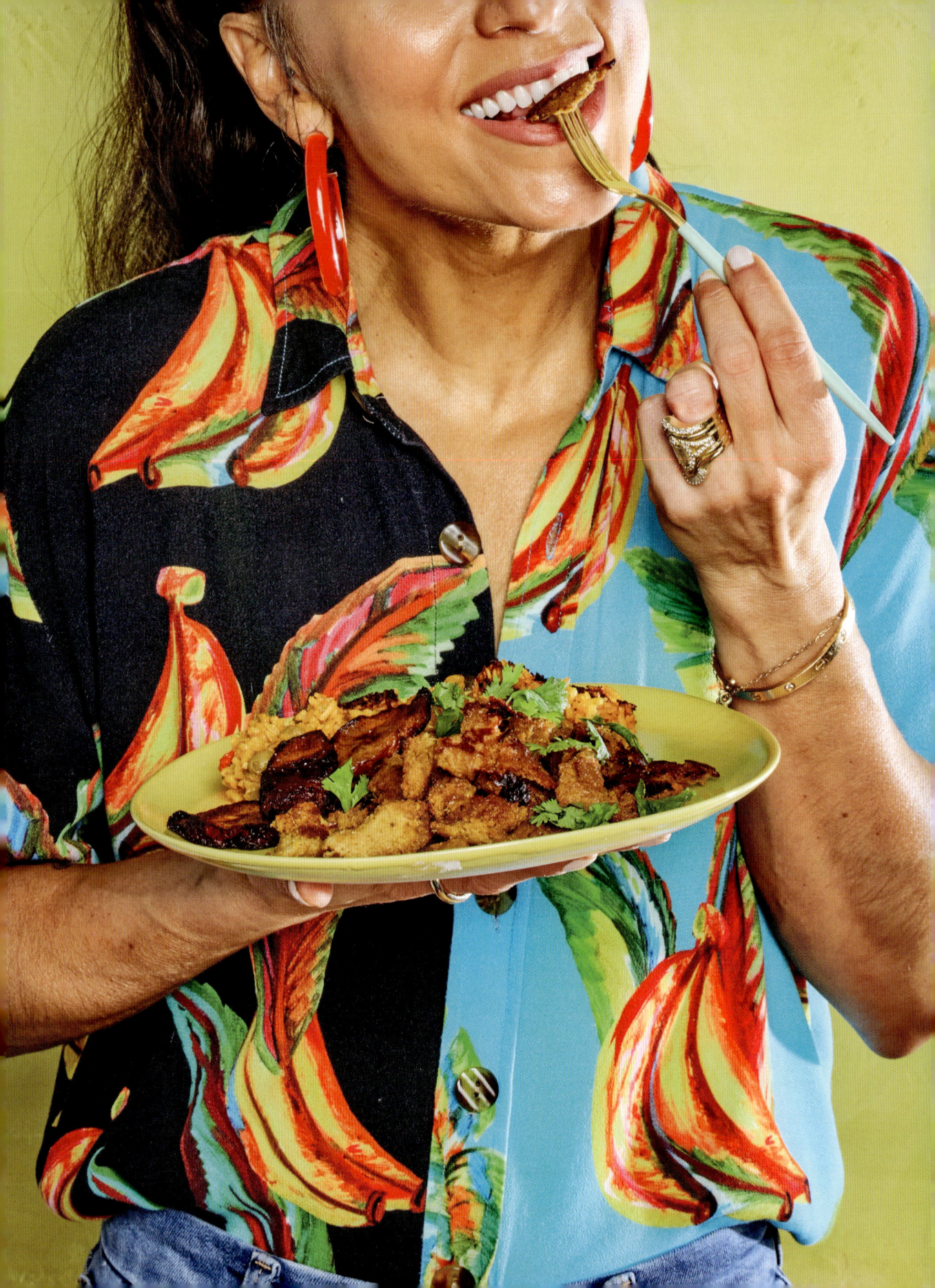

SIT-DOWN DINNERS

After a day of moving fast, I love a big meal that brings everyone to the table — and maybe even leaves me with leftovers for later in the week. This chapter is all about cooking nourishing meals that go big on flavor, protein, and staying power, and make a crowd of hungry people happy and satisfied. Because when you eat to hustle, dinner isn't just the end of the day — it's the start of what's next.

Per serving (based on 6 servings): Calories: 395 | Fat: 11g | Carbs: 52g | Fiber: 30g | Protein: 46g

This might be my kids' favorite dish in the whole book. It has a way of vanishing immediately after I make it — and why shouldn't it? Not only is it a creamy, carby crowd-pleaser, but I sneak in some protein with chickpea breadcrumbs, one of my new favorite moves. (Make a double batch and sprinkle them on everything!) This is the dish I make when unexpected company rolls through because I always have all of the ingredients on hand — this is a pantry meal at its finest (and frozen broccoli means no chopping!). When you need a big-batch meal that slaps, or when you just want something comforting that still fuels you right, this is it.

SERVES 6 TO 8+

CREAMY ZITI & BROCCOLI

Make the chickpea breadcrumbs: Preheat the oven to 350°F. Spread the chickpeas out on paper towels and pat dry, then transfer them to a rimmed baking sheet. Bake until golden brown and dry, about 50 minutes. Remove from the oven and set aside to cool. (Don't turn off the oven.)

In a food processor, combine the cooled chickpeas, garlic power, oregano, salt, and red pepper flakes, if using. Pulse 6 to 8 times to get fine crumbs. Return the crumbs to the same baking sheet and bake for 10 more minutes. Turn the oven off and let the crumbs cool on the pan in the oven, about 1 hour. Transfer the crumbs to an airtight container and store at room temperature for up to 3 days.

Make the ziti: Bring a large pot of heavily salted water to a boil over high heat. Boil the ziti, stirring often, until al dente according to package directions. About 2 minutes before the pasta is done, add the frozen broccoli to the pot. Drain the pasta and broccoli together, then return to the same pot.

Add the yogurt, nutritional yeast, lemon zest and juice, and 2 teaspoons salt. Stir to completely coat the pasta in the sauce. Taste for seasoning. Sprinkle the chickpea breadcrumbs on top and serve immediately.

Note: The ziti will absorb a lot of the sauce as it cools. To heat up leftovers, add the pasta to a skillet with a splash of water, set over medium heat, and toss until warmed through.

Chickpea Breadcrumbs
1 (15.5-ounce) can chickpeas, drained and rinsed
1 teaspoon garlic powder
1 teaspoon dried oregano
½ teaspoon kosher salt
½ teaspoon red pepper flakes (optional)

Ziti
Kosher salt
2 (8-ounce) boxes high-protein ziti (I love Kaizen, page 19)
1 (16-ounce) bag frozen broccoli florets
1 (16-ounce) container plain vegan Greek yogurt
½ cup nutritional yeast
Grated zest and juice of 1 lemon

🏋️ *Easy Lift*

⏱️⏱️⏱️ *1 Hour +*

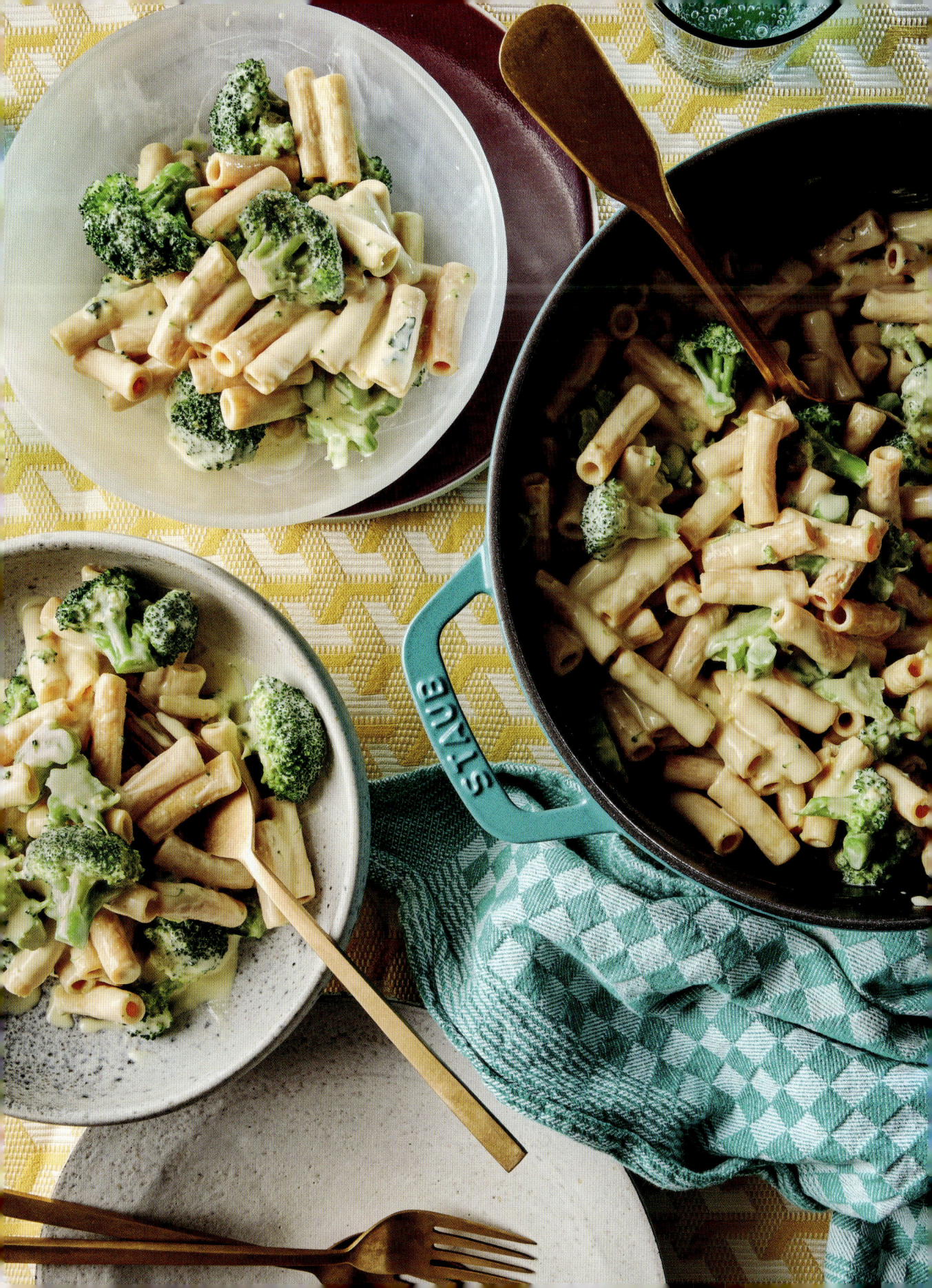

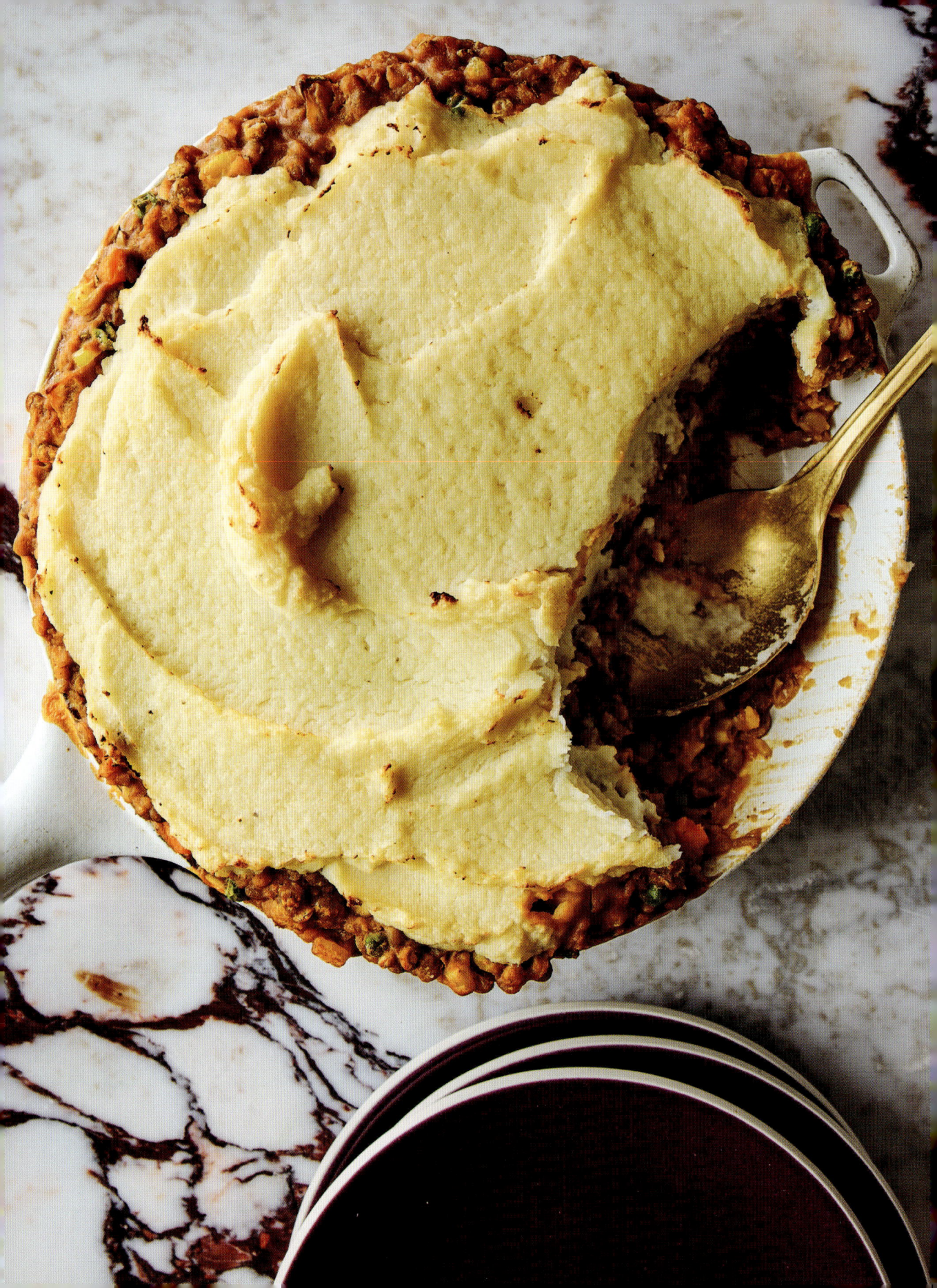

If I were Cameron Diaz in *The Holiday*, this is what I'd make for Jude Law. Hearty, protein-packed filling? Check. Cozy, comforting, and warm? Double check. A potato and cauliflower mash that keeps all the indulgence, but adds fiber, pulls back on carbs, and won't send you into a food coma? Check, check, check. This dish is pure love in a baking dish.

SERVES 6 TO 8

LENTIL SHEPHERD'S PIE

Preheat the oven to 425°F.

Make the topping: Peel the potatoes and cut them into 1-inch cubes. Cut the cauliflower into florets and add to a large pot with the potatoes, a generous amount of salt, and enough water to cover. Boil until the potatoes are fork-tender, about 20 minutes.

Meanwhile, make the filling: In a large oven-safe skillet, heat the olive oil over medium heat. Once shimmering, add the onion with a pinch of salt and pepper. Cook, stirring often, until translucent, about 5 minutes. Stir in the garlic, thyme, rosemary, paprika, and cumin. Cook until fragrant, about 1 minute. Add the tomato paste and stir until deep red, about 2 minutes.

Stir in the lentils, stock, and a pinch of salt. Bring to a simmer, then cover and reduce the heat to low. Cook, stirring occasionally, until the lentils are tender and most of the liquid is absorbed, about 20 minutes.

When the potatoes are tender, reserve 1 cup of the cooking water, then drain well. Return the potatoes and cauliflower to the pot and add the yogurt and ¼ cup of the reserved cooking water. Mash smooth adding more cooking water as needed. Season well with salt and tons of pepper.

Uncover the lentil mixture and stir in the frozen mixed vegetables. Continue to simmer, stirring often, until the vegetables are warmed through and the mixture has thickened, about 3 minutes. Remove from the heat.

Use a large spoon to dollop the topping over the filling. Smooth into an even layer, creating swoops across the surface, then spoon the melted butter evenly over the top. Set the skillet on a rimmed baking sheet, to catch any overflow. Bake the shepherd's pie until the topping is nicely browned, 10 to 15 minutes. Cool for 10 minutes to let the filling set before serving.

Topping

2 pounds russet potatoes
1 head cauliflower
Kosher salt
½ cup plain vegan Greek yogurt
Freshly ground black pepper
2 tablespoons vegan butter, melted

Filling

2 tablespoons extra-virgin olive oil
1 medium white onion, diced
Kosher salt and freshly ground black pepper
2 garlic cloves, minced
1 tablespoon thyme leaves
1 tablespoon chopped rosemary
1 teaspoon smoked paprika
1 teaspoon ground cumin
2 tablespoons tomato paste
1 cup dry green lentils, rinsed
1 cup dry yellow lentils, rinsed
4 cups vegetable stock or Liquid Gold (page 235)
1 (10-ounce) bag frozen mixed vegetables

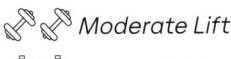 *Moderate Lift*

30 to 60 Minutes

Per serving (based on 6 servings)

Calories: 485
Fat: 15g
Carbs: 82g
Fiber: 17g
Protein: 20g

Lupini beans are having a moment at my house, where they've become an essential pantry staple. Not only are they loaded with protein, they have a great bite, too. Like lentils, lupini beans are a great entry point for anyone who thinks they're "not a bean person" — they're mild, meaty, and super satisfying. With this pot pie, they bring a subtle nuttiness and a satisfying texture to the filling, which starts with a simple vegan roux, bringing that classic buttery richness to the base. When it's all tucked beneath a flaky, golden crust, it's a guaranteed win. You're welcome!

SERVES 6 TO 8

LUPINI POT PIE

Preheat the oven to 400°F.

Make the filling: In a blender or food processor, combine the tofu, stock, and soy milk. Blend on high until smooth, about 2 minutes.

In a large sauté pan or braiser, melt the butter over medium heat. Add the flour and whisk to make a thick paste. Let the flour toast until golden brown and fragrant, about 2 minutes. Slowly pour in the tofu mixture, whisking constantly to avoid clumps. Remove from the heat. Drain and rinse the lupini beans and fold them in with the seitan, frozen vegetables, 2 teaspoons salt, 1 teaspoon pepper, thyme, and rosemary. Taste for seasoning.

Make the crust: Lightly flour a work surface, unfold the puff pastry, and lay it flat. With a lightly floured rolling pin, roll it slightly larger than the diameter of the sauté pan. (Hover the bottom of the pan above the dough to check.) Lay the crust evenly over the filling and rest the edges on the rim. Use a knife to cut 4 slits in the center of the pastry so steam can escape.

In a small bowl, whisk together the soy milk and melted butter, then brush evenly over the crust. Sprinkle the thyme and a few pinches of flaky salt across the top. Slide the pan in the oven and bake until the crust is golden brown all over, 30 to 35 minutes.

Remove from the oven and let cool for 10 minutes before serving big scoops in bowls.

Note: Little known fact, Pepperidge Farm puff pastry is actually vegan! If you want a homemade crust for your pot pie, the pie crust on page 198 works great, too.

Filling

12 ounces silken tofu, drained
2 cups vegetable stock or Liquid Gold (page 235)
½ cup unsweetened soy milk or other plant-based milk
¼ cup (½ stick) vegan butter
¼ cup all-purpose flour
1 (8-ounce) jar lupini
8 ounces seitan, store-bought or homemade (page 222), shredded
1 (10-ounce) bag frozen mixed vegetables
Kosher salt and freshly ground black pepper
1 teaspoon dried thyme
1 teaspoon dried rosemary

Crust

All-purpose flour, as needed
1 sheet frozen puff pastry, thawed (see Note)
1 tablespoon unsweetened soy milk or other plant-based milk
1 tablespoon vegan butter, melted
2 teaspoons thyme leaves or 1 teaspoon dried
Flaky sea salt

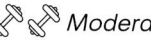 *Moderate Lift*

30 to 60 Minutes

Protein: 23g | Fiber: 4g | Carbs: 32g | Fat: 21g | Calories: 454

Per serving (based on 6 servings)

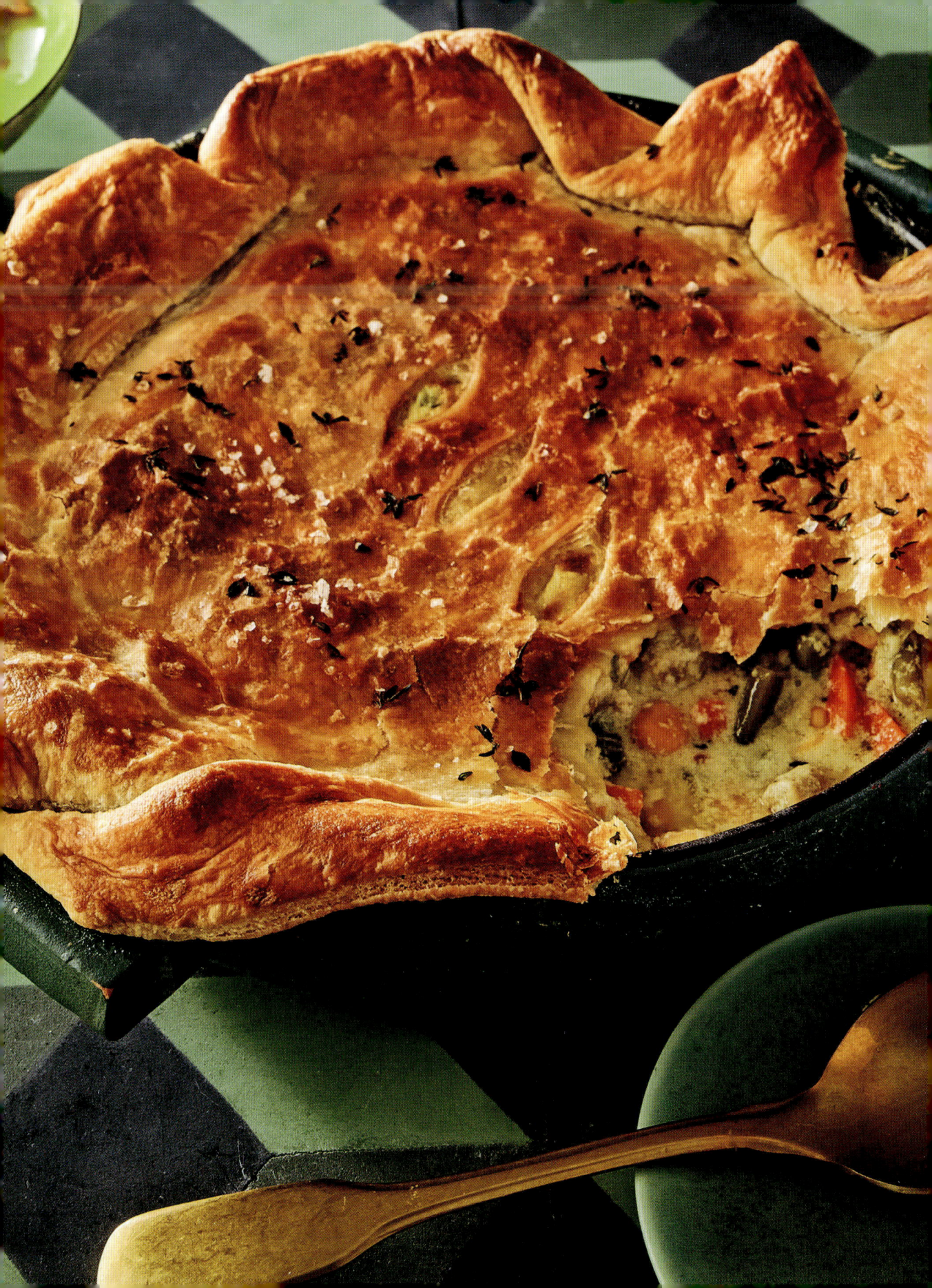

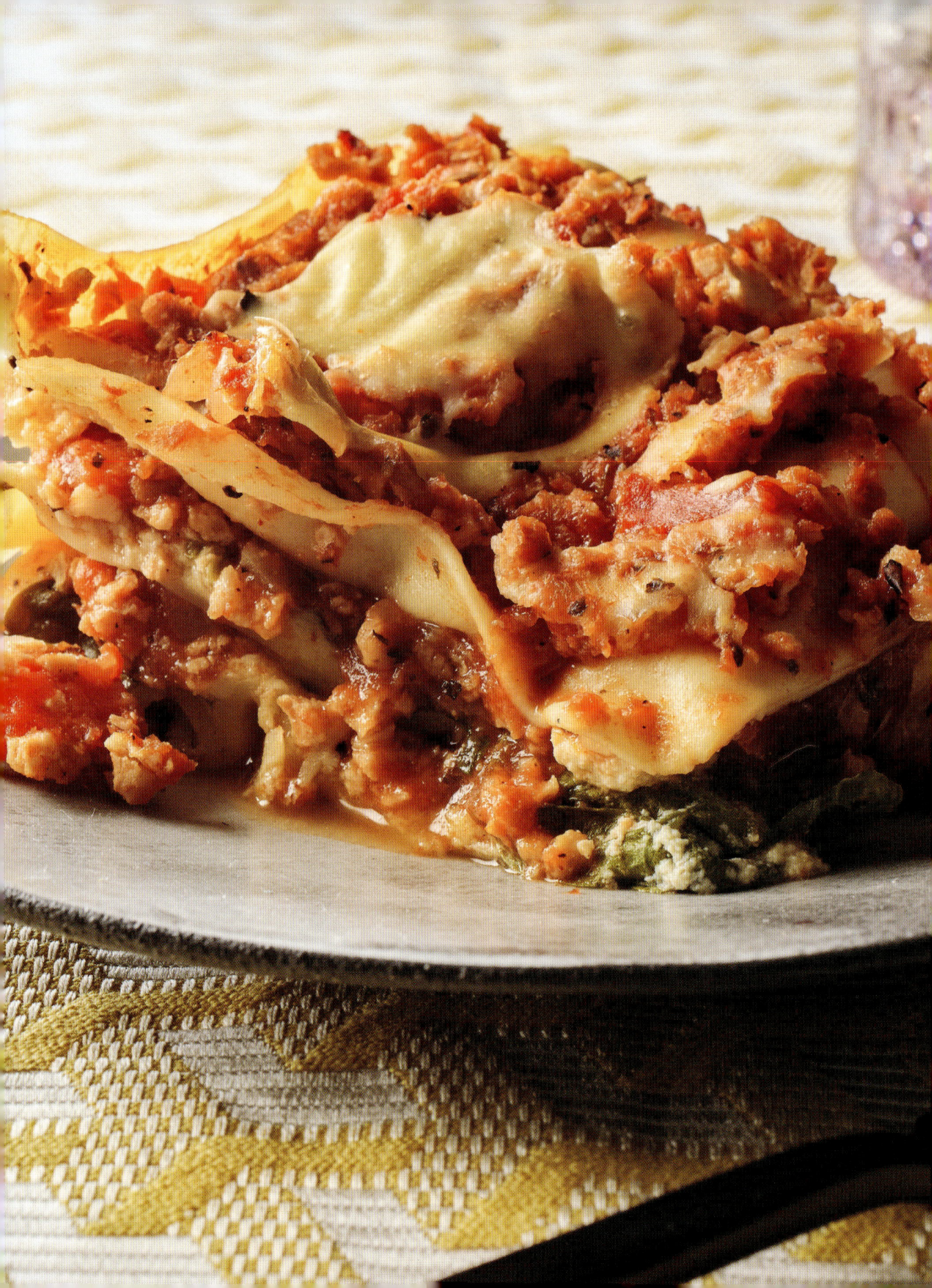

Back in college when I was studying abroad in Florence, lasagna was the first dish I made for my roommates — I even pulled off a Passover version with matzo the following year. This plant-based update is just as comforting, with layers of rich, hearty sauce, silky béchamel, and a tofu ricotta that brings the protein and the creaminess. Honestly, it's almost like a lasagna pudding, so comforting, creamy, and delicious. When I make this, my family eats it for days, even for breakfast (the best).

SERVES 12

PROTEIN-PACKED LASAGNA

Per serving

Calories: 585

Fat: 18g

Carbs: 88g

Fiber: 21g

Protein: 37g

Preheat the oven to 400°F. Lightly coat the bottom and sides of a 9 by 13-inch baking dish with olive oil.

Make the sauce: In a large Dutch oven or saucepan, heat the olive oil over medium-high heat. When the oil is shimmering, add the onion and garlic. Stir occasionally until the onions are translucent, about 5 minutes. Stir in the salt, oregano, paprika, black pepper, and a pinch of pepper flakes, if using. Add the rehydrated TVP, crushed tomatoes, diced tomatoes, basil sprig, and 1 cup water. Cover, reduce the heat to low, and simmer for 15 minutes. Taste for seasoning and adjust as needed.

Meanwhile, make the tofu ricotta: In a food processor, combine the tofu, nutritional yeast, olive oil, lemon juice, and salt. Process, stopping to scrape down the sides, to make a smooth mixture, about 1 minute. Set aside.

Extra-virgin olive oil, for the baking dish

Sauce

2 tablespoons extra-virgin olive oil

1 medium white onion, diced

2 garlic cloves, minced

2 teaspoons kosher salt, plus more as needed

1 teaspoon dried oregano

1 teaspoon smoked paprika

½ teaspoon freshly ground black pepper

Red pepper flakes (optional)

1 pound hydrated TVP MVP (page 224) or 1½ cups dry TVP (follow package instructions to hydrate)

1 (28-ounce) can crushed tomatoes

1 (14-ounce) can diced tomatoes

1 sprig fresh basil

Recipe continues...

Make the béchamel: In a medium saucepan, melt the butter over medium heat. Whisk in the flour until lightly golden and toasted, about 2 minutes. Slowly whisk in the soy milk a little at a time to avoid lumps. Simmer, whisking occasionally, until thickened, about 2 minutes. Remove from the heat and whisk in the nutmeg, salt, and pepper to taste. Set aside.

Assemble the lasagna: Spread about 2 ladlefuls of the tomato sauce across the bottom of the prepared baking dish. For the first layer, overlap lasagna noodles to cover the bottom of the pan, then spread about 2 ladlefuls of the béchamel over the noodles. Evenly sprinkle 1 cup of spinach over the bechamel. Dollop about one-third of the ricotta in small spoonfuls over the spinach and cover with about 2 ladlefuls of the tomato sauce. Repeat the process two more times (for layers 2 and 3), which will use up all the ricotta. For the final layer, use the rest of the noodles, spread the rest of the sauce, and drizzle the rest of the béchamel on top. You can add a sprinkle of vegan mozzarella if you want a cheesy finish.

Cover the baking dish loosely with aluminum foil and bake for 30 minutes. Remove the foil and bake until the top is set and the inside is bubbling, about another 15 minutes. Let the lasagna rest for 10 minutes before slicing. Serve sprinkled with chopped basil.

> **Dalina Says...**
> This lasagna brings protein to the table without losing that cozy, layered goodness. The tofu ricotta adds so much creaminess and dairy-free protein. And yes, the sauce counts as veggies!

Tofu Ricotta
- 12 ounces extra-firm tofu, drained
- 2 tablespoons nutritional yeast
- 2 tablespoons extra-virgin olive oil
- Juice of ½ lemon
- ½ teaspoon kosher salt

Béchamel
- ¼ cup (½ stick) vegan butter
- ¼ cup all-purpose flour
- 4 cups unsweetened soy milk or other plant-based milk
- Freshly grated nutmeg
- Kosher salt and freshly ground black pepper

Lasagna
- 2 (9-ounce) boxes no-boil lasagna noodles
- 3 cups baby spinach
- Shredded vegan mozzarella (optional)
- Chopped fresh basil, for serving

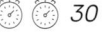 *Heavy Lift*

30 to 60 Minutes

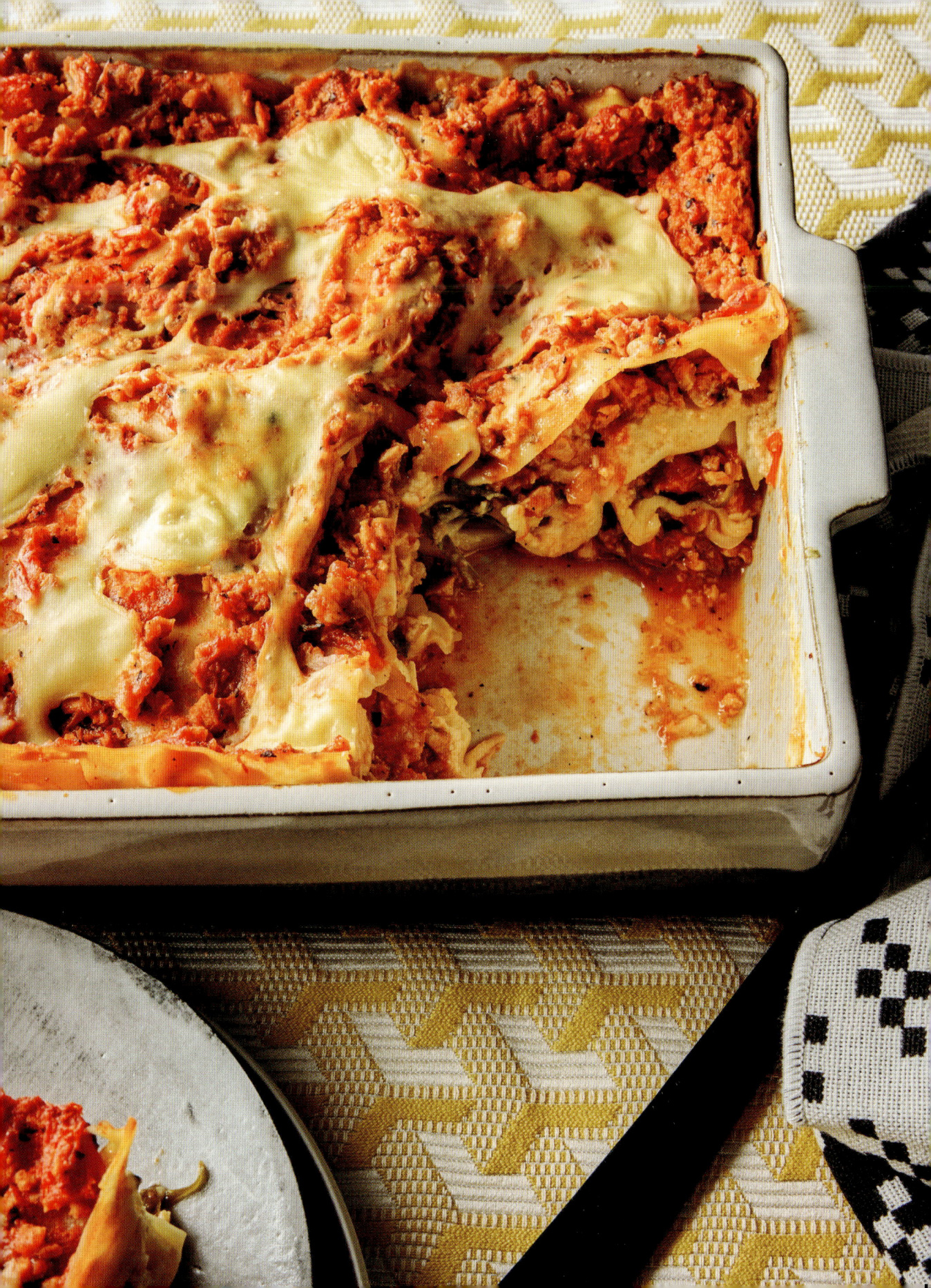

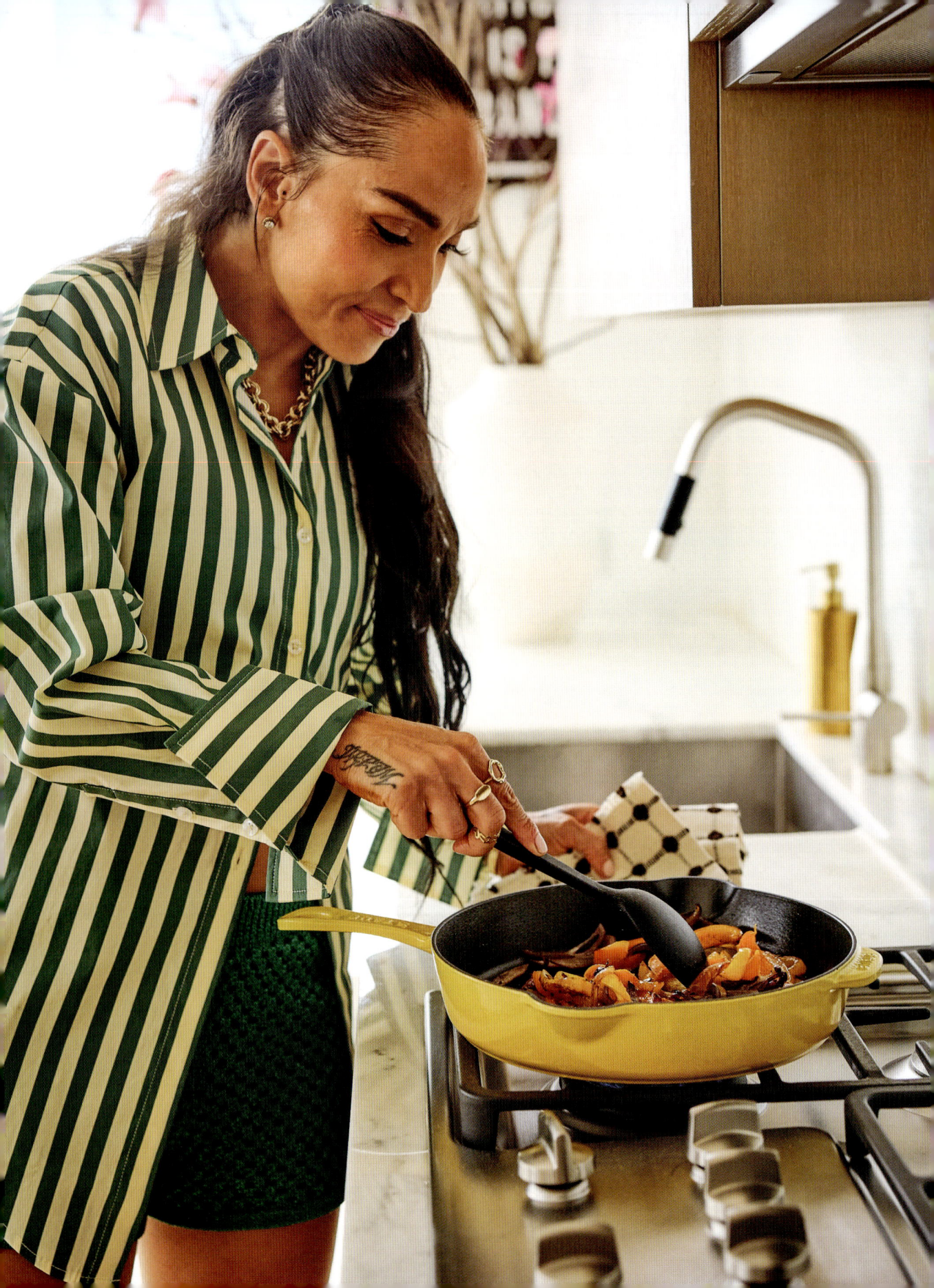

The second a sizzling skillet of fajitas hits a table in a restaurant, you just know that everyone not at that table is rethinking their order. This version keeps all the smoky, limey magic of a classic fajita plate but swaps in protein-packed seitan for that perfect chew. The best part, it's a build-your-own situation, making it super kid-friendly. So, load up those tortillas with all the fixings and make it exactly how you like it.

SERVES 4

SEITAN FAJITAS

Preheat the oven to 200°F. Stack the tortillas, wrap in aluminum foil, and place in the oven to warm up.

In a large nonstick skillet, heat 1 tablespoon of the avocado oil over medium heat. When the oil easily swirls around the skillet, add the seitan in an even layer. Sear, without stirring, until the bottom is nicely charred, about 6 minutes, then remove from the heat. Add the lime juice and 2 tablespoons of the chili powder. Quickly stir to coat the seitan as the lime juice boils off. Taste for seasoning; depending on the salt content of your chili powder, you might want to add a pinch of kosher salt. Transfer the seitan to a large serving platter.

Wipe out the skillet and set over high heat with the remaining 1 tablespoon avocado oil. When the oil starts to release wisps of smoke, add the bell peppers and onion in an even layer. Sear, without stirring, until the bottoms are nicely charred but the peppers are still crisp, about 3 minutes. Remove from the heat. Add the remaining 1 tablespoon chili powder and stir to coat. Transfer to the platter with the seitan.

In the same skillet (no need to wipe it out), combine the black beans, ¼ cup water, and a pinch of salt. Set over high heat and bring to a boil, using a wooden spoon to stir and scrape up all the tasty browned bits from the bottom of the skillet. When the liquid reduces by about half, about 4 minutes, transfer the beans to a small serving bowl.

To serve, make a fajita station with the platter surrounded by warm tortillas, black beans, a bowl of sour cream, and plenty of hot sauce.

- 8 high-protein tortillas, such as Hero
- 2 tablespoons avocado oil
- 1 pound seitan, store-bought or homemade (page 222), shredded
- Juice of 2 limes, plus wedges for serving
- 3 tablespoons chili powder or taco seasoning
- Kosher salt
- 2 large bell peppers, any color, seeded and sliced
- 1 large red onion, halved and sliced
- 1 (15.5-ounce) can black beans, drained and rinsed
- Store-bought or homemade vegan sour cream (page 146) and hot sauce, for serving

 Easy Lift
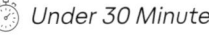 *Under 30 Minutes*

Per serving
Calories: 511
Fat: 14g
Carbs: 68g
Fiber: 32g
Protein: 48g

Tangy, creamy, and ridiculously easy — this dairy-free sour cream is a game changer. It's got the same smooth, velvety texture as the classic but with a protein boost from silken tofu — and without stabilizers, gums, or any other additives.

MAKES 1 CUP

VEGAN SOUR CREAM

In a blender or food processor, blend together the tofu, lemon juice, avocado oil, and salt on medium speed until smooth. Transfer to an airtight container and refrigerate until ready to use, or up to 5 days.

8 ounces silken tofu, drained
Juice of ½ lemon
1 tablespoon avocado oil
½ teaspoon kosher salt

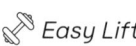 *Easy Lift*

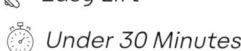 *Under 30 Minutes*

Per ¼ cup

Calories: 69

Fat: 5g

Carbs: 2g

Fiber: <1g

Protein: 4g

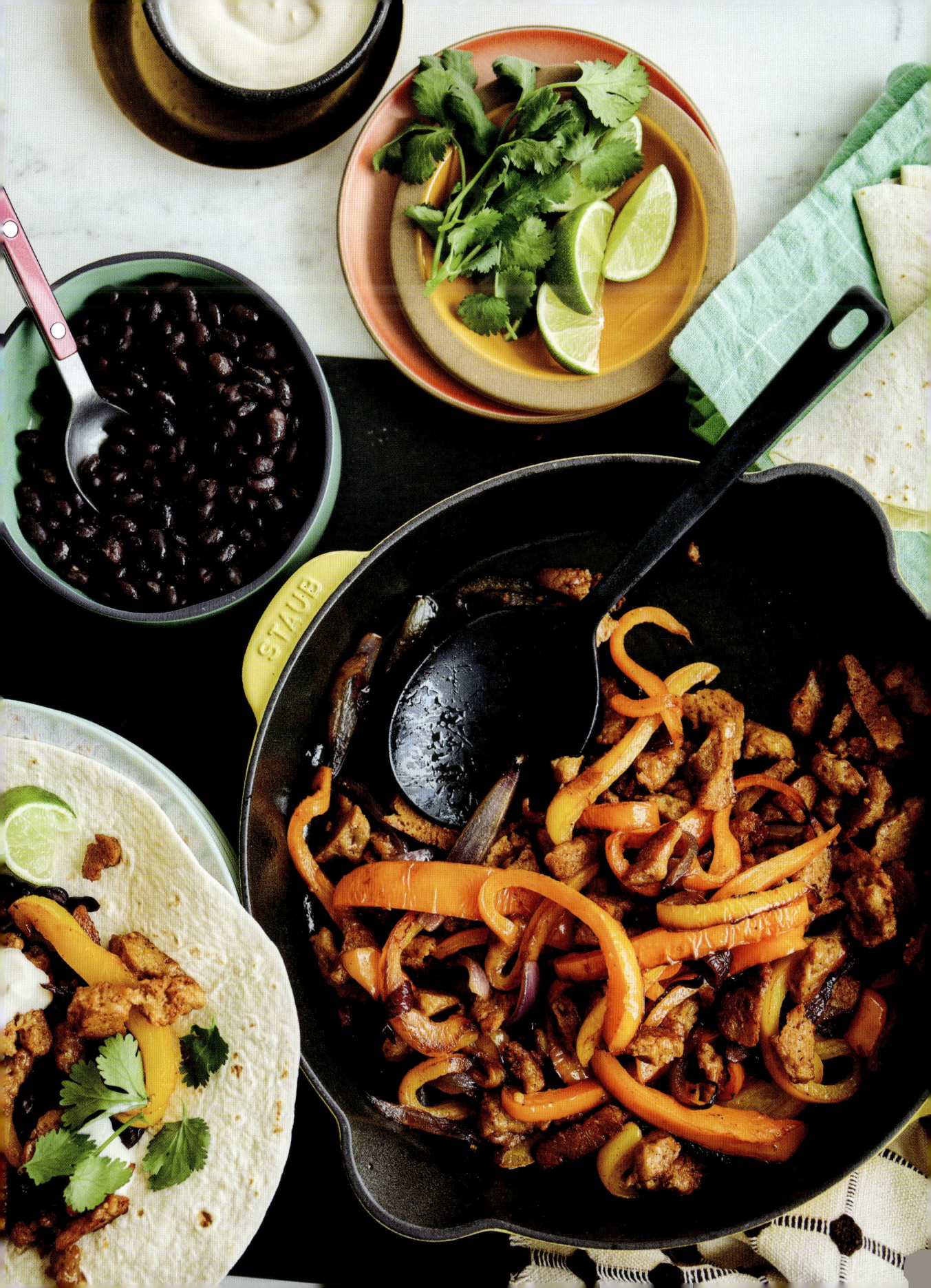

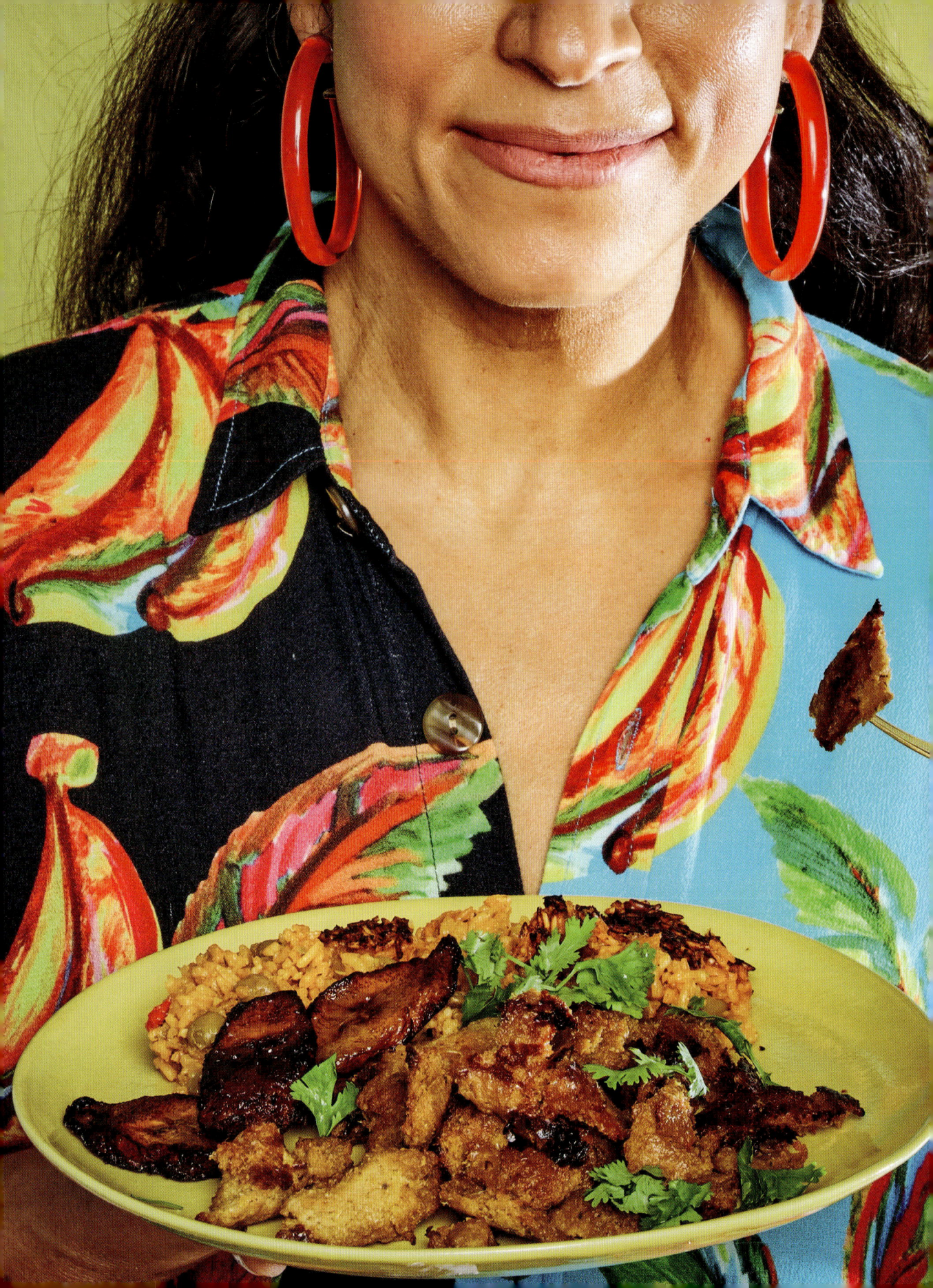

This dish is straight from my childhood — big Christmas dinners, Tuesday night family meals, special occasions, you name it. Pernil is a marinated, slow-roasted, crispy pork shoulder that's popular in Puerto Rico and other Latin American countries. I used to go with my dad to his friend's butcher shop to pick up ingredients, but now I'm giving pernil a plant-based remix. An easy arroz con gandules (a naturally complete rice-and-beans protein) and some sweet plantains help round out the perfect plate. But the star is always the vegan pernil with all of its crispy, garlicky, homey vibes and flavors that transport me right back to my little Boricua roots. ¡Wepa!

SERVES 6 TO 8

VEGAN PERNIL PLATE

Preheat the oven to 400°F. Line a rimmed baking sheet with parchment paper.

In a blender, combine the orange pieces, garlic, onion, avocado oil, coconut sugar, oregano, cumin, salt, pepper, paprika, and 2 cups water. Blend on high, stopping to scrape down the sides as needed, until smooth, about 2 minutes.

Tear the seitan into strips, like shredded meat. In a large saucepan, combine the seitan and liquid from the blender. Set over medium heat and bring to a simmer. Stir occasionally until most of the liquid has evaporated, about 10 minutes.

Transfer the seitan mixture to the prepared baking sheet and spread into an even layer. Roast until the tops are charred, about 20 minutes, then flip the pernil and rotate the baking sheet. Bake until the pernil is charred all over, another 20 to 25 minutes.

On each plate, serve generous scoops of arroz con gandules and pernil. Top with a few pieces of maduros and garnish with cilantro before serving.

2 large navel oranges, peeled and broken into segments
8 garlic cloves
1 medium white onion, cut into pieces
¼ cup avocado oil
¼ cup coconut sugar
1 tablespoon dried oregano
1 tablespoon ground cumin
1 tablespoon kosher salt
1 teaspoon freshly ground black pepper
1 teaspoon smoked paprika
2 pounds seitan, store-bought or homemade (page 222)
Arroz con Gandules (page 150) and Maduros (page 151), for serving
Chopped fresh cilantro, for serving

Heavy Lift
30 to 60 Minutes

Pernil, per serving (based on 6 servings)

Calories: 370
Fat: 17g
Carbs: 30g
Fiber: 2g
Protein: 27g

Protein: 11g | Calories: 486 | Fat: 12g | Carbs: 80g | Fiber: 10g

Arroz con Gandules, per serving (based on 6 servings)

This dish has the perfect balance of fluffy, fragrant rice and tender pigeon peas (gandules), which are small, slightly nutty legumes that add texture without overpowering the rice. We season with sazón — a powerhouse spice blend that brings a pop of color and deep, savory flavor — and fold in alcaparrado, a briny mix of olives and capers that gives the rice a punch of salty, tangy goodness. But let's be real — we all know it's all about the pegao, that crispy, golden crust on the bottom of the pot. My abuela and dad used to fight me for the last crunchy bits.

SERVES 6 TO 8

ARROZ CON GANDULES (RICE WITH PIGEON PEAS)

In a medium bowl, cover the rice with cold water. Swish aggressively and carefully tilt the bowl to drain. Repeat a few more times until the water runs clear. Strain the rice in a sieve and set aside.

In a food processor, combine the onion, bell pepper, cilantro, garlic, and avocado oil. Process, stopping to scrape the sides as needed, until a rough paste forms, about 1 minute.

Scrape the mixture into a large saucepan and set over medium-high heat. Cook, stirring often, until the mixture starts to brown and most of the liquid has evaporated, about 6 minutes. Stir in the sazón, salt, and pepper, then add the rice. Stir to coat in the oil and continue to toast the rice, stirring occasionally, until some of the grains are translucent, about 3 minutes.

Stir in the stock, alcaparrado, and bay leaves. Scatter the pigeon peas over the top. Bring to a boil, cover, and reduce the heat to low. Simmer until the liquid is absorbed and the rice is tender, 20 to 25 minutes. (Bonus points if you get a good crust on the bottom of the rice! Dig a spoon deep down to check a little bit.) Remove from the heat and let steam for 15 minutes before serving.

- 2 cups medium-grain white rice
- 1 medium white onion, roughly chopped
- 1 medium green bell pepper, seeded and roughly chopped
- 1 large bunch cilantro, stems and leaves roughly chopped
- 8 garlic cloves
- ¼ cup avocado oil
- 2 (1.4-ounce) packets sazón con culantro y achiote (sazón with cilantro and achiote)
- 2 teaspoons kosher salt
- 1 teaspoon freshly ground black pepper
- 3 cups vegetable stock or Liquid Gold (page 235)
- 1 (7-ounce) jar alcaparrado, drained
- 2 dried bay leaves
- 1 (15-ounce) can pigeon peas, drained and rinsed

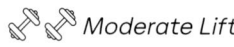 *Moderate Lift*

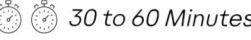 *30 to 60 Minutes*

If you're not throwing a couple of these caramelized beauties onto your pernil plate, you're doing it wrong. Maduros bring the perfect hit of sweetness to balance out the savory goodness of pernil and arroz con gandules.

SERVES 6 TO 8

MADUROS (FRIED SWEET PLANTAINS)

Peel the plantains by cutting off both ends, cutting a shallow slit down the length of the plantain, then removing the peel. Cut each plantain diagonally into ½-inch-thick slices.

In a nonstick skillet, heat the avocado oil over medium heat. When the oil shimmers, work in batches to fry the plantains, taking care not to crowd the pan. Fry until golden brown, about 2 minutes per side. Transfer to paper towels and immediately season with salt. Fry the remainder, adding more oil as needed.

2 small ripe (mostly black) plantains
2 tablespoons avocado oil, plus more as needed
Kosher salt

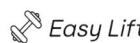 *Easy Lift*

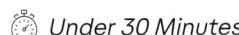 *Under 30 Minutes*

Maduros, per serving (based on 6 servings) | Calories: 114 | Fat: 5g | Carbs: 19g | Fiber: 1g | Protein: 1g

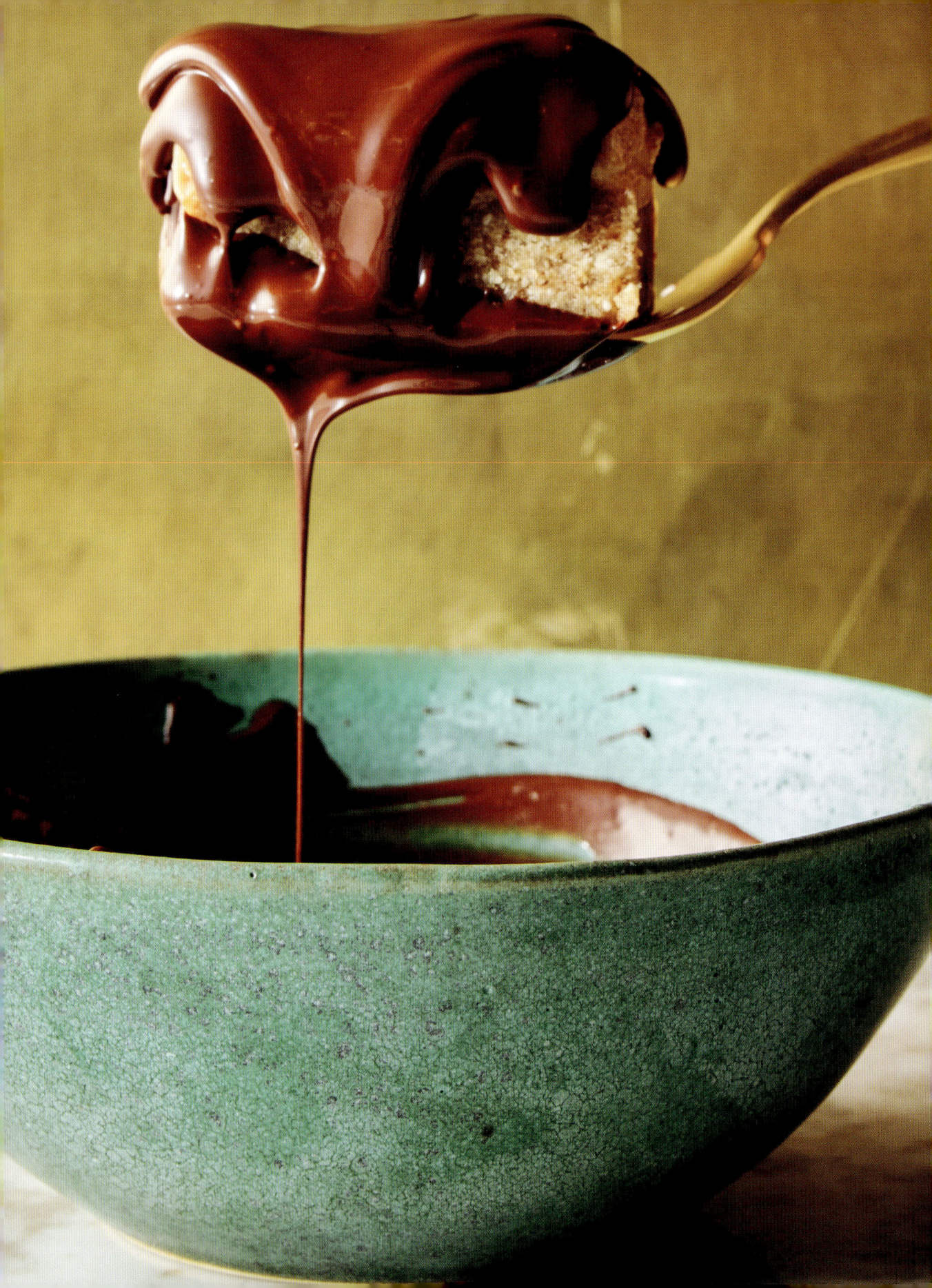

KEEP CALM AND SNACK ON

Anyone who follows me on social media knows I'm a firm believer in the power of a good purse snack! Life moves fast, and I like to be ready for whatever comes next — which means having something on hand to keep my energy up and hunger in check. (It's even more important for me because I'm diabetic — staying ahead of those blood sugar dips is nonnegotiable.) These small but mighty bites are packed with protein and just enough fuel to hold you (or little ones) over between meals. Whether you need a quick pre-workout boost, an afternoon pick-me-up, or something to stash in your bag for later, this chapter has you covered.

Protein: 9g | **Fiber: 1g** | **Carbs: 59g** | **Fat: 8g** | **Calories: 344** | **Per bar**

Back in my golden days of VHS players and sleepovers, these were *the* snack. My cousins and I would make giant trays of them — you know the ones made from melted marshmallows and that crackling rice cereal! — then park ourselves in front of the TV, watching *Grease* on repeat until we passed out. This version stays true to the sticky, chewy classic but sneaks in a little protein powder — because grown-up me still loves a good nostalgia bite, especially when it's a hard working one.

MAKES 9 BARS

SWEET CRISPY TREATS

Lightly coat an 8 by 8-inch baking pan with 1 tablespoon of the coconut oil. Set aside.

In a large pot, heat the remaining 2 tablespoons coconut oil over low heat and add the condensed milk. Use a rubber spatula to stir until combined. Add the marshmallows and salt and stir until melted and smooth, about 10 minutes.

Remove from the heat and stir in the protein powder. Add the cereal and gently fold until completely coated and sticky.

Coat your hands in the coconut oil pooled at the bottom of the baking pan, then scrape the mixture into the pan. Use your oily hands to lightly press it into an even layer, being careful not to compact the mixture too much so the treats stay light. Let rest at room temperature for 1 hour to set, then cut into 9 pieces. Any leftovers can be stored in a zip-top bag at room temperature for up to 3 days.

- 3 tablespoons refined coconut oil
- ½ cup sweetened condensed coconut or oat milk
- 1 (10-ounce) bag vegan marshmallows, such as Dandies
- 1 teaspoon kosher salt
- 1 cup vanilla protein powder
- 5 cups crisp rice cereal

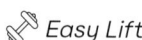 *Easy Lift*

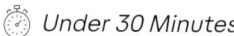 *Under 30 Minutes*

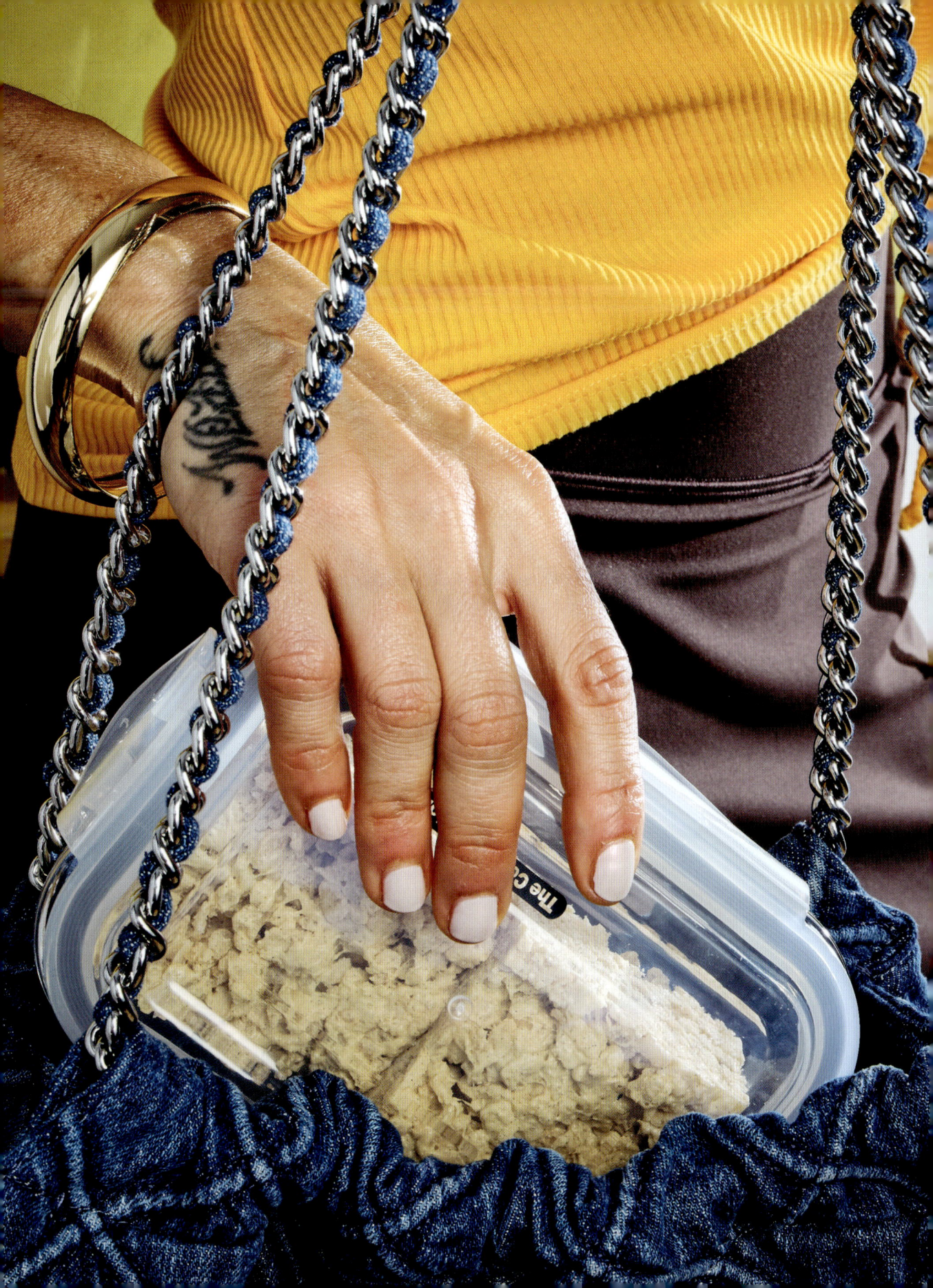

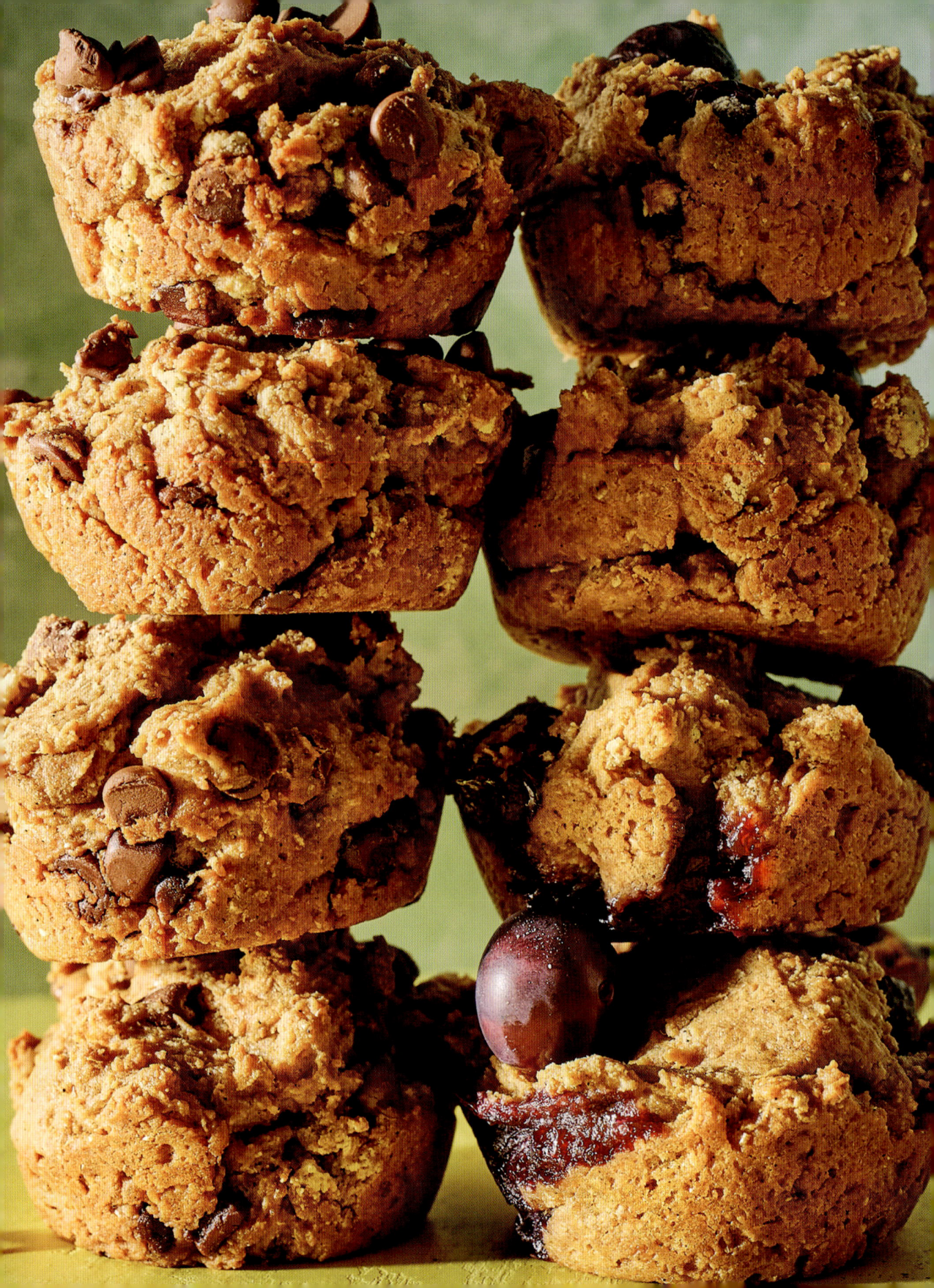

There's a lot of '90s nostalgia in this book, and these take me straight back. My mom wasn't big on buying packaged snacks, so I was the kid with mystery treats in foil and baggies. But every time I went to a friend's house, I wanted all the good stuff — especially those little mini muffins (you know the ones!). This is my "I'm an adult, I eat what I want" version, only with a little more balance. Still sweet, still snackable, just way more fuel for your day. I'm offering two varieties to suit your mood.

MAKES 24 MINI MUFFINS

MINI ENERGY MUFFINS

Preheat the oven to 350°F. Brush the cups of a mini muffin tin with a light layer of coconut oil.

In a large bowl, whisk the ¼ cup coconut oil with the soy milk, coconut sugar, maple syrup, and lemon juice. Set a mesh strainer over the bowl and sift the flour, protein powder, baking powder, and salt into the batter. Use a rubber spatula to stir until almost combined, then add the blueberries or chocolate chips and finish folding.

Fill each muffin cup to the top (work in batches if your muffin tin only makes 12). Bake until a toothpick inserted in the center comes out clean, about 15 minutes. Let cool for 5 minutes in the tin, then transfer to a wire rack to finish cooling. (Let the muffin tin finish cooling and brush with more coconut oil if baking in batches). Store in a zip-top bag at room temperature for up to 4 days.

¼ cup refined coconut oil, melted, plus more for the pan
1 cup unsweetened soy milk or other plant-based milk
½ cup coconut sugar
2 tablespoons pure maple syrup
Juice of ½ lemon
1 cup whole wheat flour
1 cup vanilla protein powder
1½ teaspoons baking powder
1 teaspoon kosher salt
½ cup blueberries or mini vegan chocolate chips

🏋 Easy Lift
⏱ Under 30 Minutes

Per serving (3 muffins), blueberry	Per serving (3 muffins), chocolate chip
Calories: 257	Calories: 310
Fat: 9g	Fat: 9g
Carbs: 33g	Carbs: 33g
Fiber: 3g	Fiber: 2g
Protein: 12g	Protein: 12g

Dalina Says...

When thinking of "snacks" always try to reach for those with 2 to 3 macros in them to help you feel satisfied. And always remember this is meant to carry you over until your next meal—so it doesn't have to be big but it can carry tons of nutrition. These snack bites hit perfectly with 12g of protein plus a few grams of fiber packed into each one.

Kale's publicist was really working overtime during the 2010s, but let's be real — kale chips still hit when they're seasoned right. That earthy, crispy goodness needs big flavors, and everything bagel seasoning brings it into the present day. It's the kale chip glow-up we all deserve!

SERVES 4

SEASONED KALE CHIPS

Preheat the oven to 250°F and set the racks in the upper and lower third of the oven. Line two rimmed baking sheets with parchment paper.

Pull the kale from the stems and tear the leaves into chip-sized pieces. Gather the kale in a clean kitchen towel and pat completely dry.

In a large bowl, combine the kale with the coconut oil, nutritional yeast, 2 tablespoons of the everything bagel seasoning, and the hemp seeds, paprika, and cayenne. Toss to completely coat. Evenly spread the kale on the prepared baking sheets, leaving a little space between each piece so they crisp up. Sprinkle the remaining 3 tablespoons everything bagel seasoning on top.

Bake for 6 minutes, then switch the baking sheets from top to bottom and rotate front to back. Bake until the kale is crisp and just starting to brown, another 4 to 6 minutes.

Let cool completely on the baking sheets (the kale chips will continue to crisp as they cool) and serve immediately. Any leftovers can be stored in a zip-top bag or airtight container at room temperature for up to 2 days.

- 1 large bunch curly kale
- 3 tablespoons refined coconut oil, melted
- ¾ cup nutritional yeast
- 5 tablespoons everything bagel seasoning
- 1 tablespoon hemp seeds
- 1 teaspoon smoked paprika
- ½ teaspoon cayenne pepper

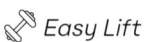 *Easy Lift*

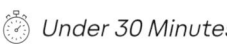 *Under 30 Minutes*

Per serving — Calories: 265 | Fat: 18g | Carbs: 14g | Fiber: 3g | Protein: 13g

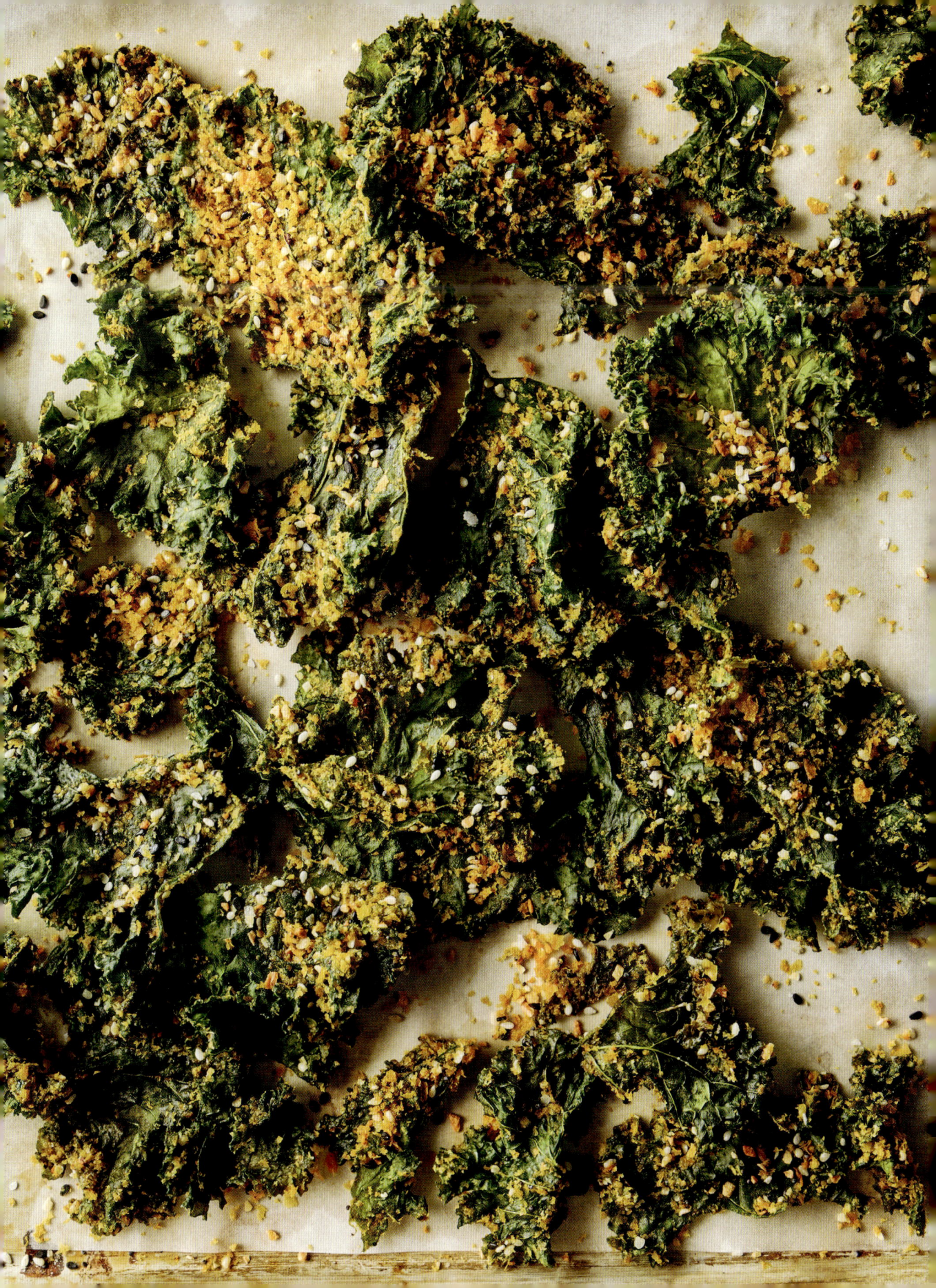

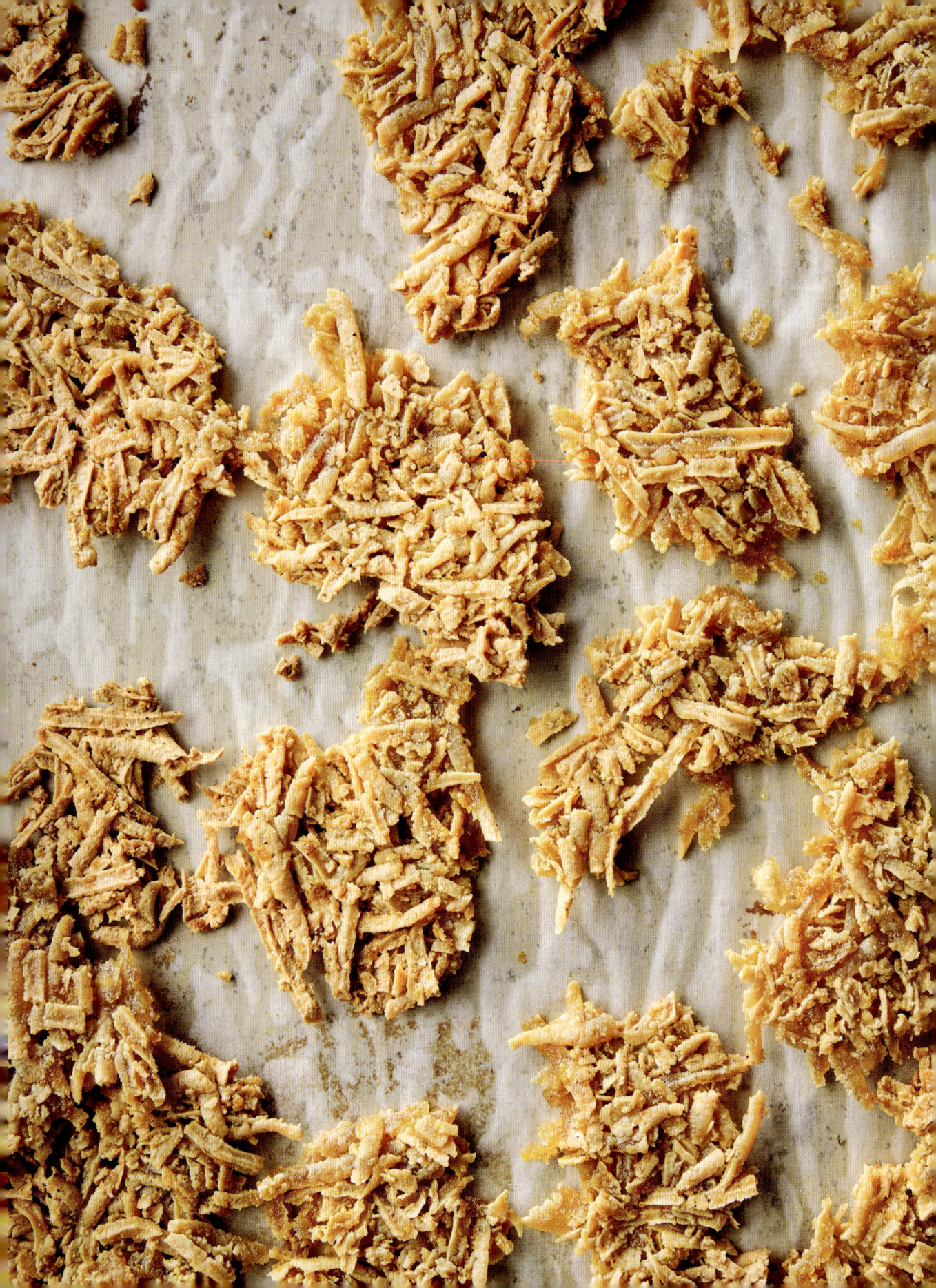

Who needs pork rinds when you've got tofu that can do this? These "chicharrones" are the ultimate snack — light, crispy, and shockingly addictive. Baking gives them the perfect crunch, but if you're feeling a little extra, fry them for next-level crispiness. Sprinkle on some flaky salt, and they're perfect for munching solo, pairing with your favorite dips, or crumbling over a salad. Trust me, mija, you'll find every excuse to make this snack-worthy crunchfest.

SERVES 4

TOFU CHICHARRONES

Preheat the oven to 350°F. Line a rimmed baking sheet with parchment paper.

Using the grater blade on a food processor (or the large holes of a box grater), grate the block of tofu. (You might have to cut it into small pieces to fit in the food processor.) In a large bowl, toss the tofu with the nutritional yeast, olive oil, onion powder, garlic powder, kosher salt, and pepper.

Spread the mixture evenly on the prepared baking sheet (you'll fill the entire sheet pan), then lightly press to form one large, cohesive rectangle that covers the entire baking sheet. Bake, rotating the baking sheet every 30 minutes. until the tofu is completely dry and starting to crisp around the edges, 1 to 1½ hours. Sprinkle flaky sea salt over the surface and cut the tofu into bite-sized pieces. Let cool completely on the baking sheet.

This is optional, but for extra crispy chicharrones, fill a large saucepan with about 1 inch of vegetable oil. Set over medium heat until the oil is just beginning to release faint wisps of smoke. Lower a few pieces of the baked tofu into the oil and fry until very crisp, about 2 minutes, flipping them halfway through. Transfer to paper towels to drain and season with a pinch of flaky salt. Repeat with the remaining pieces.

The chicharrones can be served immediately or stored at room temperature in a loosely covered container for up to 2 days.

- 1 (16-ounce) package extra-firm tofu, drained
- 2 tablespoons nutritional yeast
- 2 tablespoons extra-virgin olive oil
- 1 teaspoon onion powder
- 1 teaspoon garlic powder
- 1 teaspoon kosher salt
- ½ teaspoon freshly ground black pepper
- Flaky sea salt
- Vegetable oil (optional)

Easy Lift

1 Hour +

Per serving
Calories: 173
Fat: 13g
Carbs: 4g
Fiber: 2g
Protein: 13g

Protein: 10g | Fiber: 4g | Carbs: 24g | Fat: 7g | Calories: 196 | Per bar

There's this café in Ocean City, New Jersey, called Goji, and they make these incredible vegan candy bars. Drew loves them so much he bought a bunch of them wholesale and stuffed them into our freezer — literally pushing aside bags of pumped breast milk to make space! Priorities, right? These bites — my love letter to Snickers, which are tragically not vegan — are my homemade take on that obsession, a little salty, a little sweet, and dangerously good straight from the fridge.

MAKES 16 MINI BARS

VEGAN CANDY BAR BITES

Make the base: In a food processor, combine the almond flour, coconut oil, and salt. Process until the mixture comes together, about 1 minute, using a silicone spatula to scrape down the sides as needed.

Line an 8 by 4-inch loaf pan with parchment paper, leaving some overhang to lift the candy out later. Transfer the dough to the pan and press into an even layer. Transfer to the freezer to cool.

Meanwhile, make the caramel: In the same food processor (no need to clean it), combine the peanut butter powder and milk. Process until smooth, about 1 minute. Add the dates, maple syrup, coconut oil, and salt. Process again to make a gooey caramel, about 2 minutes. Pour the caramel over the base and sprinkle the peanuts over top. Freeze for 1 hour to set.

Make the coating: Remove the baking sheet from the freezer and let the candies slightly thaw, about 15 minutes. Melt the chocolate in the microwave in 30-second bursts, stirring between each one, until melted, about 2 to 3 minutes total.

Use the parchment to transfer the candy to a cutting board, then cut into 16 mini bars, about 1 by 2 inches each. Working one at a time, dip a candy in the chocolate and flip to coat on all sides. Use a fork to lift and let the excess drip off, then transfer back to the parchment. Repeat with the remaining candies. Refrigerate for about 10 minutes to set the chocolate.

The candies can be refrigerated in an airtight container for up to 1 week or frozen for up to 1 month.

Base
2 cups almond flour
2 tablespoons maple syrup
1 tablespoon coconut oil
¼ teaspoon kosher salt

Caramel
½ cup peanut butter powder
½ cup unsweetened soy milk or plant-based milk
5 medjool dates, pitted and finely chopped
1 teaspoon coconut oil
¼ teaspoon kosher salt
⅓ cup salted roasted peanuts

Coating
16 ounces vegan chocolate chips

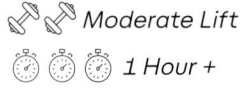 *Moderate Lift*

1 Hour +

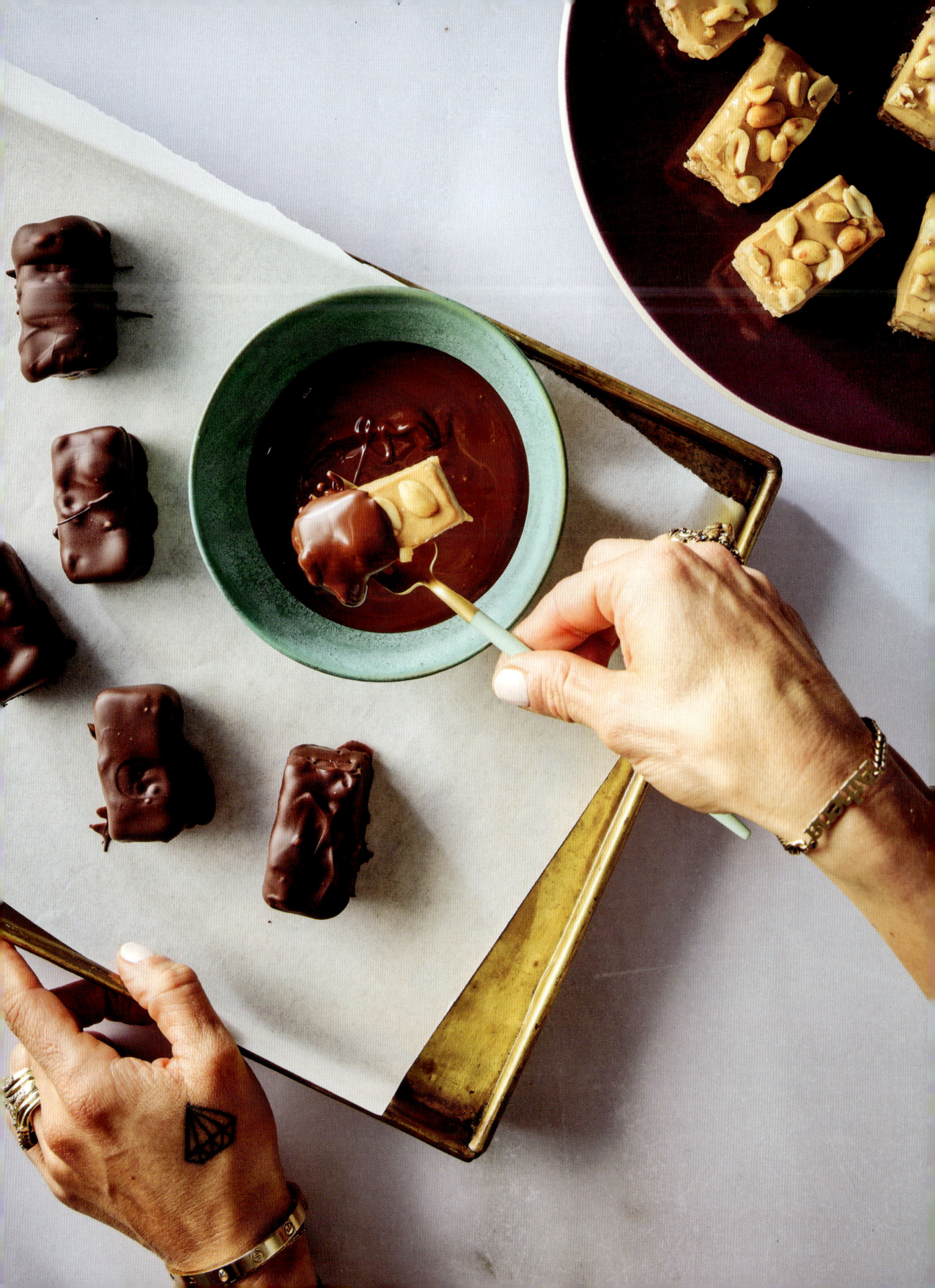

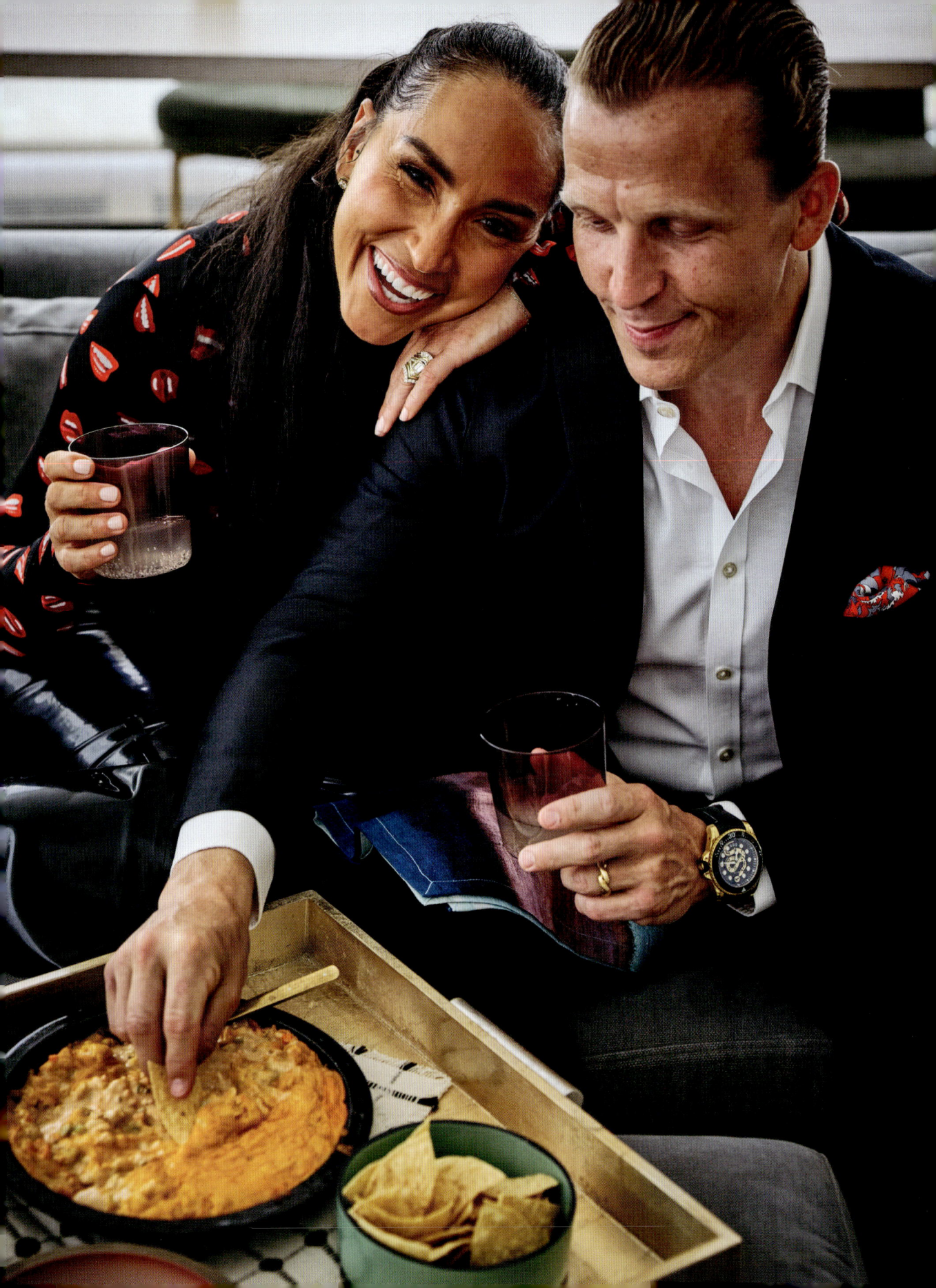

COUCH POTATO CRAVINGS

Sometimes, you just need to kick back, grab a snack, and enjoy the show. Whether it's game day, an awards-night watch party, or just a well-earned night on the couch, these bites bring the indulgence without wrecking your macros. We're talking bold flavors, crave-worthy textures, and plenty of protein to keep you satisfied. So, get comfy and dig in — because snack time should hit just as hard as prime time.

Per Serving — Calories: 301 | Fat: 11g | Carbs: 43g | Fiber: 18g | Protein: 14g

These wings plus a homemade lemony hummus dip? Nonnegotiable. The dip is so bright and lemony, you'll swear you're sailing straight to a Mediterranean coastline. And the artichokes are a dream for the purists who prefer to skip the meat replacements. The quinoa breading brings the perfect crunch while sneaking in some extra protein. Tangy, crispy, and totally addictive — you might want to double the batch. Note that I like using an air fryer to make these but they get just as crisp in a hot oven.

SERVES 4

AIR FRYER ARTICHOKE WINGS WITH LEMONY HUMMUS DIP

Make the hummus: In a blender or food processor, combine the chickpeas, lemon zest and juice, garlic, tahini, salt, and ¼ cup cold water. Blend on high until completely smooth. Transfer to an airtight container and refrigerate until ready to serve, or up to 5 days.

Make the wings: Cut each artichoke heart in half lengthwise and transfer, cut side down, to paper towels to drain.

In a large shallow bowl, whisk together the soy milk and flaxseed. Let sit for 10 minutes to thicken. In another large shallow bowl, mix the quinoa, salt, pepper, paprika, and avocado oil. Working one at a time, dip each artichoke half in the soy milk mixture to coat on all sides. Transfer to the quinoa mixture and lightly press to adhere. Transfer to a plate while coating the rest.

Preheat an air fryer to 400°F. Arrange the wings in a single layer, working in batches if needed, and bake, flipping halfway, until the coating is golden brown and crisp, 10 to 15 minutes. (You can also roast the wings on a parchment paper–lined rimmed baking sheet in a 450°F oven for 10 to 15 minutes, flipping halfway through the baking time.) Serve hot with the lemon hummus for dipping.

Hummus
1 cup cooked chickpeas (page 232)
Grated zest and juice of 1 lemon
1 garlic clove
1 tablespoon tahini
1 teaspoon kosher salt

Wings
1 (14-ounce) can whole artichoke hearts, drained
¾ cup unsweetened soy milk or other plant-based milk
¼ cup ground flaxseed
1 cup cooked and cooled quinoa (see Grains for Days, page 231)
1 teaspoon kosher salt
1 teaspoon freshly ground black pepper
1 teaspoon smoked paprika
1 teaspoon avocado oil

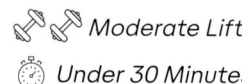 *Moderate Lift*

Under 30 Minutes

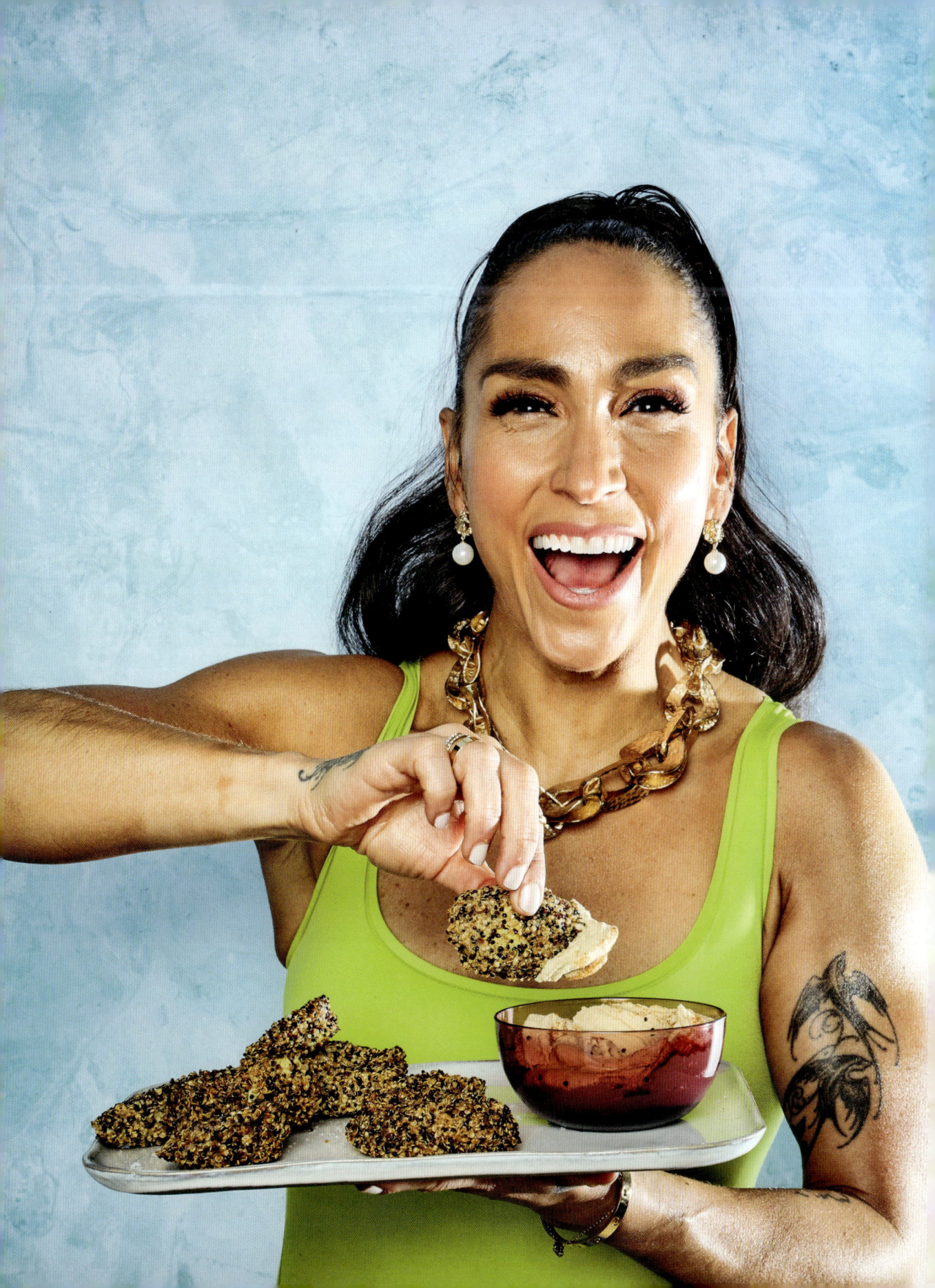

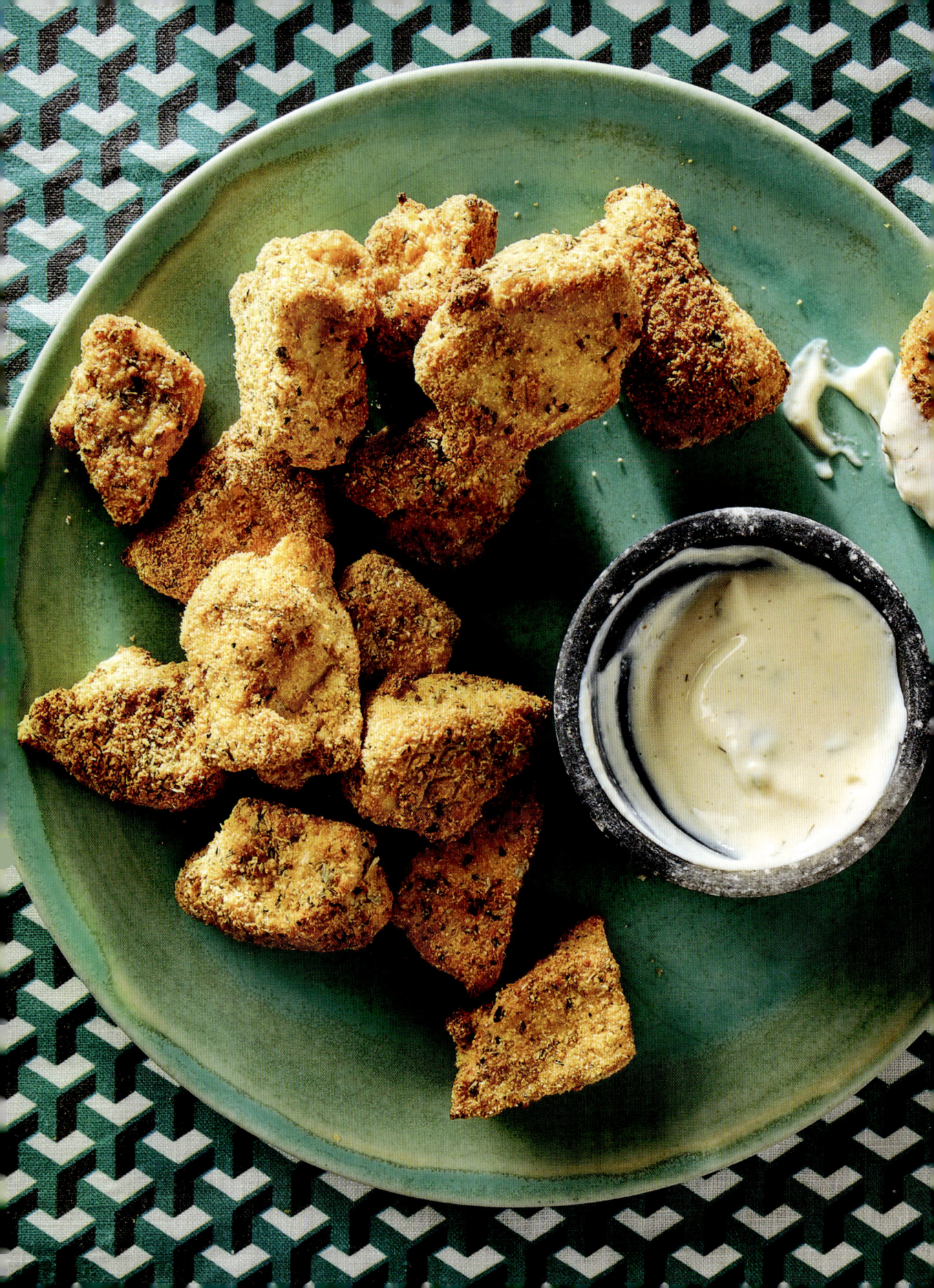

These tofu bites are the ultimate answer to any nugget craving — crispy, golden, and totally dunkable. They hit that nostalgic chicken nugget spot but in a plant-based, protein-packed way. Plus, they're ridiculously easy to throw together, making them a weeknight win. Serve them up with ranch (because obviously), or mix it up with Buffalo sauce, BBQ sauce, or even a spicy agave drizzle if you're feeling wild.

SERVES 4

CRISPY AIR-FRIED TOFU NUGGETS

Wrap the tofu in paper towels and set on a plate. Set another plate on top with a few cans of beans or tomatoes to weigh it down. Let it sit to drain for about 10 minutes. Meanwhile, in a small bowl, whisk the breadcrumbs, nutritional yeast, garlic powder, onion powder, oregano, and salt together.

Unwrap the drained tofu and cut it in half lengthwise to make two thinner pieces. Break into craggy 1-inch pieces and drop into a large bowl. Add the cornstarch and toss to completely coat the tofu. Add 2 tablespoons of the soy milk and toss again to make a sticky paste. Add about half of the seasoning mix in big pinches, then toss the tofu again. Repeat this process with the remaining 1 tablespoon soy milk and the rest of the seasoning. Press any stray seasoning onto the tofu pieces.

Preheat an air fryer to 400°F. Arrange the tofu pieces in a single layer, working in batches if needed, and bake, flipping halfway through the baking time, until the coating is golden brown and crisp, 10 to 15 minutes. (You can also roast the nuggets on a parchment paper–lined rimmed baking sheet in a 450°F oven for 10 to 15 minutes, flipping halfway through the baking time.) Serve hot with plenty of ranch for dunking.

16 ounces extra-firm tofu, drained
2 tablespoons plain breadcrumbs
2 tablespoons nutritional yeast
1 tablespoon garlic powder
1 tablespoon onion powder
1 tablespoon dried oregano
1½ teaspoons kosher salt
2 tablespoons cornstarch
3 tablespoons unsweetened soy milk or other plant-based milk
Tofu Ranch Dressing (page 121), for serving

🏋 *Easy Lift*
⏱ *Under 30 Minutes*

Per serving
Calories: 159
Fat: 6g
Carbs: 12g
Fiber: 3g
Protein: 13g

These crispy-on-the-outside and saucy-on-the-inside pizza bites are taking me straight back to my after-school routine — just me, the couch, and Oprah. But this version is a total upgrade. A spicy filling brings the heat and heartiness (shhh, they're packed with lentils, too), while the golden, buttery shell gives major garlic bread energy.

MAKES 16 BITES

PIZZA BITES

Preheat the oven to 400°F. Line a rimmed baking sheet with parchment paper.

In a blender, combine the bell pepper, onion, garlic, tomato paste, salt, red pepper flakes, and ½ cup water and blend to make a smooth sauce. Transfer to a medium saucepan and set over medium heat. Let the sauce come to a simmer, stirring often, and reduce by half, about 10 minutes. Stir in the lentils and remove from the heat. Let cool for 15 minutes. Meanwhile, let the pizza dough sit at room temperature so it's easy to roll.

On a lightly floured surface, divide the dough into 16 equal-sized pieces (1 ounce each). Working one at a time, use a lightly floured rolling pin to roll each piece into a roughly 3-inch round. Place a heaping tablespoon of the lentil mixture in the center, then lift the edges over the filling and pinch shut. Roll, seam side down, to make a tight ball. Repeat with the remaining dough and filling, evenly spacing the balls on the prepared baking sheet.

In a small bowl, mix the melted butter and garlic powder. Brush the balls evenly with the butter mixture, then transfer to the oven. Bake until the dough is golden brown, 15 to 20 minutes. Transfer to a serving plate and garnish with parsley before serving.

1 red bell pepper, seeded and roughly chopped
1 small white onion, roughly chopped
4 garlic cloves
2 tablespoons tomato paste
1 teaspoon kosher salt
½ teaspoon red pepper flakes
1 cup cooked green lentils (page 233)
1 pound Packed Pizza Dough (page 219) or store-bought pizza dough
All-purpose flour, for rolling
2 tablespoons vegan butter, melted
½ teaspoon garlic powder
Chopped fresh parsley, for serving

Moderate Lift

30 to 60 Minutes

Per serving (3 bites) — Calories: 82 | Fat: 9g | Carbs: 33g | Fiber: 4g | Protein: 21g

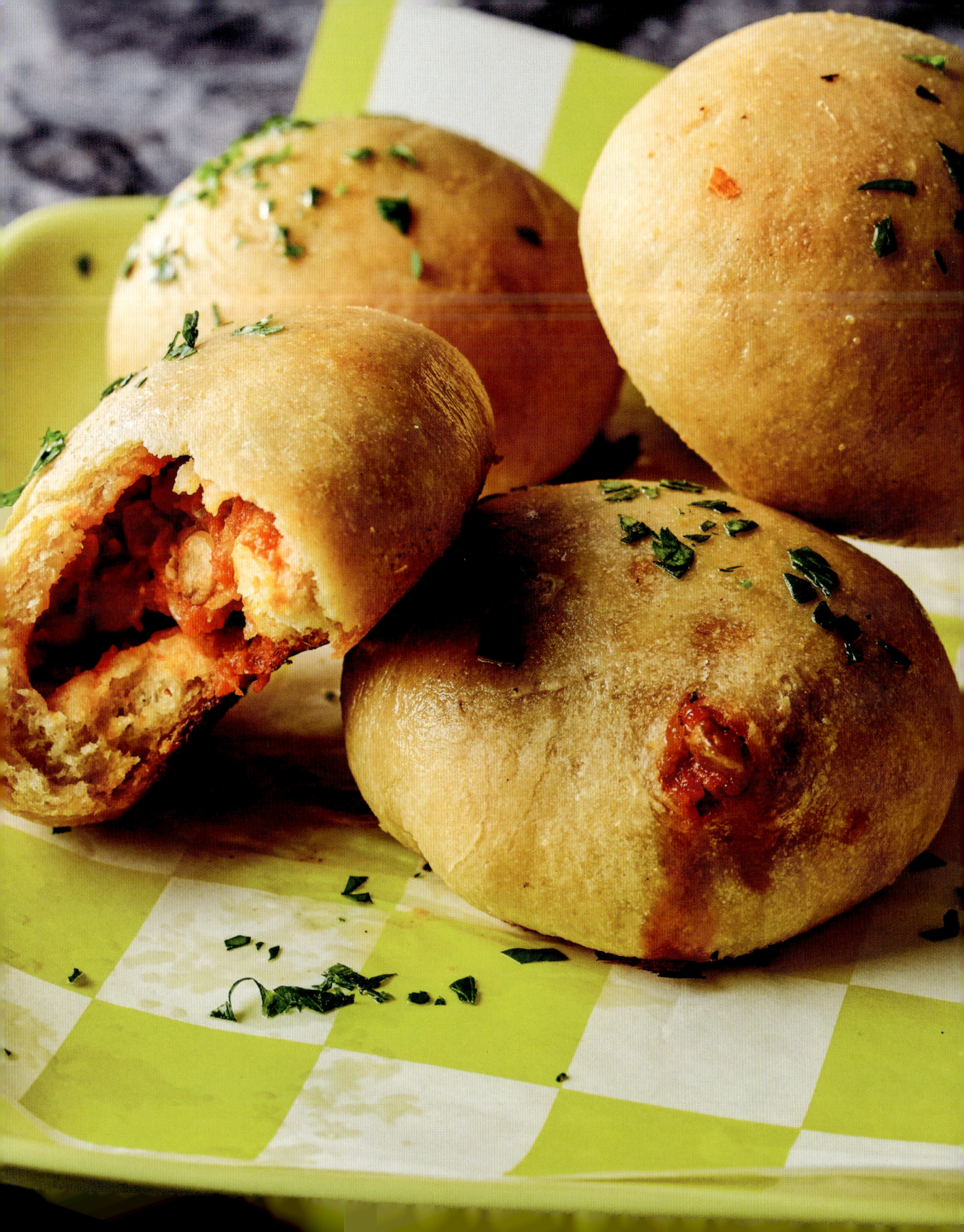

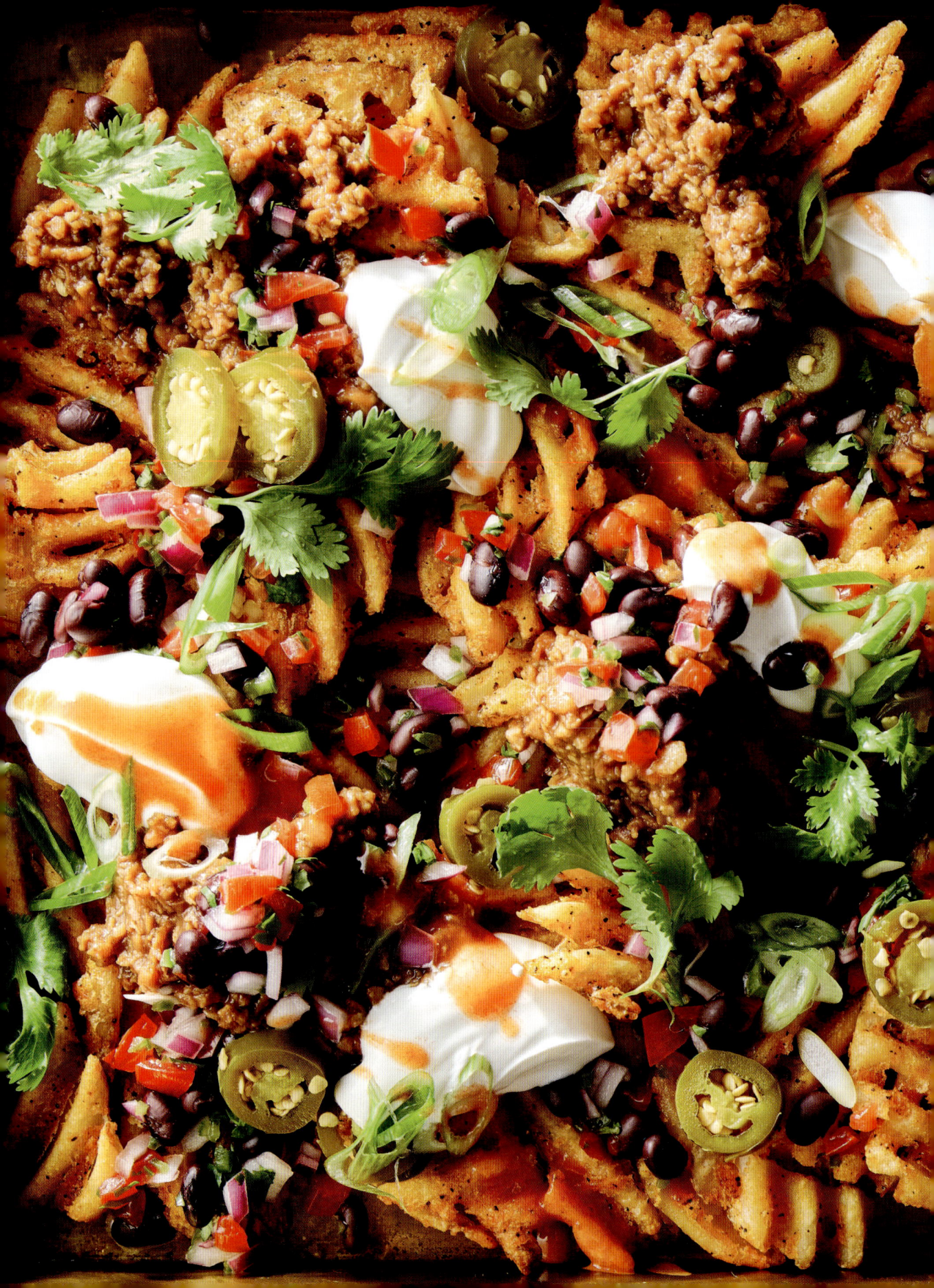

These nacho fries are a hands-down crowd favorite in my house, and it's easy to see why. Crispy waffle fries are a gift to humanity (although, I'll take potatoes in any form). Here, they get the ultimate upgrade with layers of protein, fiber, and all the loaded nacho toppings you could want. It's indulgent, satisfying, and, yes, a complete meal — because who says comfort food can't also deliver on nutrition?

SERVES 4

STACKED NACHO FRIES

Preheat the oven and bake the waffle fries according to the package instructions.

Meanwhile, in a medium bowl, combine the tomato, onion, jalapeño, cilantro, lime juice, and salt. Stir to combine, then fold in the black beans. In a small saucepan, combine the refried beans, TVP, and chili powder. Set over low heat, stirring occasionally, until warmed through.

Arrange the warm fries on a serving plate (or keep on the sheet pan). Spoon the refried bean mixture evenly over the fries, then top with the black bean salsa. Finish with your choice of toppings, like sour cream, pickled jalapeños, scallions, cilantro, and hot sauce. Serve immediately.

```
Dalina Says...
If the easiest way for you to work more vegeta-
bles into your diet is to reach for frozen, do
it—there is absolutely no shame in using frozen
vegetables (and starches) to help you save time
and money. Even though Robin uses frozen fries
here (love it), these nacho fries are still
loaded with nutrition.
```

Nachos

1 (22-ounce) bag frozen waffle fries
1 vine-ripened tomato, diced
¼ small red onion, diced
1 jalapeño, minced
2 tablespoons finely chopped fresh cilantro
Juice of 1 lime
½ teaspoon kosher salt
½ cup rinsed canned black beans or homemade black beans (page 232)
½ cup refried beans
1 cup hydrated TVP MVP (page 224)
2 tablespoons chili powder

Toppings

Vegan sour cream, store-bought or homemade (page 146)
Sliced pickled jalapeños
Thinly sliced scallions
Fresh cilantro leaves
Hot sauce

 Easy Lift

Under 30 Minutes

Per serving

Calories: 453

Fat: 14g

Carbs: 71g

Fiber: 14g

Protein: 21g

Tempeh gets its time to shine! This should be the number one thing you bookmark when you need a potluck showstopper — creamy, spicy, and ridiculously satisfying. Traditional Buffalo dip is a dairy-loaded gut bomb, but this version keeps all the bold flavor while bringing in gut-friendly fiber and protein, thanks to tempeh. No bloating, no couch coma — just pure, dippable deliciousness. Pair it with tortilla chips, celery sticks, or whatever crunchy vehicle you've got on hand, and watch it disappear before halftime.

SERVES 4

TEMPEH BUFFALO DIP

Preheat the oven to 350°F.

In a small skillet, combine the tempeh and enough water to cover. Set over high heat and boil for about 10 minutes. (This removes the bitter flavor from the tempeh.) Drain the tempeh and set aside until cool enough to handle.

In a large bowl, whisk together the yogurt, ranch, and Buffalo sauce until smooth. Fold in the scallions, celery, carrot, pepper, and salt. Crumble the tempeh into small pieces and fold in.

Transfer the mixture to a 9-inch pie plate. Evenly sprinkle the cheddar cheese on top. Bake until the cheese is melted and the edges are bubbling, about 15 minutes. Serve immediately with tortilla chips for scooping.

8 ounces tempeh
1 cup plain vegan Greek yogurt
½ cup Tofu Ranch Dressing (page 121)
½ cup store-bought Buffalo sauce, plus more to taste for optional garnish
2 scallions, thinly sliced, plus more for serving
1 celery stalk, diced
1 medium carrot, peeled and diced
1 teaspoon freshly ground black pepper
½ teaspoon kosher salt
1 cup shredded vegan cheddar cheese
Tortilla chips, for serving

 Easy Lift

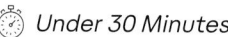 *Under 30 Minutes*

Per serving · Calories: 377 · Fat: 24g · Carbs: 40g · Fiber: 13g · Protein: 28g

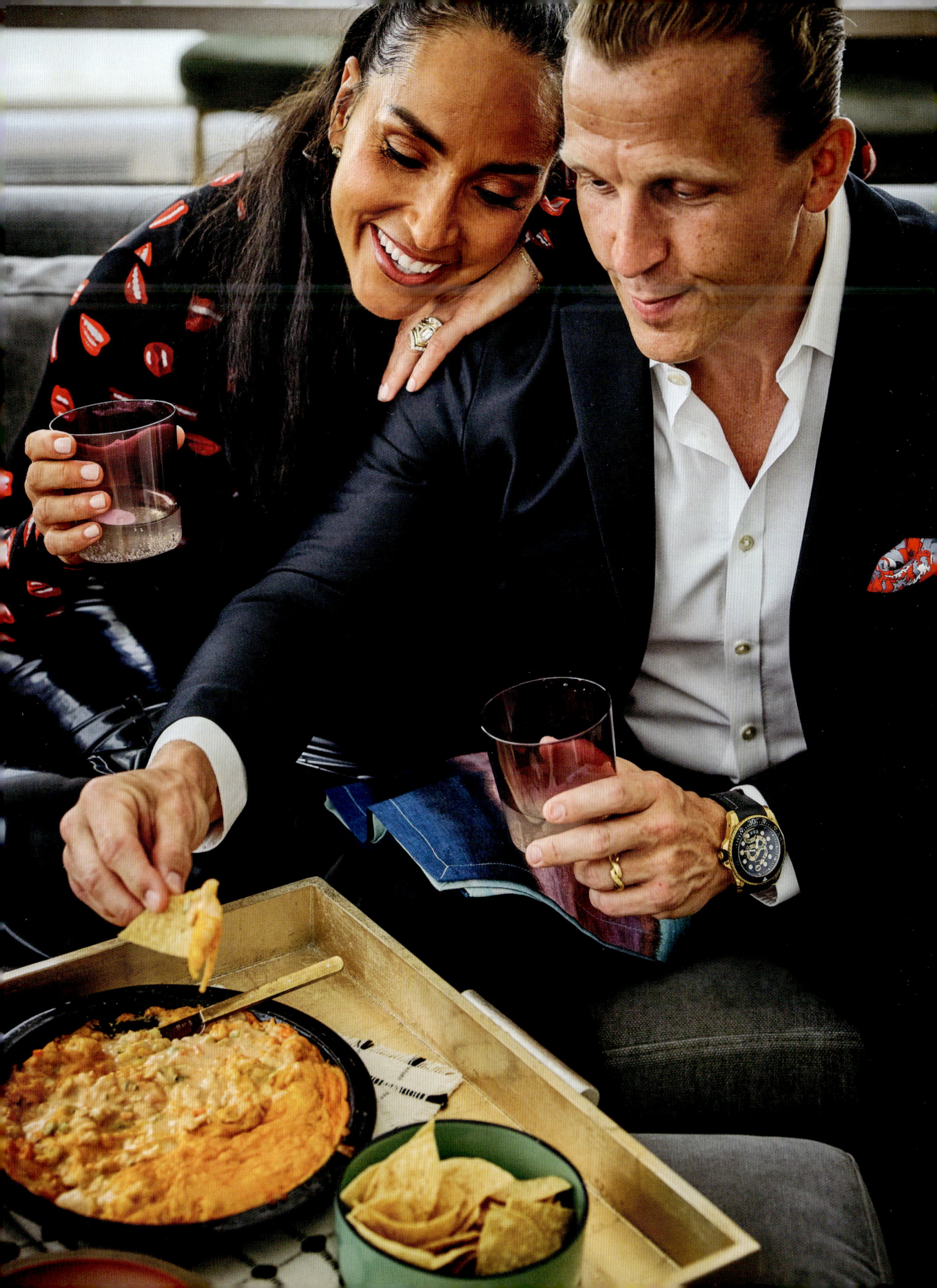

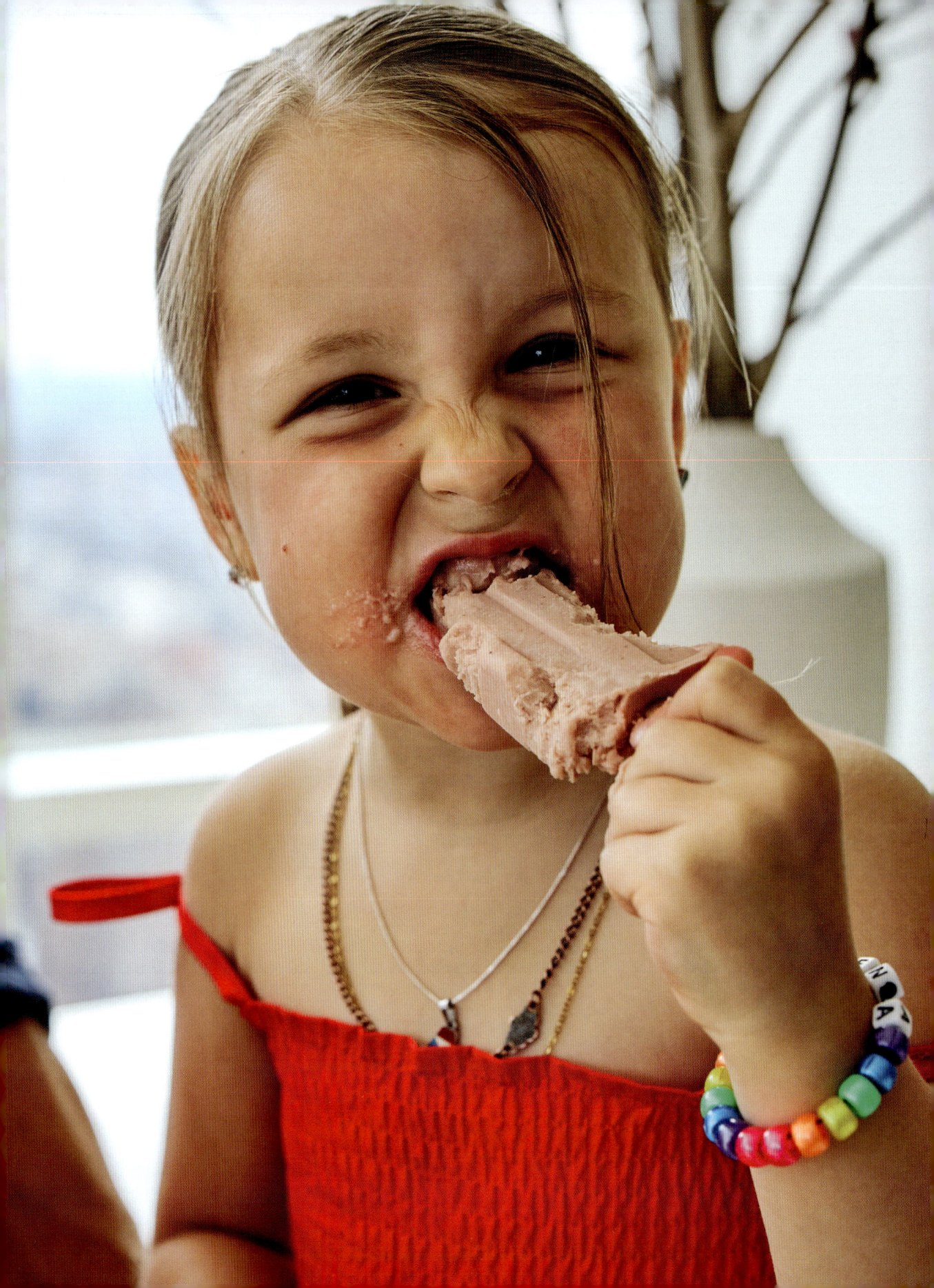

DESSERTS WITH MUSCLE

Dessert is the grand finale, the sweet reward, the victory lap at the end of a long day. And just like the rest of your meals, it deserves intention. This chapter proves that a little sweetness can still work hard for you, delivering that perfect ending without the energy crash. We're talking rich, satisfying, crave-worthy cookies, pies, and bars that hit the spot and fuel your goals by keeping protein front and center. Because why choose between indulgence and intention when you can have both?

This was my #1 pregnancy craving when I was expecting Atlas. Every night, Drew would make me a plate, and I'd sit there, happily dunking apple slices into that dreamy, peanut buttery dip. It's sweet, a little salty, totally satisfying — and bonus, it's actually good for you. Kids love it, adults love it, and it's the kind of snack that works for everything from after school to a late-night treat.

SERVES 1

APPLE CHOCOLATE "NACHOS"

In a small microwave-safe bowl, combine the coconut oil and chocolate. Microwave on high in 30-second bursts, stirring each time, until melted.

Meanwhile, in a small serving bowl, whisk together the yogurt, peanut butter powder, salt, cinnamon, and 1 tablespoon water to combine into a smooth dip.

Set the dip in the center of a large serving plate and arrange the apple slices evenly around the dip. Drizzle the chocolate mixture over the apple slices. Transfer the plate to the refrigerator to chill for 10 minutes before serving.

- 1 teaspoon refined coconut oil, softened or melted
- 1 ounce dark or vegan milk chocolate, chopped
- ½ cup plain vegan Greek yogurt
- 1 tablespoon peanut butter powder
- ½ teaspoon kosher salt
- ½ teaspoon ground cinnamon
- 1 Fuji, Gala, or Honeycrisp apple, cored and thinly sliced

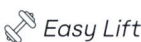 *Easy Lift*

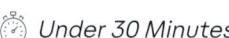 *Under 30 Minutes*

Per serving — Calories: 382 | Fat: 22g | Carbs: 43g | Fiber: 10g | Protein: 19g

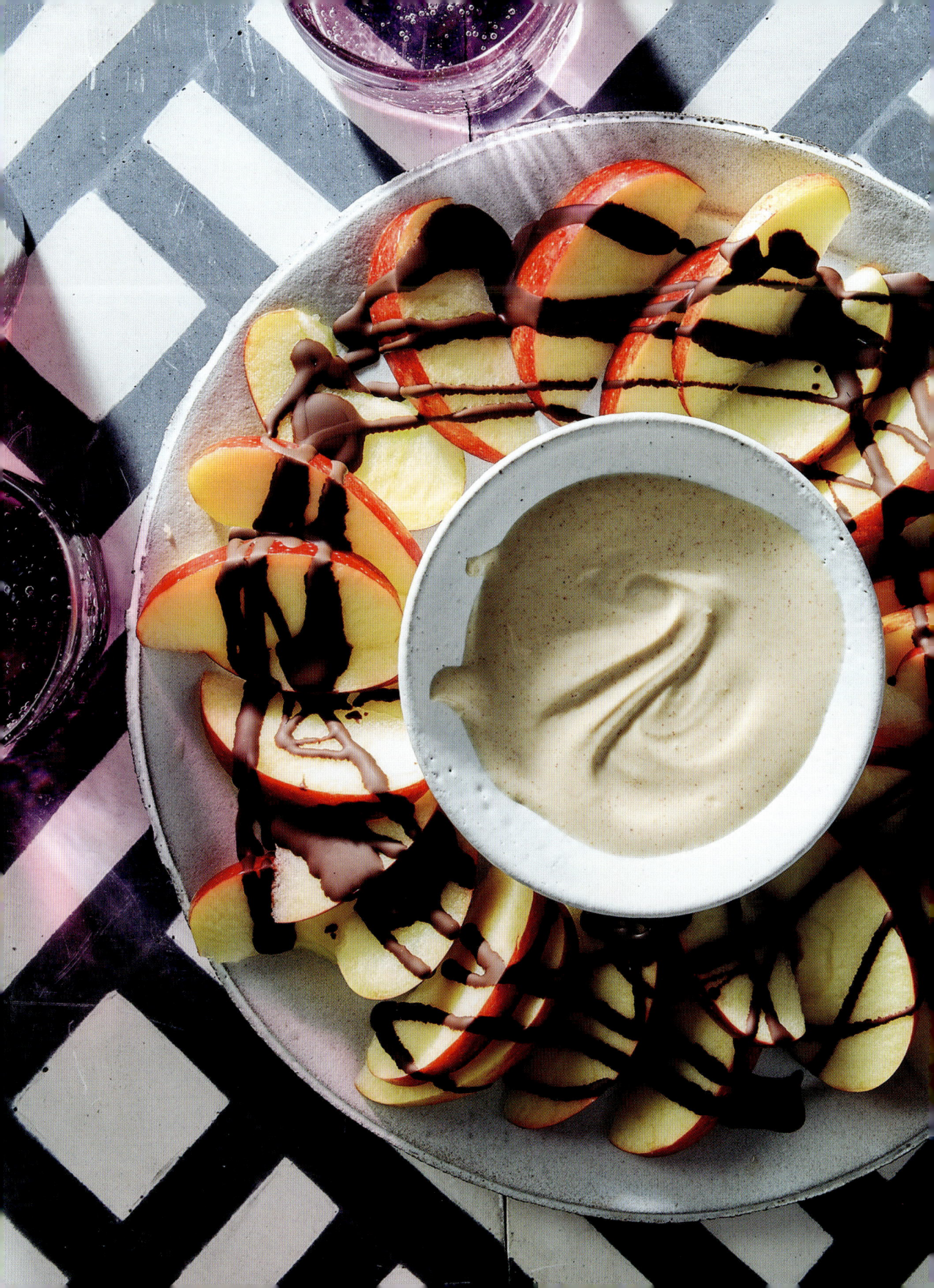

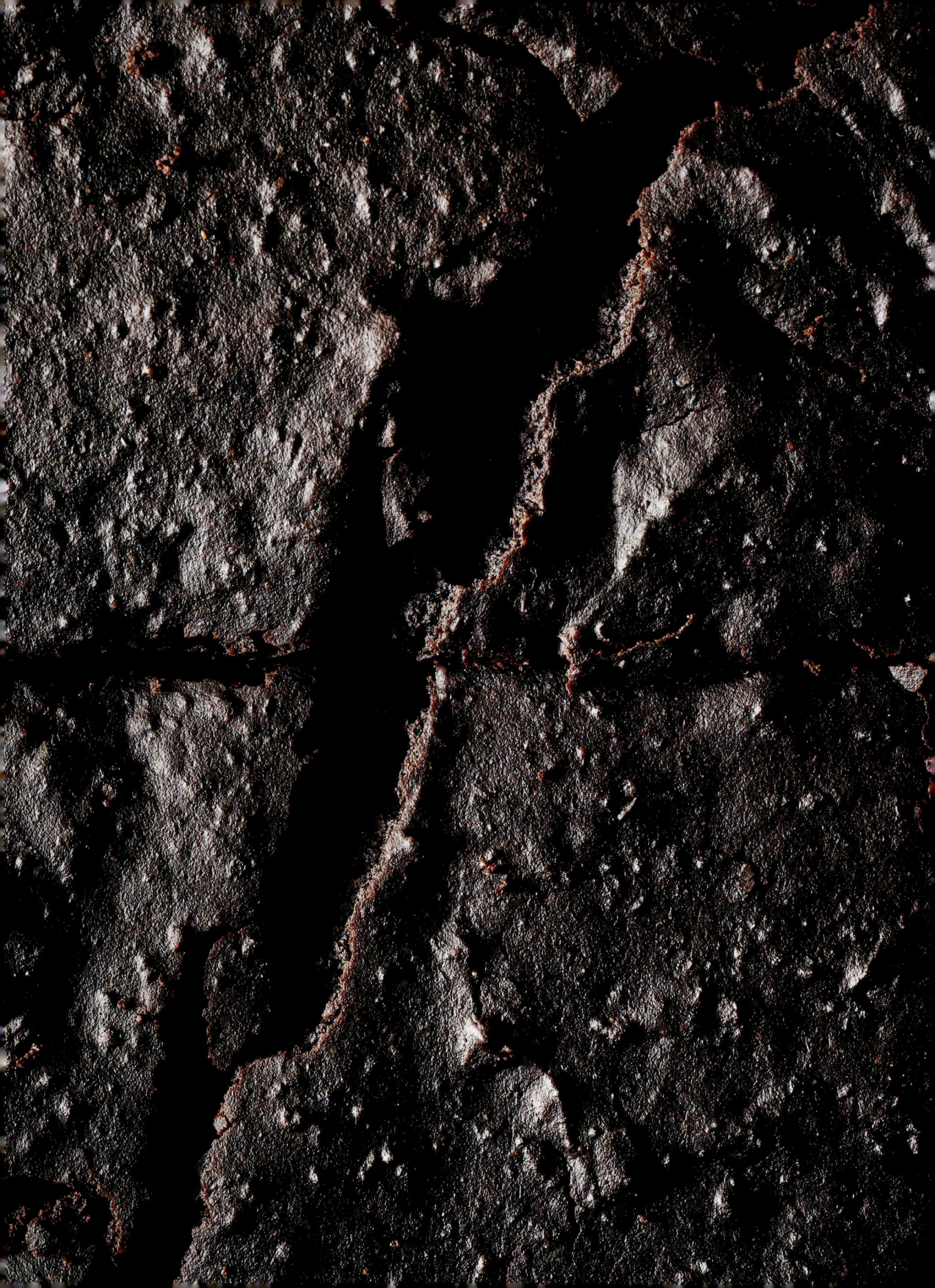

This is for my spicy girls. These brownies have a rich, fudgy center, but with a little surprise hit of cayenne heat at the end. My sister — who was the first vegan in the family — started making them for every occasion, and I followed her lead. The black beans blend right in but add tons of fiber and keep everything extra moist. If you're sensitive to spice, cut the cayenne in half (or even quarter it), but if you like a kick, trust me, the heat balances out the deep chocolate perfectly.

MAKES 9 BROWNIES

BLACK BEAN BROWNIES

Preheat the oven to 350°F. Lightly coat an 8 by 8-inch baking pan with nonstick spray.

In a small bowl, whisk the flaxseed with 5 tablespoons water. Let it sit for 5 minutes to gel.

In a food processor, combine the flax mixture, beans, protein powder, coconut sugar, cocoa powder, maple syrup, coconut oil, baking powder, baking soda, salt, cinnamon, cayenne, and vanilla. Process, scraping down the sides as needed, until smooth, about 2 minutes.

Scrape into the prepared baking pan and smooth into an even layer. Bake until a toothpick inserted in the center comes out with a few moist crumbs, 25 to 30 minutes. Let cool in the pan for at least 30 minutes before slicing into 9 pieces and serving. Leftovers can be refrigerated in an airtight container for up to 5 days.

Nonstick cooking spray
2 tablespoons flaxseed meal
1 (15.5-ounce) can black beans, drained and rinsed
½ cup chocolate protein powder
½ cup coconut sugar
¼ cup Dutch-process cocoa powder
¼ cup pure maple syrup or agave syrup
3 tablespoons refined coconut oil
1½ teaspoons baking powder
1 teaspoon baking soda
1 teaspoon kosher salt
1 teaspoon ground cinnamon
1 teaspoon cayenne pepper or chipotle powder
1 teaspoon pure vanilla extract

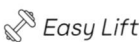 *Easy Lift*

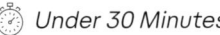 *Under 30 Minutes*

Per brownie

Calories: 203

Fat: 6g

Carbs: 32g

Fiber: 5g

Protein: 10g

I love a kitchen clean-out recipe. This one was born when I was doing a purge of my kitchen cupboards and realized I had way too many cans of chickpeas hanging around. Instead of making yet another batch of hummus, I went dessert mode. These soft, chewy, protein-packed cookies have the perfect crispy edges and melty chocolate pockets. If you're drowning in chickpeas (or, let's face it, just craving a chocolate chip cookie!), this is your sign to bake a batch.

MAKES 12 COOKIES

CHICKPEA CHOCO-CHIP COOKIES

Preheat the oven to 350°F. Line two rimmed baking sheets with parchment paper.

In a small bowl, whisk the flaxseed with 5 tablespoons water. Let sit for 5 minutes to gel.

In a food processor, combine the flax mixture with the chickpeas, flour, protein powder, almond butter, maple syrup, vanilla, salt, baking powder, and baking soda. Process, using a silicone spatula to scrape down the sides and bottom of the bowl as needed, until smooth, about 2 minutes. Scrape the mixture into a large bowl and add the chocolate chips. Fold until combined.

Use a ¼-cup scoop to portion the dough onto the prepared baking sheets, 6 scoops on each spaced about 2 inches apart. Sprinkle a little flaky salt on each cookie. Bake until the cookies are set around the edges, 12 to 15 minutes. Let cool completely on the baking sheet to allow the cookies to firm up before serving (they're pretty soft coming out of the oven). Leftovers can be refrigerated in an airtight container for up to 5 days.

2 tablespoons flaxseed meal
1 (15.5-ounce) can chickpeas, drained and rinsed
⅔ cup all-purpose flour
½ cup vanilla protein powder
½ cup unsalted almond or peanut butter
¼ cup pure maple syrup
2 teaspoons pure vanilla extract
1 teaspoon kosher salt
½ teaspoon baking powder
½ teaspoon baking soda
1 cup vegan chocolate chips
Flaky sea salt

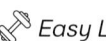 *Easy Lift*

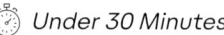 *Under 30 Minutes*

Per cookie — Calories: 257 | Fat: 11g | Carbs: 29g | Fiber: 5g | Protein: 10g

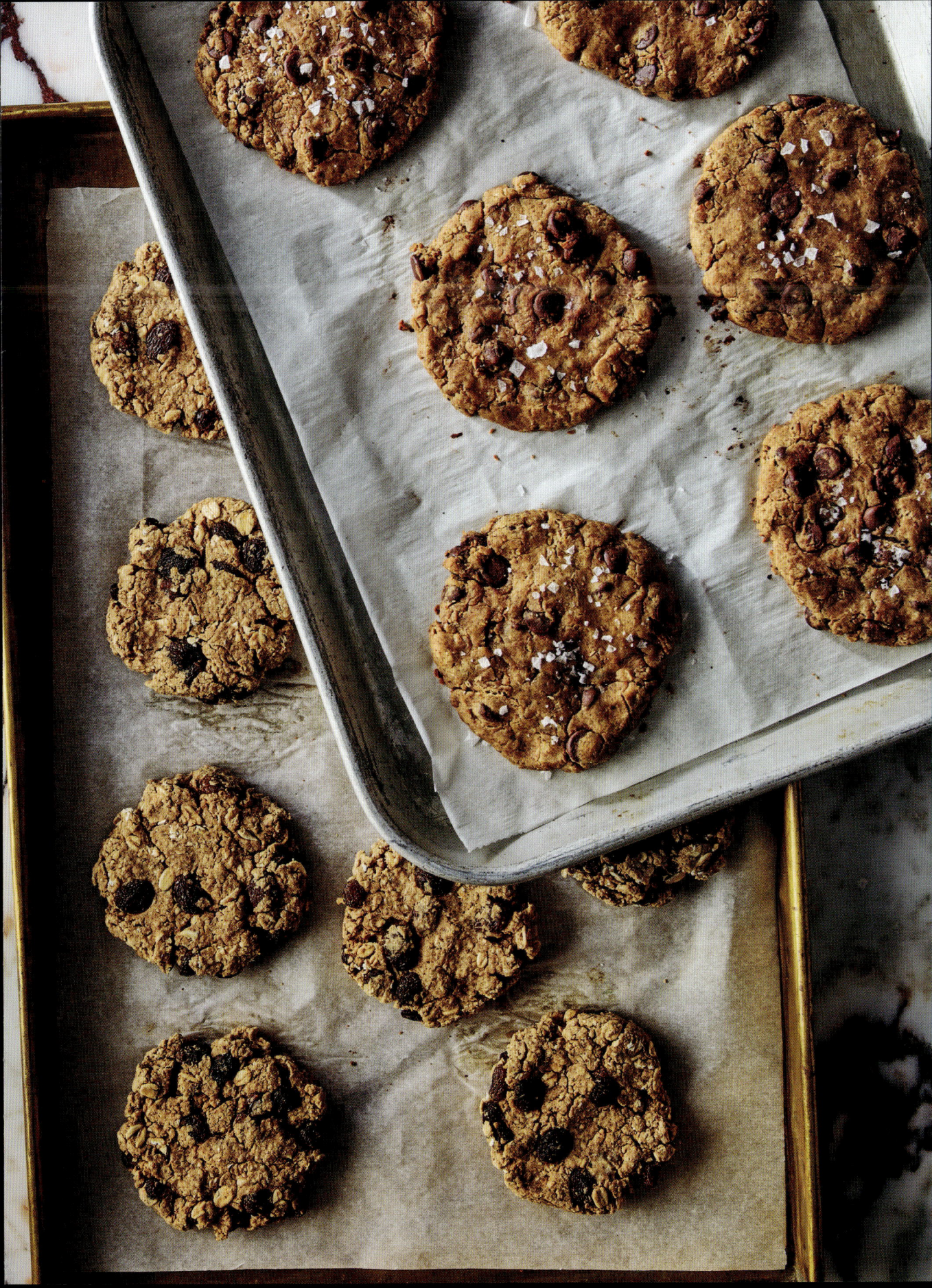

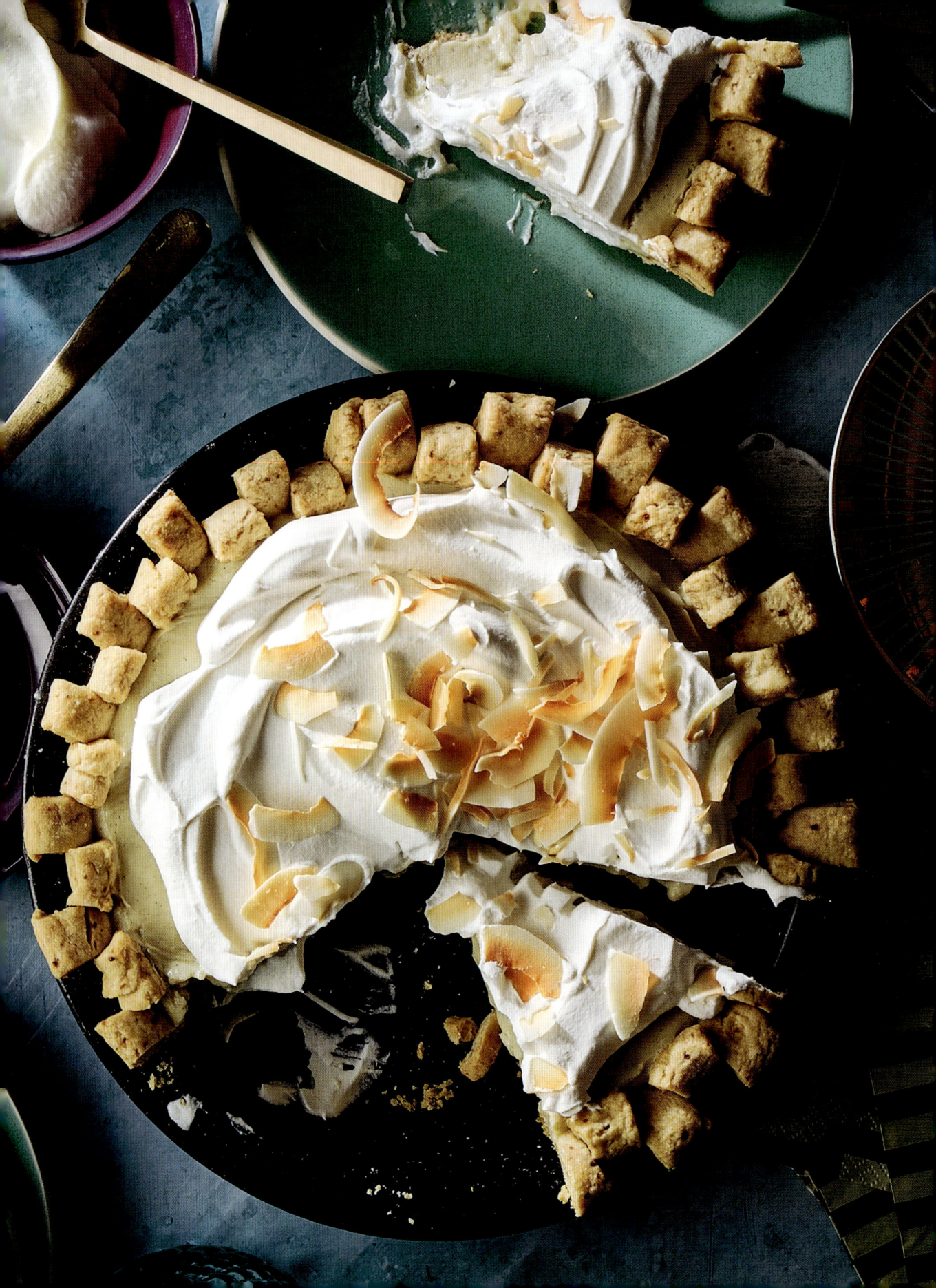

These pies! What?! The first time Drew tried this and the Chocolate Silk Pie (page 198), he nearly fainted. "Are you sure there's protein in this? *You're sure this is good for me?*" The answer is yes, and yes. The coconut filling is silky, the crust is buttery (without the butter), and when you top it with a cloud of vegan whip and toasted coconut, it's basically a tropical vacation in pie form. Make this when you want to impress — birthday, dinner party, whatever. The work is worth it.

SERVES 8

COCO-LICIOUS CREAM PIE

Bake the store-bought pie crust according to the package directions; or make, bake, and cool a homemade pie crust following the instructions on page 198.

In a blender or food processor, combine the soy milk, tofu, sugar, protein powder, cornstarch, coconut oil, and salt. Blend on medium, stopping to scrape the sides as needed, until completely smooth, about 2 minutes.

Pour the mixture into a medium saucepan and set over medium heat. Whisk occasionally until the mixture comes to a boil and thickens into a pudding, about 5 minutes. Remove from the heat and add the shredded coconut, butter, and coconut extract. Continue to whisk until the butter is melted.

Pour the filling into the crust. Press plastic wrap directly on the surface of the pie. Refrigerate for at least 4 hours, until set, or up to 3 days. Slice and serve the pie with vegan whip and toasted coconut flakes.

- Vegan pie crust, store-bought or homemade (page 198)
- 2 cups unsweetened soy milk or other plant-based milk
- 12 ounces silken tofu, drained
- ½ cup granulated sugar
- ½ cup vanilla protein powder
- ¼ cup cornstarch
- 2 tablespoons refined coconut oil
- 2 teaspoons kosher salt
- 1 cup unsweetened shredded coconut
- ¼ cup (½ stick) vegan butter, cubed
- 1 teaspoon coconut extract
- Vegan Whip (page 234), for serving
- Toasted coconut flakes, for serving

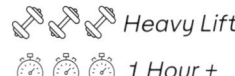 *Heavy Lift*

🕐 🕐 🕐 *1 Hour +*

Per serving

Calories: 406

Fat: 25g

Carbs: 36g

Fiber: 3g

Protein: 11g

These sticky-sweet rolls take me straight back to summers in the Poconos, driving through Amish country and picking up the biggest cinnamon rolls I'd ever seen. This is my plant-based love letter to those — soft, swirled with cinnamon sugar, and draped in a tangy-sweet glaze. They're equally exciting on slow weekend mornings or waiting for you at the finish line after a long marathon training run.

MAKES 9 ROLLS

GOOEY CINNAMON ROLLS

Preheat the oven to 350°F. Lightly coat an 8 by 8-inch baking pan with nonstick spray.

Make the rolls: In a large bowl, whisk together the flour, protein powder, baking powder, and salt. Add the yogurt and stir into a shaggy dough. Knead the dough in the bowl until it's smooth and just slightly sticky. Cover the bowl with a kitchen towel and let the dough rest for 30 minutes.

Lightly flour a clean work surface. Turn out the dough and roll into a roughly 12 by 14-inch rectangle. Brush half of the butter evenly over the surface. In a small bowl, use your fingers to rub the coconut sugar and cinnamon together, then evenly sprinkle over the butter. Drizzle the rest of the butter over the top. Starting from a long side, roll the dough into a log. Cut crosswise into 9 equal pieces and evenly space in the prepared baking pan.

Bake until a toothpick inserted into the center of a roll comes out clean, about 30 minutes. Let cool for 30 minutes to set.

Meanwhile, make the glaze: In a medium bowl, whisk together the yogurt and powdered sugar until you have a nice spreadable consistency, adding a splash of soy milk as needed to help smooth it out. Slather the glaze over the warm rolls and serve immediately.

Nonstick cooking spray

Rolls

2 cups all-purpose flour, plus more as needed
½ cup vanilla protein powder
1 tablespoon baking powder
1 teaspoon kosher salt
1½ cups plain vegan Greek yogurt
¼ cup (½ stick) vegan butter, melted
3 tablespoons coconut sugar
1 tablespoon ground cinnamon

Glaze

⅔ cup plain vegan Greek yogurt
½ cup powdered sugar
Unsweetened soy milk or other plant-based milk, as needed

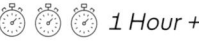 *Moderate Lift*

⏱️⏱️⏱️ *1 Hour +*

Protein: 10g | Fiber: 2g | Carbs: 35g | Fat: 7g | Calories: 243
Per roll

> **Dalina Says...**
>
> Even though this recipe has added protein powder in it, you'd never know—it still gives all the gooey, cinnamon roll vibes. The Greek yogurt in the dough adds a little protein and keeps the dough super soft.

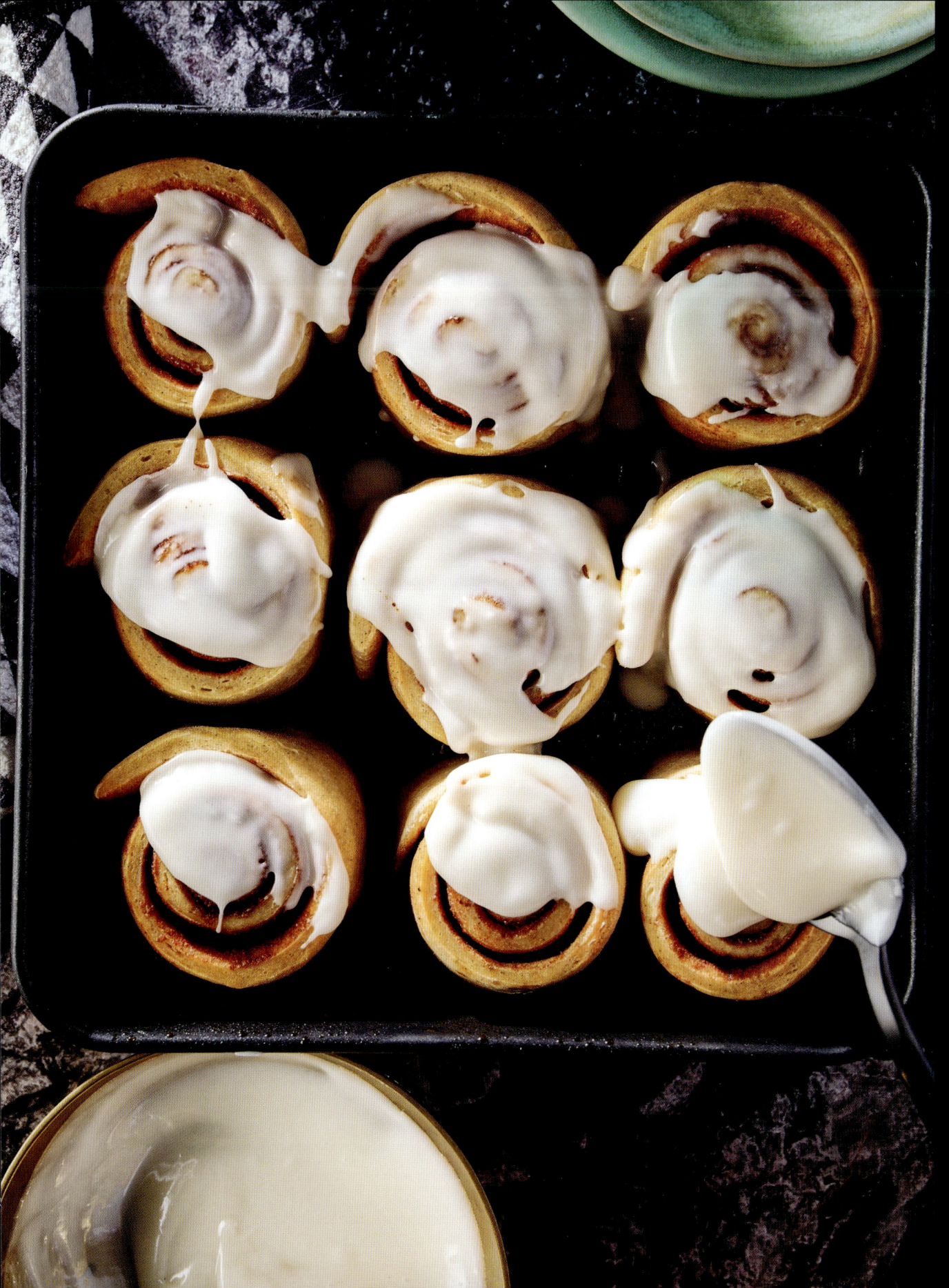

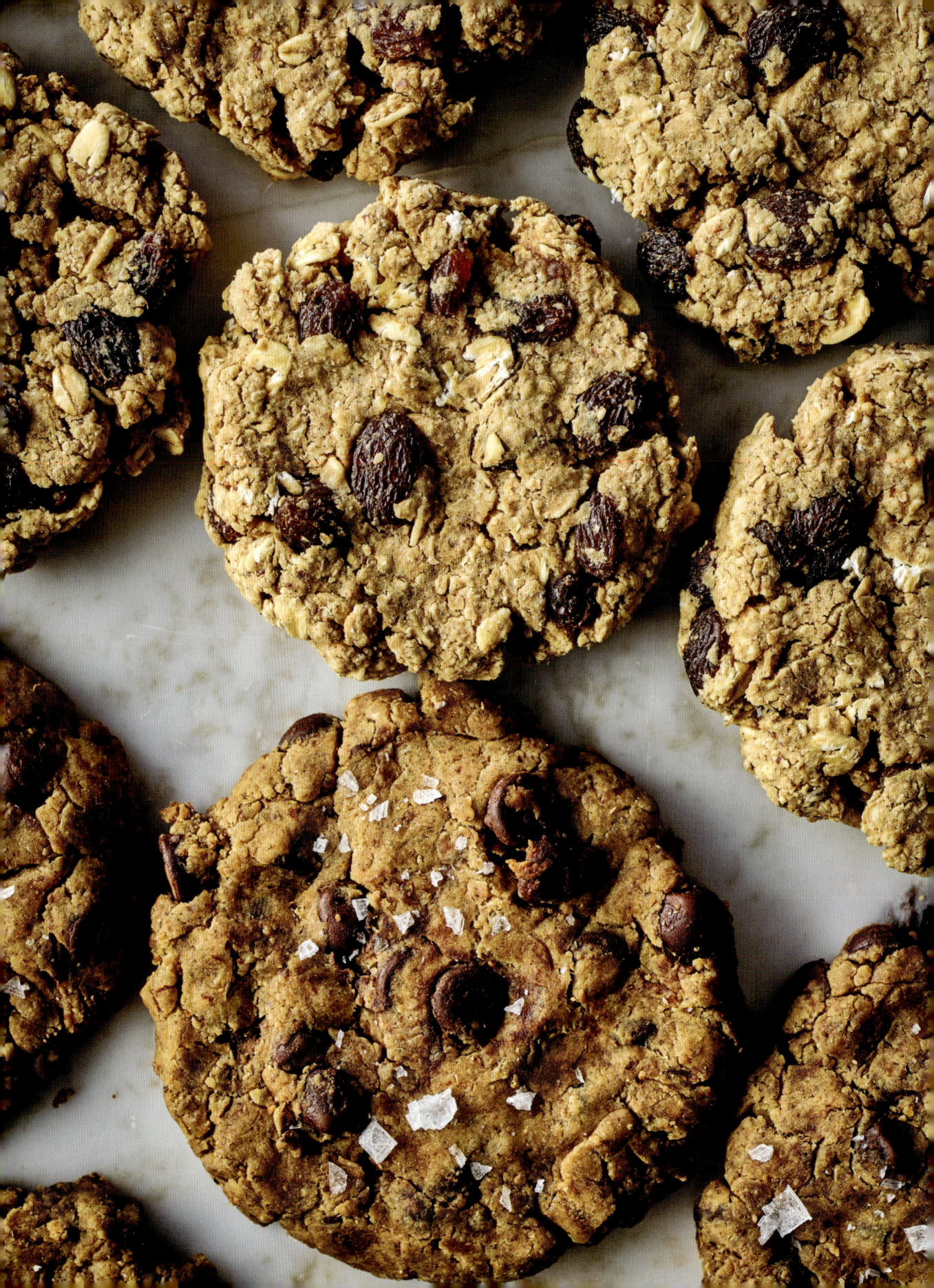

Beans in cookies? Just trust me. The combo of cannellini beans and oats means these cookies are protein packed, fiber filled, and actually keep you full. Plus, they're chewy in all the right ways, scented with warm cinnamon and vanilla, and totally satisfying. Basically, they're what an oatmeal-raisin cookie was born to be.

MAKES 12 COOKIES

OATMEAL-RAISIN POWER COOKIES

Preheat the oven to 350°F. Line a rimmed baking sheet with parchment paper.

In a large bowl, whisk the flaxseed with 5 tablespoons water. Let sit for 5 minutes to gel.

In a food processor, process 1 cup of the oats to make a fine oat flour, about 3 minutes. Add the beans, soy milk, protein powder, coconut oil, salt, cinnamon, vanilla, baking powder, and baking soda to the food processor. Process, scraping down the sides as needed, until smooth, about 2 minutes. Scrape the mixture into the large bowl with the flax mixture. Add the raisins and remaining 1 cup oats. Fold until combined.

Use a 3-tablespoon scoop to portion the dough onto the prepared baking sheet, spaced about 2 inches apart. Bake until the cookies are set, 12 to 15 minutes. Let cool completely on the baking sheet to allow the cookies to set before serving. Leftovers can be refrigerated in an airtight container for up to 5 days.

- 2 tablespoons ground flaxseed
- 2 cups old-fashioned oats
- 1 (15.5-ounce) can cannellini beans, drained and rinsed
- ¾ cup unsweetened soy milk or other plant-based milk
- ½ cup vanilla protein powder
- 3 tablespoons refined coconut oil
- 1 teaspoon kosher salt
- 1 teaspoon ground cinnamon
- 1 teaspoon pure vanilla extract
- ½ teaspoon baking powder
- ½ teaspoon baking soda
- 1 cup raisins

 Easy Lift

 Under 30 Minutes

Per cookie
Calories: 190
Fat: 5g
Carbs: 27g
Fiber: 5g
Protein: 10g

Turning frozen bananas into ice cream has been a vegan trick forever, but this version levels it up even more with protein-full peanut butter (and some jelly magic). It's creamy, naturally sweet, and swirled with just enough nutty and berry goodness to make you forget all about traditional ice cream. No churn, no drama — just blend, freeze, scoop, and enjoy. (Do note that you need to freeze the bananas the day before you plan to make the ice cream, and that the ice cream needs to set for at least a few hours before scooping.)

MAKES 2 PINTS (1 QUART)

PB&J SWIRL NICE CREAM

Peel and thinly slice the bananas. Transfer the pieces to an airtight container and freeze overnight.

The next day, break up the frozen banana pieces and scatter in a food processor or blender. Process until a crumbly mixture forms, about 20 seconds. Scrape down the sides and pour in the coconut cream, protein powder, and maple syrup. Process again, scraping down the sides as needed, until the nice cream is smooth, about 30 seconds.

In a small bowl, whisk the peanut butter powder with ¼ cup of the soy milk. In another small bowl, whisk the protein powder with the remaining ¼ cup soy milk.

The nice cream can be packed in one quart-sized container, two pint containers, or a loaf pan. Drizzle a little of the peanut butter and protein powder mixtures over the bottom of the container(s), then alternate with layers of nice cream and peanut butter and strawberry drizzles, finishing with strawberry and peanut butter drizzles on top. Cover and freeze until set, at least 4 hours, or overnight. The nice cream can be stored in the freezer for up to 3 months.

- 4 large, ripe bananas
- 1 cup unsweetened coconut cream
- ½ cup vanilla protein powder
- 2 tablespoons pure maple syrup or agave syrup
- 2 tablespoons peanut butter powder
- ½ cup unsweetened soy milk or other plant-based milk
- 2 tablespoons strawberry protein powder

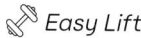 *Easy Lift*

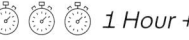 *1 Hour +*

Protein: 14g
Fiber: 4g
Carbs: 44g
Fat: 14g
Calories: 364

Per 1 cup

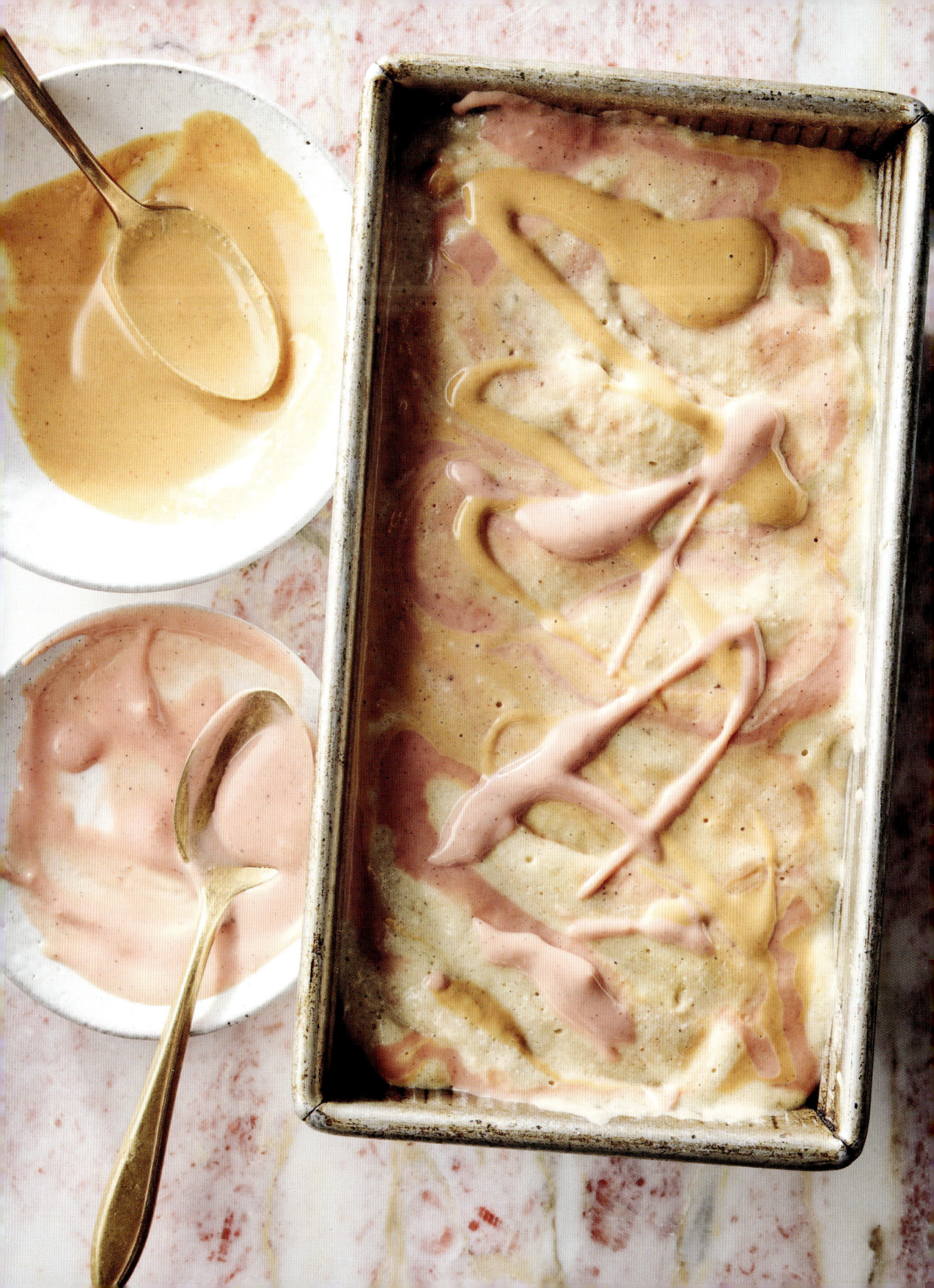

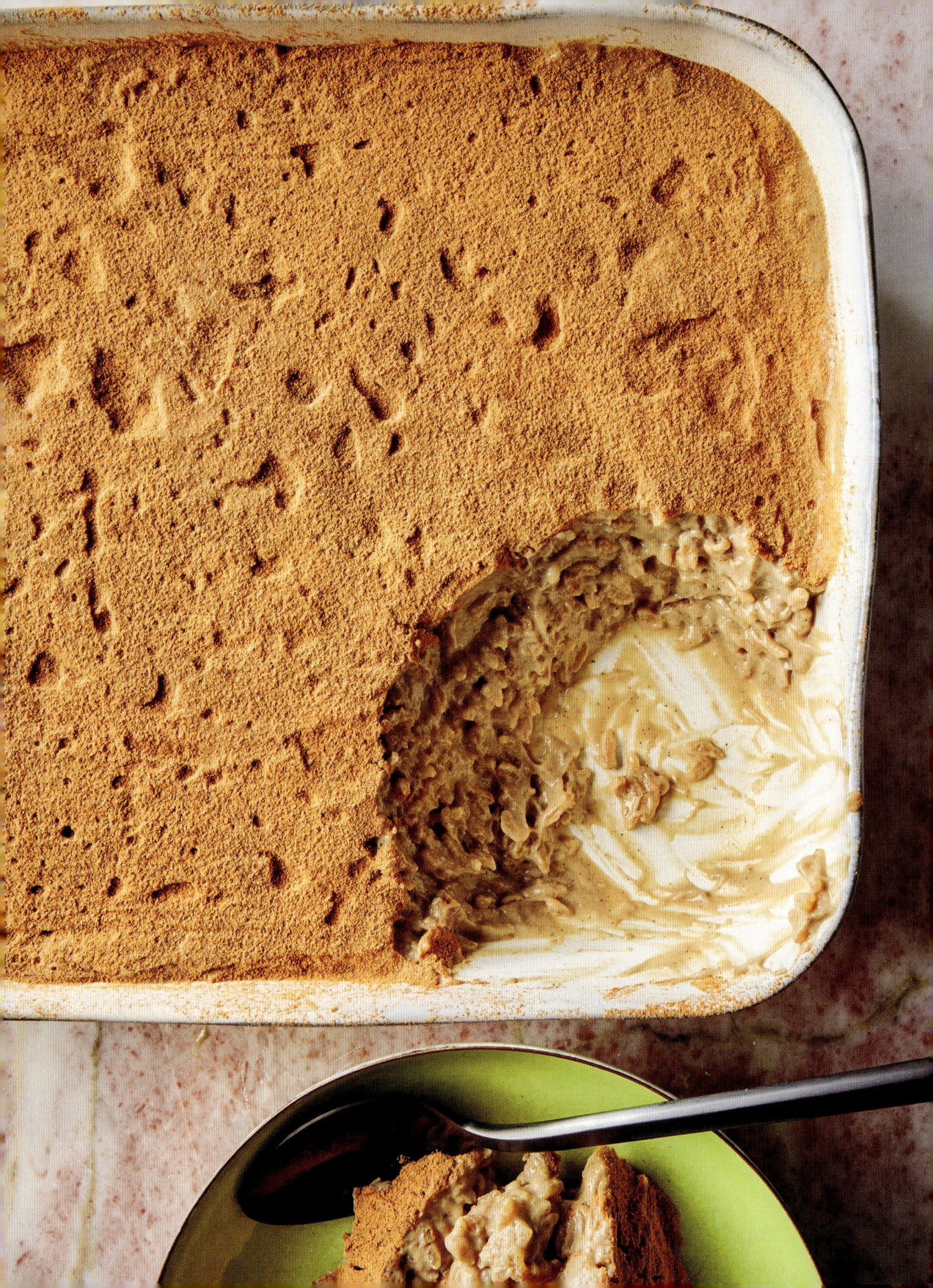

This one's for my dad. Rice pudding was his dessert, and this is my high-protein, plant-based version that still keeps all the creamy, cinnamon-y goodness of the original. It's rich, nostalgic, and somehow even better the next day. You'll cook it low and slow on the stovetop until the rice is tender, then it heads to the fridge, where it sets up into the velvety texture that makes every spoonful feel like a little victory lap.

SERVES 8 TO 10

POWER-PACKED RICE PUDDING

In a large Dutch oven, whisk together the soy milk, rice, coconut sugar, protein powder, butter, and salt to combine. Set over high heat and bring to a boil, whisking occasionally to prevent the rice from sticking. Reduce the heat to low and switch to a wooden spoon. Simmer, stirring often, until the pudding is thick and the rice is soft, about 30 minutes.

Transfer the rice pudding to a 9 by 13-inch baking dish or a large bowl and smooth into an even layer. Press plastic wrap directly on the surface of the pudding and refrigerate for at least 2 hours or overnight.

Just before serving, remove the plastic and blanket the top with ground cinnamon. Serve cold.

8 cups (2 quarts) unsweetened soy milk or other plant-based milk
1 cup long-grain rice
1 cup coconut sugar
1 cup vanilla protein powder
2 tablespoons vegan butter
2 teaspoons kosher salt
Ground cinnamon

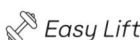 *Easy Lift*

 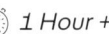 1 Hour +

Per serving (based on 8 servings)

Calories: 356
Fat: 9g
Carbs: 63g
Fiber: 9g
Protein: 13g

My Christmas and Hanukkah holiday decorations go up pretty much the second the last trick-or-treater has gone to bed, but there's still room for some fall flavors in my let's-get-to-Christmas world. This mousse is my go-to — a creamy, spiced, pumpkin-y dream with a nut brittle that's packed with protein and feels like a hug in dessert form. Hallmark movie girlies, this one's for you.

SERVES 4

PUMPKIN SPICE MOUSSE WITH MAPLE BRITTLE

Make the mousse: In a large bowl, combine the pumpkin puree, yogurt, maple syrup, pumpkin spice, salt, and vanilla. Use a handheld mixer (or a whisk and your biceps) to beat the mixture on medium until light and fluffy, 2 to 3 minutes. Spoon into small serving glasses, cover with plastic wrap, and refrigerate for at least 2 hours to chill, or up to 3 days.

Meanwhile, make the brittle: Preheat the oven to 275°F. Line a rimmed baking sheet with parchment paper.

In a small bowl, toss together the pecans, pumpkin seeds, hemp seeds (if using), maple syrup, cinnamon, and salt. Spread evenly on the prepared baking sheet. Bake until the mixture is toasted and caramelized, about 20 minutes. (It'll still be gooey but will firm up as it cools.) Remove from the oven and let cool on the baking sheet for 1 hour before breaking into pieces. Store the nut brittle in an airtight container at room temperature until ready to use or up to 3 days.

Top each pudding cup with a dollop of vegan whip and a shard or sprinkle of the nut brittle. Serve immediately.

Mousse

1 (15-ounce) can pumpkin puree
1 cup plain vegan Greek yogurt
6 tablespoons pure maple syrup
2 tablespoons pumpkin pie spice
1 teaspoon kosher salt
1 teaspoon pure vanilla extract

Brittle

½ cup chopped raw pecans or walnuts
2 tablespoons raw pumpkin seeds
1 tablespoon hemp seeds (optional)
3 tablespoons pure maple syrup
½ teaspoon ground cinnamon
¼ teaspoon kosher salt
Vegan Whip (page 234), for serving

Moderate Lift

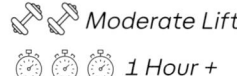 *1 Hour +*

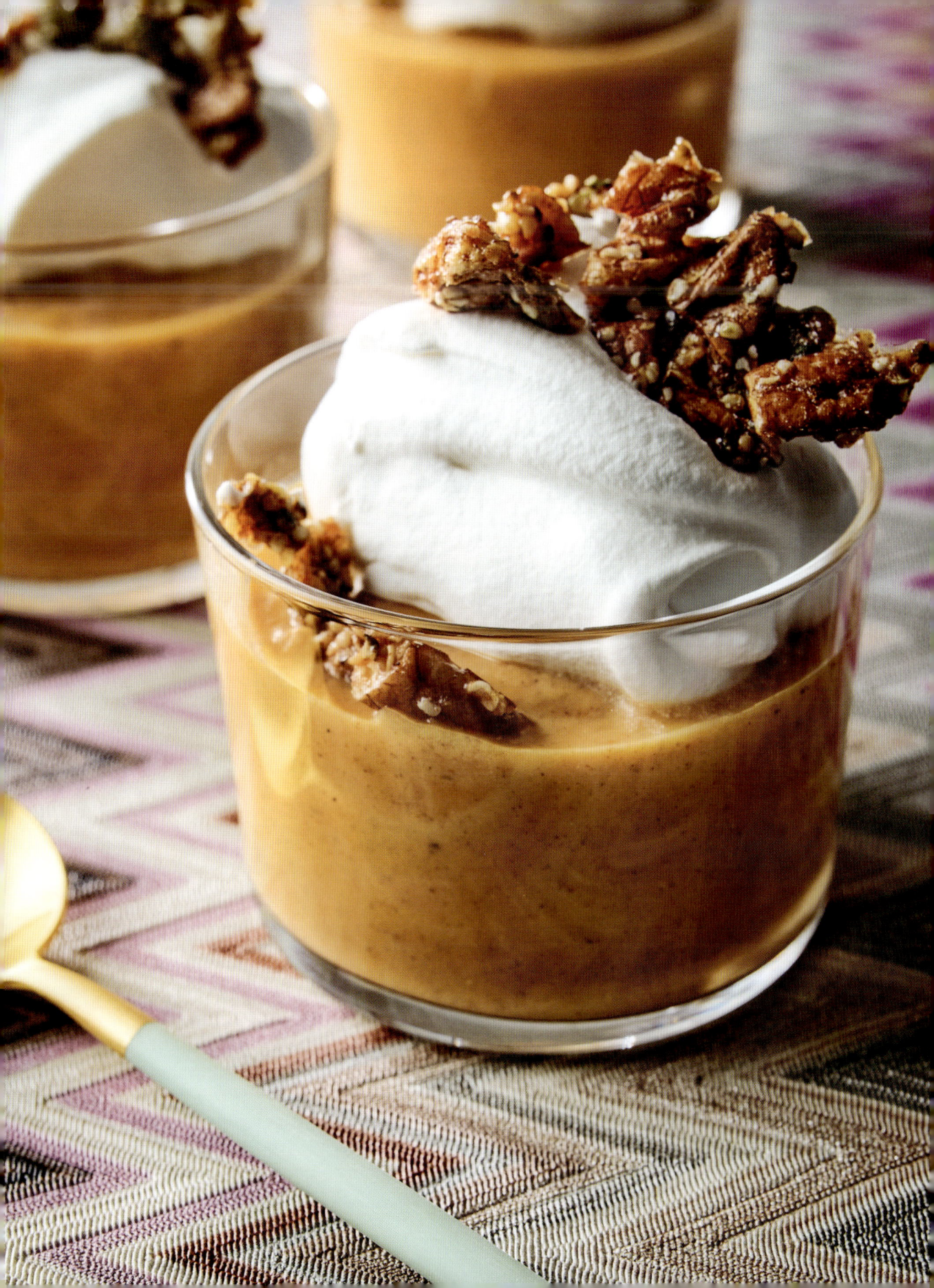

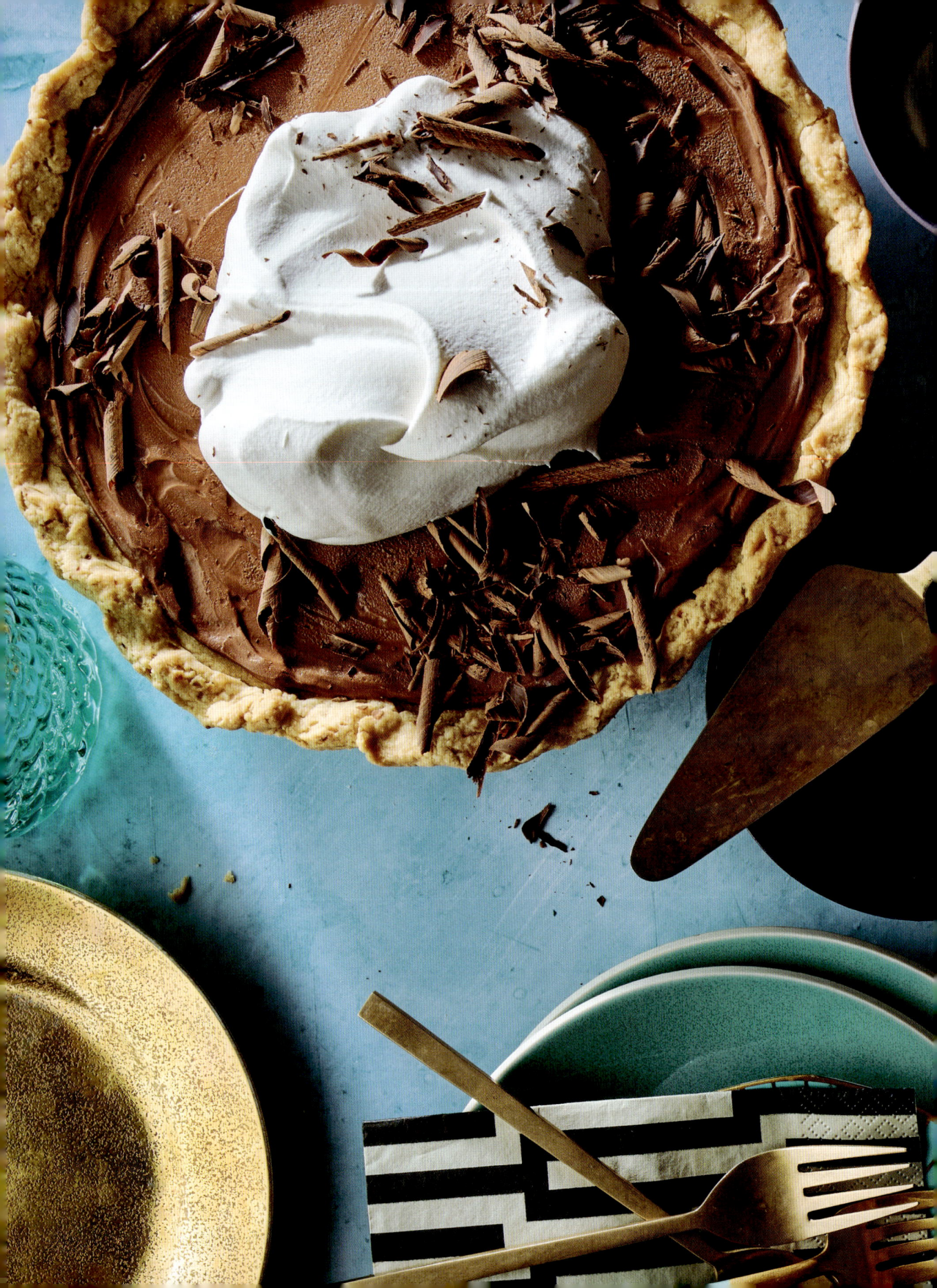

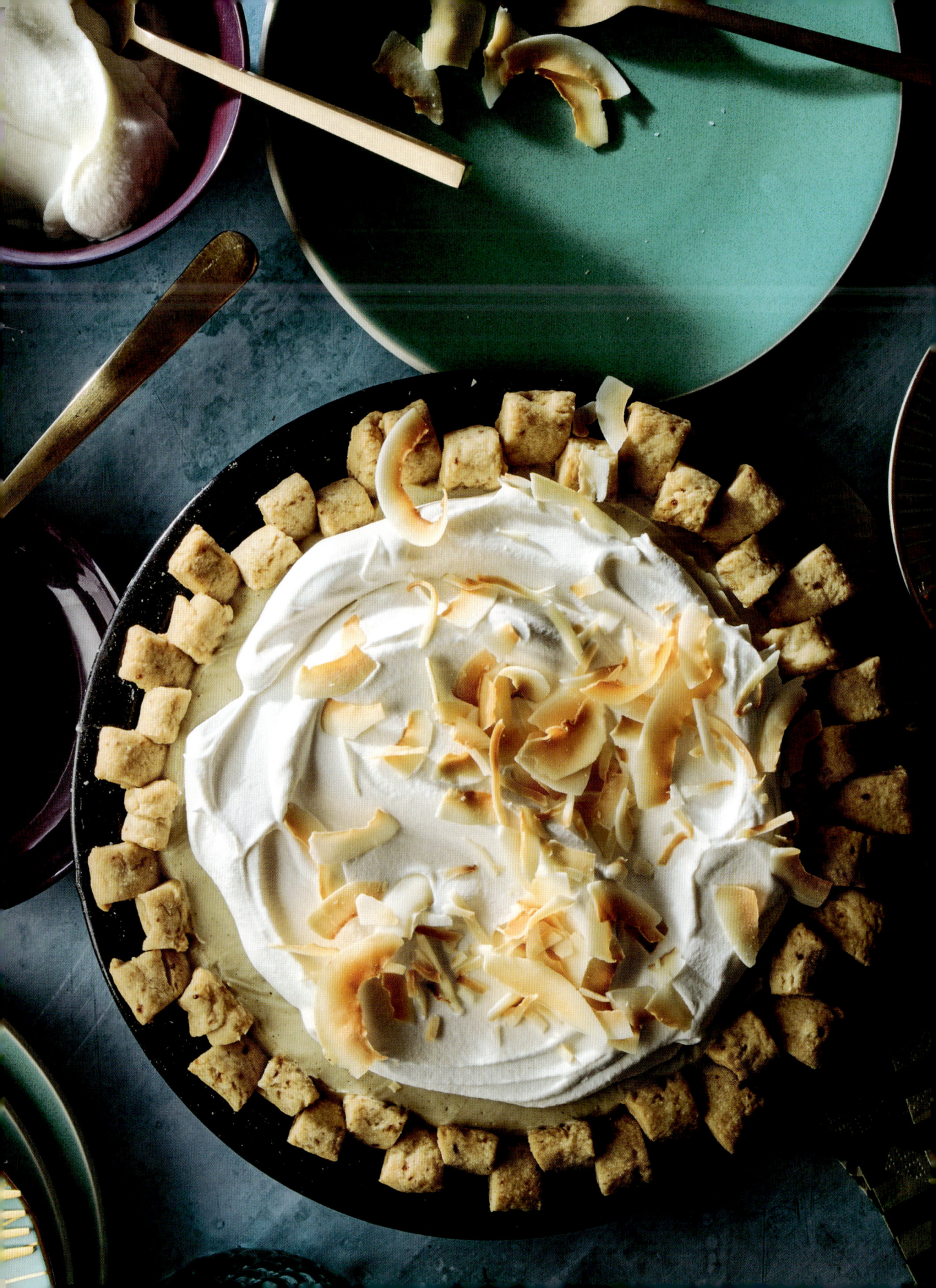

This might be my favorite dessert in the book. It's rich and chocolatey, but without that sugar overload. The silken tofu keeps it impossibly smooth, and the whole thing has the kind of velvety, melt-in-your-mouth texture that makes people go *wait*, this is vegan?! It's the perfect end to any meal — and even better straight from the fridge the next morning. For a quicker dessert, use a store-bought vegan pie crust.

SERVES 8

CHOCOLATE SILK PIE

Make the pie crust: In a large bowl, whisk together the flour, coconut sugar, and salt. Add the shortening and butter. Use a fork to press the fat into the flour, making a crumbly, sandy mixture. Drizzle in 3 tablespoons ice water and use the fork to stir until the dough comes together. Add 1 more tablespoon water if needed to help it pull together. (This can also be done in a food processor by gradually pulsing in each set of ingredients to form a crumbly mixture and then a cohesive dough.)

Turn the dough onto a lightly floured work surface. Knead once or twice to make a cohesive ball, then use a lightly floured rolling pin to roll into a 12-inch round adding more flour as needed to keep the dough from sticking. Loosely roll the dough around the rolling pin and transfer to a 9-inch pie plate. Lift and adjust the dough to help it touch the bottom and sides of the plate. Fold any excess dough under and crimp the edge of the crust with a fork or by pinching it between your fingers. Transfer to the freezer for 30 minutes to set.

Preheat the oven to 350°F.

Line the pie crust with aluminum foil, gently pressing it into all the nooks and crannies. Fill the pie plate to the brim with pie weights or dried beans. Bake the crust until the bottom and edges are golden brown, 40 to 45 minutes. Let the crust cool completely, then remove the weights and foil.

Pie Crust

1½ cups all-purpose flour, plus more for rolling
1 tablespoon coconut sugar
½ teaspoon kosher salt
¼ cup vegetable shortening, chilled
¼ cup (½ stick) vegan butter, cubed and chilled
3 to 4 tablespoons ice water

Filling

2 cups vegan chocolate chips
2 tablespoons refined coconut oil
2 (12-ounce) packages silken tofu
1 cup coconut sugar
½ cup chocolate protein powder
2 tablespoons unsweetened soy milk or other plant-based milk
1½ teaspoons kosher salt

Per serving — Calories: 406 · Fat: 18g · Carbs: 52g · Fiber: 1g · Protein: 14g

Make the filling: In a medium microwave-safe bowl, combine the chocolate chips and coconut oil. Microwave on high in 30-second bursts, stirring between each one, until the chocolate is melted. In a blender or food processor, combine the melted chocolate, tofu, coconut sugar, protein powder, soy milk, and salt. Blend on medium, stopping to scrape down the sides as needed, until completely smooth, about 2 minutes.

Pour the filling into the prebaked crust. Press plastic wrap directly on the surface of the pie. Refrigerate for at least 4 hours, until set, or overnight.

Garnish the pie: Top the pie with vegan whip and use a vegetable peeler to peel chocolate curls from a bar directly onto the pie. Slice and serve or refrigerate for up to 3 days.

Garnish
Vegan Whip (page 234), for serving
Chocolate shavings, for serving

Heavy Lift

1 Hour +

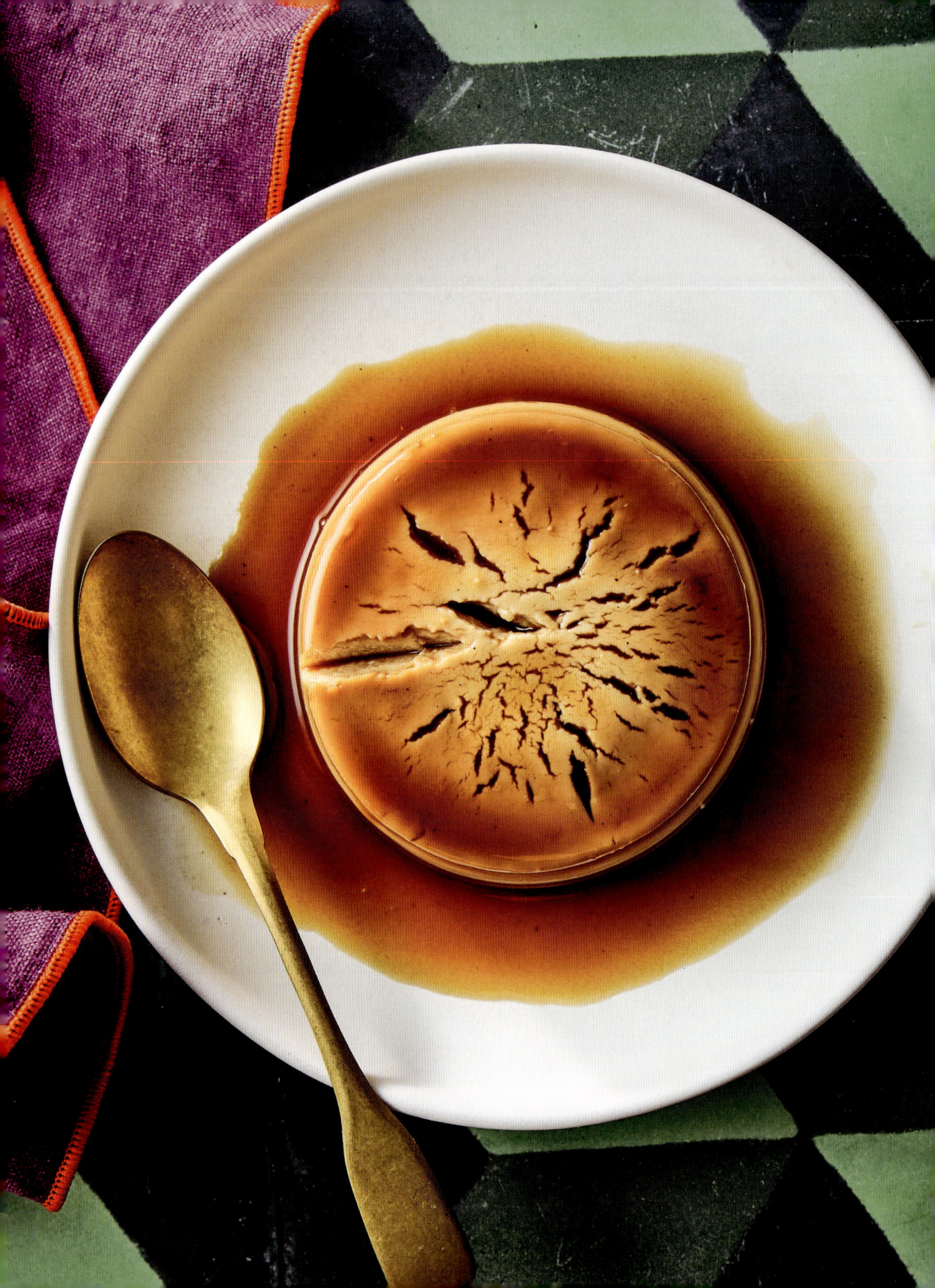

This is straight up for my abuelas. The Cuban side of my family made the most incredible flan — caramelized just right, smooth as silk, and somehow always with that perfect deep brown top. This version is my tribute to them, and when my mom tried it, she said it would make Abuela Carmita proud. That's the highest honor I could imagine.

SERVES 4

SILKY CARAMEL FLAN

Make the caramel sauce: In a small saucepan, combine the coconut sugar, salt, vanilla, and 2 tablespoons water. Set over high heat. Let the sugar dissolve and start to boil, then swirl the saucepan to mix in any remaining sugar. Continue to simmer until the surface starts to bubble all over, then swirl once more. Remove from the heat and spoon a generous 1 tablespoon of the caramel in the bottom of each of four 8-ounce ramekins. Place the ramekins in the refrigerator to let the caramel set while making the flan. Wash and dry the saucepan.

Make the flan: In a blender, combine the tofu, yogurt, soy milk, coconut sugar, cornstarch, agar agar, salt, and vanilla and blend on high until smooth, about 1 minute. Pour the mixture into the clean small saucepan. Set over medium-high heat. Whisk often until the mixture thickens into a runny pudding and starts bubbling around the edges, about 3 minutes. Immediately scrape the mixture back into the blender. Crack the lid so steam can escape and blend on medium to break up any clumps, about 1 minute.

Pour a scant 1 cup of the mixture into each ramekin. Tap the ramekins on the counter a few times to release any air bubbles. Let cool for 15 minutes, then cover with plastic wrap, pressing onto the surface of the flan, and refrigerate for at least 2 hours, until set, or overnight.

To serve, dip the bottom of each ramekin in a bowl of hot water to help release the flan. Set a small serving plate on top of the ramekin and flip. Lift the ramekin up, letting the caramel pool around the plate. Serve immediately.

Caramel Sauce

¼ cup coconut sugar
½ teaspoon kosher salt
½ teaspoon pure vanilla extract

Flan

8 ounces silken tofu, drained
1½ cups plain vegan Greek yogurt
¼ cup unsweetened soy milk or other plant-based milk
¼ cup coconut sugar
3 tablespoons cornstarch
1 tablespoon agar agar powder
1 teaspoon kosher salt
1 teaspoon pure vanilla extract

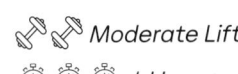 *Moderate Lift*

 *1 Hour +*

Per serving

Calories: 226

Fat: 5g

Carbs: 42g

Fiber: 1g

Protein: 14g

Protein: 13g | Calories: 389 | Fat: 26g | Carbs: 30g | Fiber: 1g | Per pop

I wish the ice cream truck had rolled up with these back in the day. They remind me of the soft pudding pops I'd dig out of my cousins' freezer, but my pops are packed with protein and totally plant based. Want to switch it up? Try chocolate or vanilla protein powder instead of the strawberry.

MAKES 6 POPS

STRAWBERRY PROTEIN POPS

Put a set of popsicle molds in the freezer to chill.

In a medium saucepan, whisk together the protein powder, sugar, cornstarch, and salt to combine. Whisk in the coconut milk a little at a time to make a smooth mixture. Whisk in the smashed strawberries, if using.

Set over low heat. Use a spatula to stir constantly until the mixture thickens into a loose pudding, about 8 minutes. Remove from the heat and stir in the vanilla. Transfer to a medium bowl and press plastic wrap directly onto the surface of the pudding. Refrigerate for 2 hours to firm up (the mixture needs to be firm for the sticks to hold).

Spoon the pudding into the chilled popsicle molds. Insert sticks and cover. Freeze for at least 4 hours, until set, or overnight. The popsicles can be stored in the freezer for up to 3 months.

- 1 cup strawberry protein powder
- ½ cup granulated sugar
- ¼ cup cornstarch
- 1 teaspoon kosher salt
- 3 cups full-fat coconut milk (measured from two 13.5-ounce cans)
- 1 teaspoon pure vanilla extract
- 1 cup strawberries, hulled and smashed (optional)

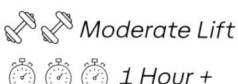 *Moderate Lift*

🕑🕑🕑 1 Hour +

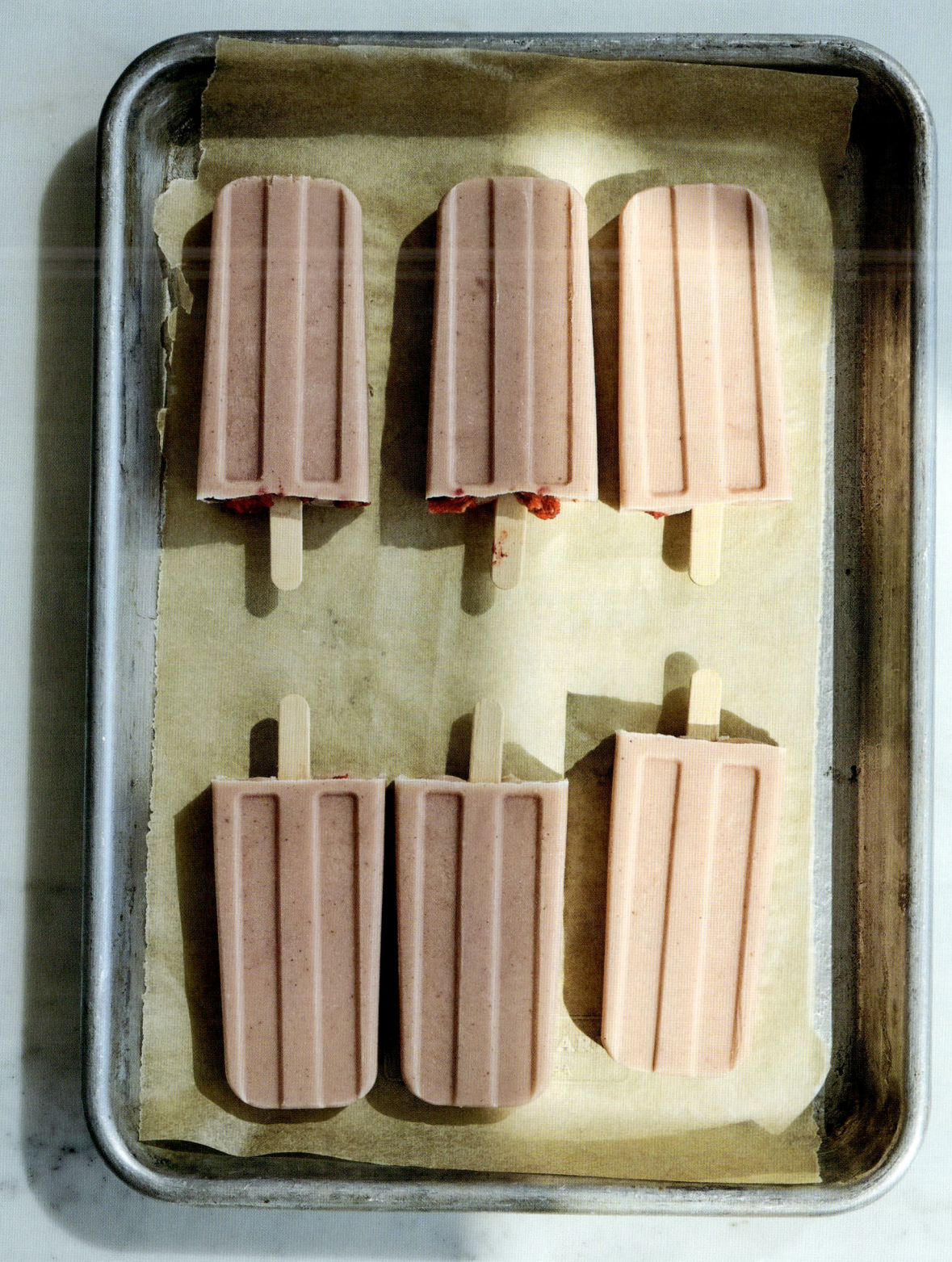

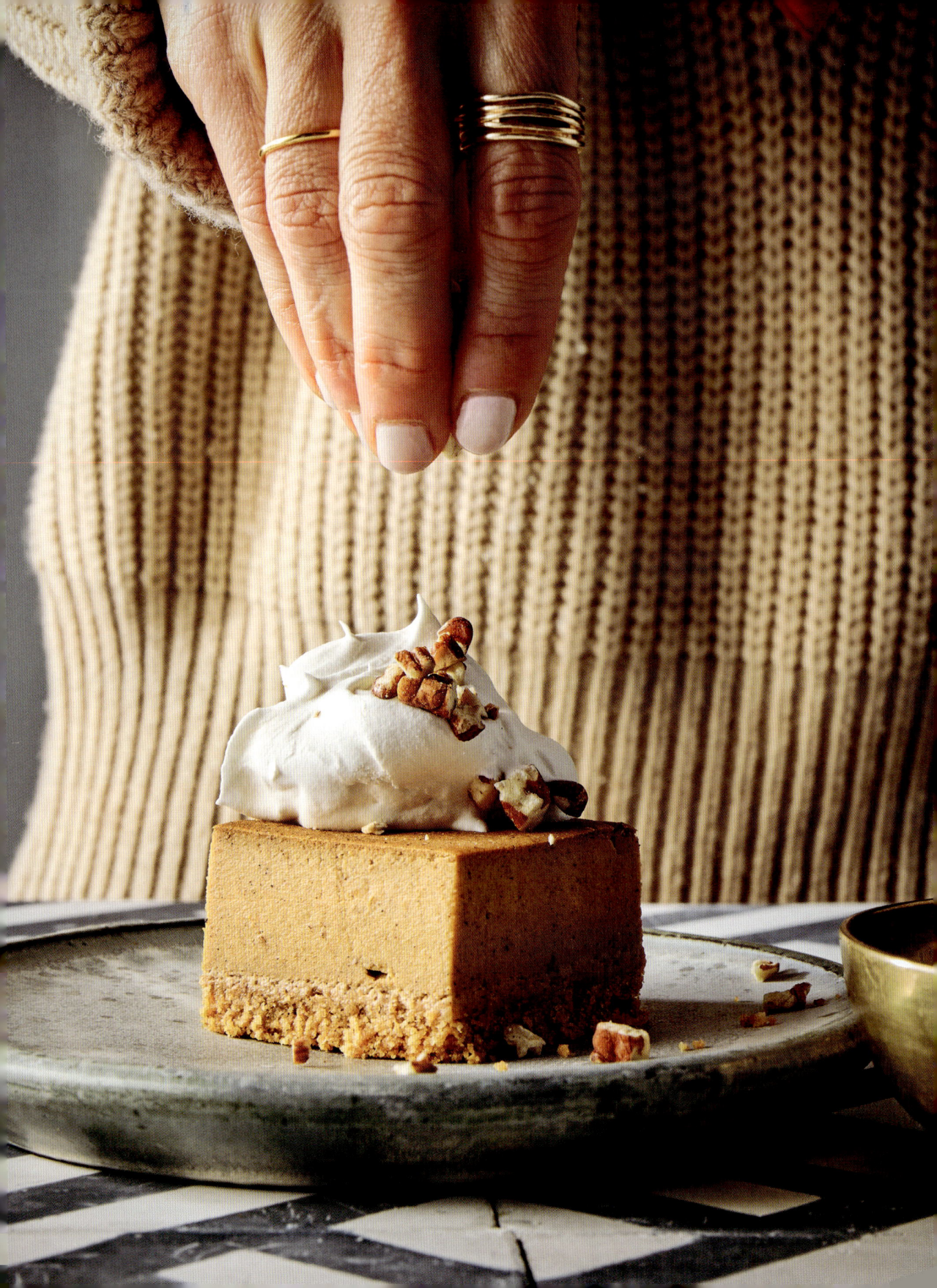

Yes, these bars scream Thanksgiving, but I make them year-round because why should cozy, spiced sweet potato goodness be seasonal? The filling is silky, the crust has that perfect crunch, and when you top the bars with vegan whip and a sprinkle of toasted pecans it's absolute perfection.

MAKES 9 BARS

SWEET POTATO PIE BARS

Preheat the oven to 350°F. Line an 8 by 8-inch baking pan with parchment paper, leaving some overhang on each side.

Make the crust: In a food processor, pulse the graham crackers about 10 times to create fine crumbs. Pour in the melted butter and pulse until a rough dough forms. Press evenly into the bottom of the prepared baking pan.

Make the topping: Pierce the sweet potatoes all over with a fork and set on a microwave-safe plate. Microwave on high for 5 minutes. If the sweet potatoes aren't tender, continue to microwave in 2-minute increments. Cut lengthwise to let the steam escape and let cool slightly. Once cool, scoop out the flesh from the skins and add to a food processor (snack on the skins or discard).

Add the tofu, protein powder, cornstarch, pumpkin pie spice, and salt. Process, scraping down the sides as needed, until smooth, about 2 minutes. Scrape the mixture over the crust and smooth into an even layer.

Bake until the center is set (give it a jiggle to test), 30 to 35 minutes. Let cool completely in the pan, then use the parchment to lift it to a cutting board. Slice into 9 bars. Top each bar with a dollop of vegan whip and a sprinkle of chopped pecans before serving. Leftovers can be refrigerated in an airtight container for up to 5 days.

Crust
- 18 whole graham crackers (from 2 sleeves)
- ½ cup (1 stick) vegan butter, melted

Topping
- 4 medium sweet potatoes
- 16 ounces silken tofu
- ½ cup vanilla protein powder
- ¼ cup cornstarch
- 2 tablespoons pumpkin pie spice
- 1 teaspoon kosher salt
- Vegan Whip (page 234), for serving
- Chopped toasted pecans, for serving

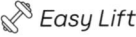 *Easy Lift*

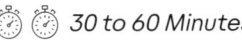 *30 to 60 Minutes*

Per bar — Calories: 359 | Fat: 15g | Carbs: 46g | Fiber: 4g | Protein: 10g

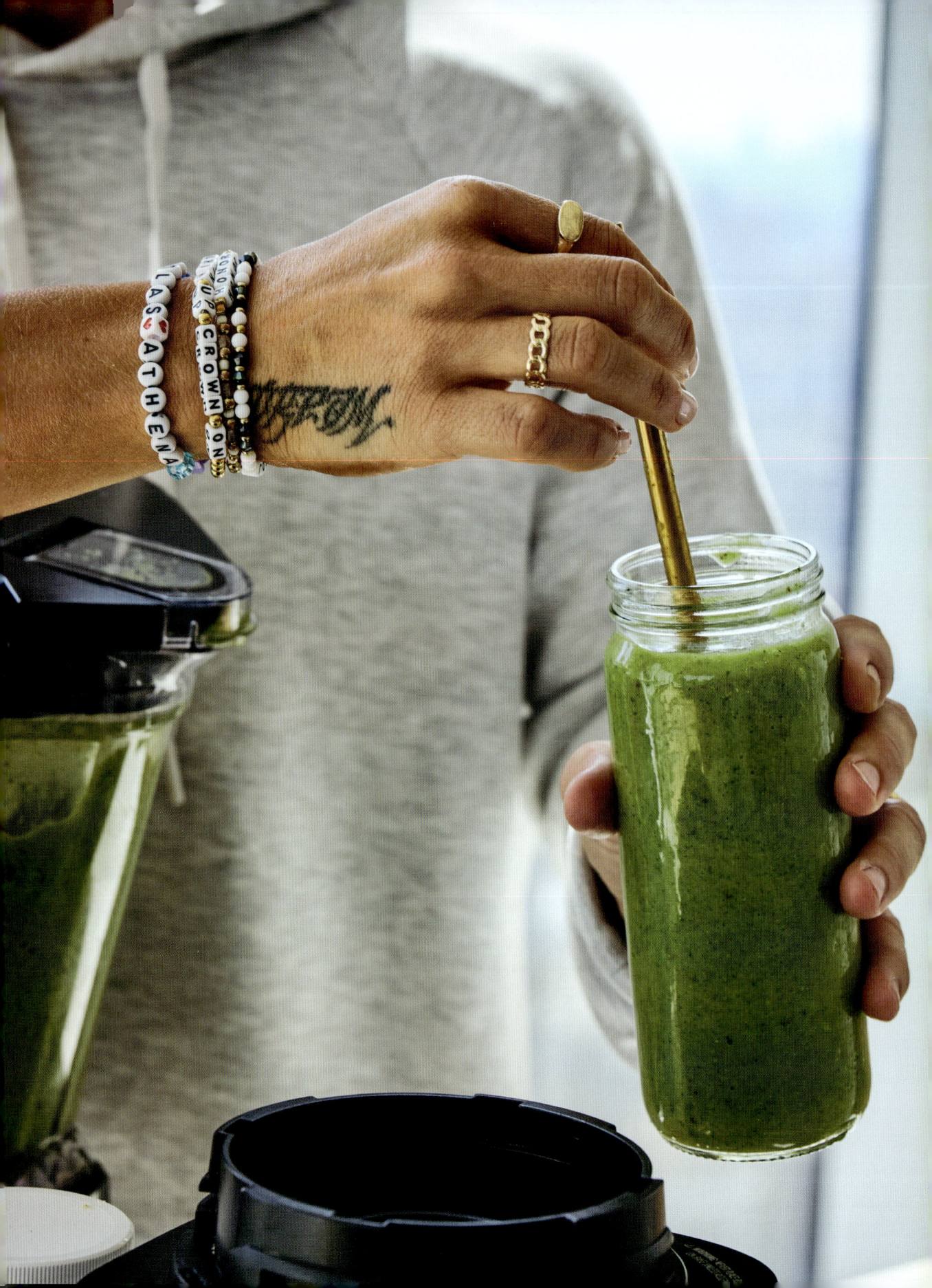

SUNDAYS ARE FOR MEAL PREP

Sundays are for setting yourself up to win. A little time in the kitchen now means fewer decisions, less stress, and zero excuses later. This chapter is all about meal prep that works — big-batch basics, mix-and-match proteins, and ready-to-go staples that keep your week running smoothly. Because when life gets busy (and it will), having a plan — and a fridge full of fuel — makes all the difference.

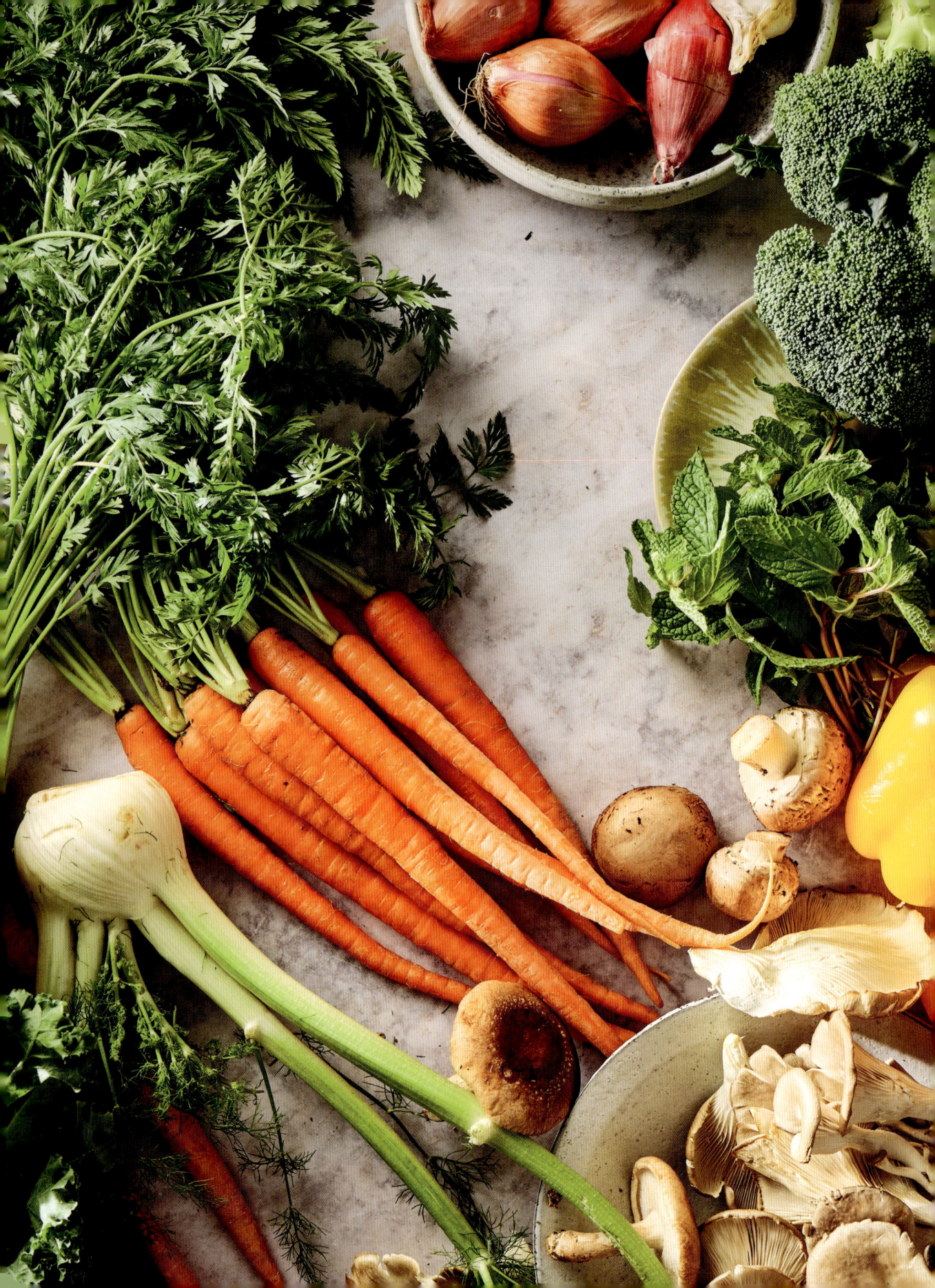

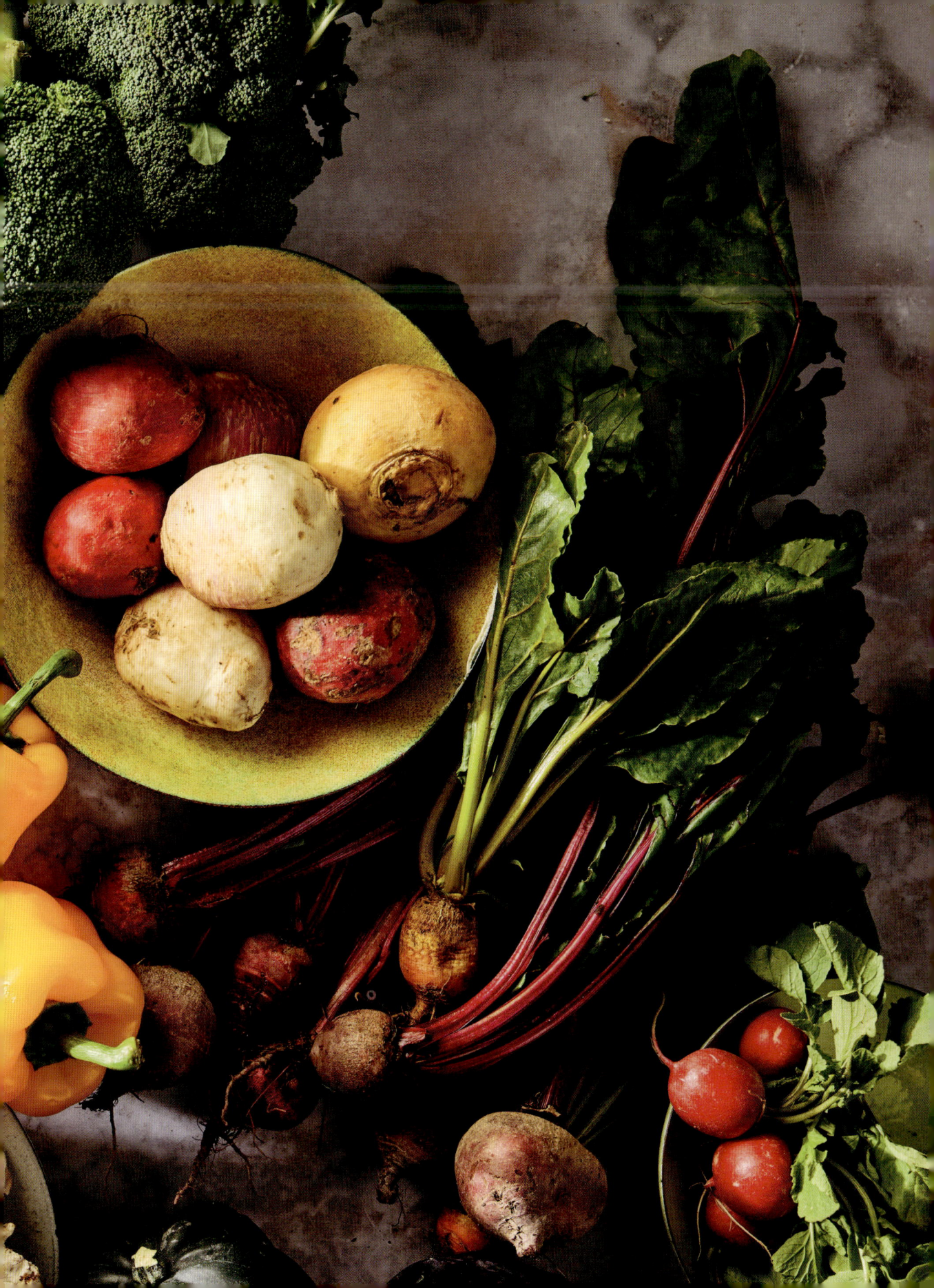

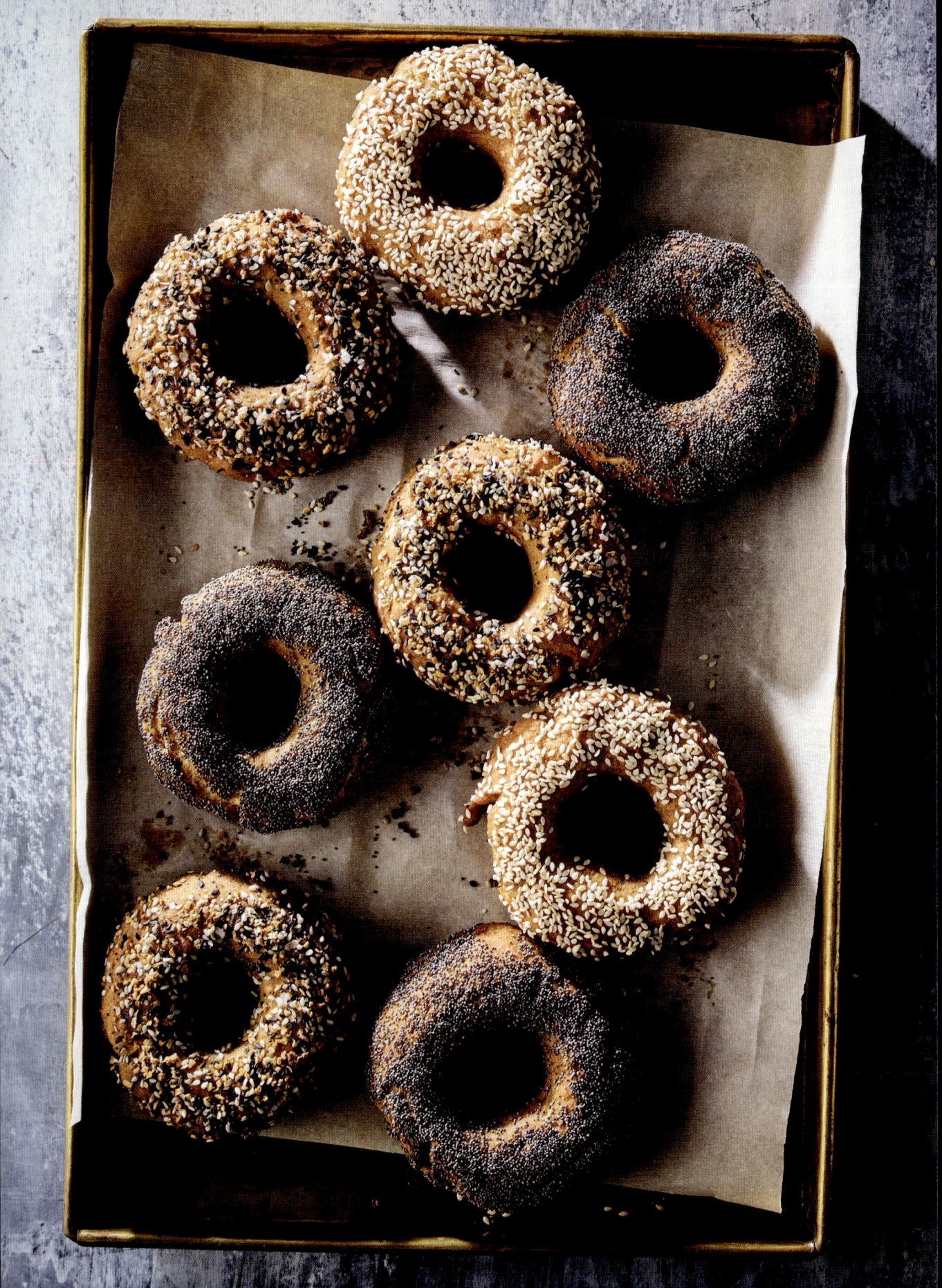

Bagels, but better. Lupini beans are incorporated into the dough to not only sneak in extra protein but add the starch that gives these a stretchy chew that's just a chef's kiss. Making them is easier than you think: once the dough is shaped into rings, the bagels get a quick boil before baking. That boiling step is key — it sets the crust early, locks in moisture, and gives you that signature shiny, chewy exterior that separates a real-deal bagel from just round bread. Then it's into the oven to bake to golden perfection. Go wild with toppings — sesame, poppy, everything seasoning, flaky salt — to get that classic bagel shop vibe without having to leave the house.

MAKES 8 BAGELS

BAGELS WITH A BOOST

Preheat the oven to 450°F.

In the bowl of a stand mixer fitted with the dough hook, combine the all-purpose flour, whole wheat flour, vital wheat gluten, baking powder, and salt and process briefly to mix. In a blender, combine the lupini beans, soy milk, vegan butter, and 2 teaspoons of the coconut sugar. Blend on high, stopping to scrape down the sides, to make a smooth mixture, about 2 minutes. Pour the liquid into the stand mixer. Mix on low speed until the dough comes together, about 5 minutes, then increase the speed to medium until the dough is smooth and barely sticky, about 2 minutes. (This dough can also be mixed in a large bowl, turned out onto a lightly floured work surface, and kneaded by hand until smooth, about 5 minutes.) Cover with a clean kitchen towel and let rest for 15 minutes.

In a large pot, combine 3 quarts water with the baking soda and remaining 2 tablespoons coconut sugar. Set over high heat and bring to a boil. Line a rimmed baking sheet with parchment paper and set nearby.

Divide the dough into 8 equal pieces. Working with one piece at a time, roll each into a smooth ball, then press with your palm to flatten. Push your thumb through the center to make a hole, then stretch and rotate to make a bagel shape with a slightly wider hole. (The bagels will swell in the water.)

2 cups all-purpose flour, plus more as needed
1 cup whole wheat flour
1 cup vital wheat gluten flour
2 tablespoons baking powder
1 tablespoon kosher salt
1 (16-ounce) jar lupini beans, drained and rinsed
1 cup unsweetened soy milk or other plant-based milk
2 tablespoons vegan butter, cubed
2 tablespoons plus 2 teaspoons coconut sugar
2 tablespoons baking soda
Everything bagel seasoning, toasted sesame seeds, poppy seeds, or flaky sea salt, for topping

Moderate Lift
30 to 60 Minutes

Per bagel
Calories: 332
Fat: 6g
Carbs: 44g
Fiber: 4g
Protein: 24g

Recipe continues...

Once all the bagels are shaped, lower half of them into the water bath. The bagels will sink, then float to the surface. Boil, flipping halfway, until the dough is puffy and soaked through, about 2 minutes. Transfer the bagels to the prepared baking sheet and top with your choice of seasonings while the surface is still wet. Repeat with the remaining bagels.

Slide the baking sheet into the oven. Bake until the bagels are golden brown and firm, 20 to 25 minutes. Transfer to a wire rack to cool for at least 10 minutes, or completely, before serving. The cooled bagels can be stored in a zip-top bag at room temperature for up to 5 days or frozen for up to 4 months. Thaw in the refrigerator overnight before serving.

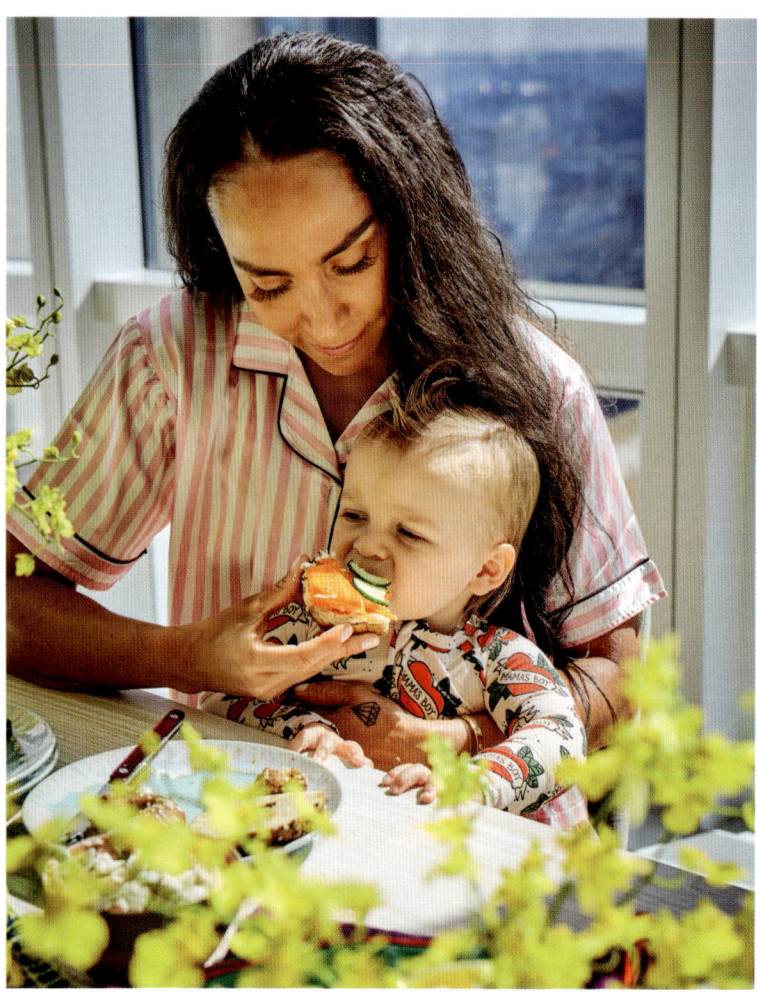

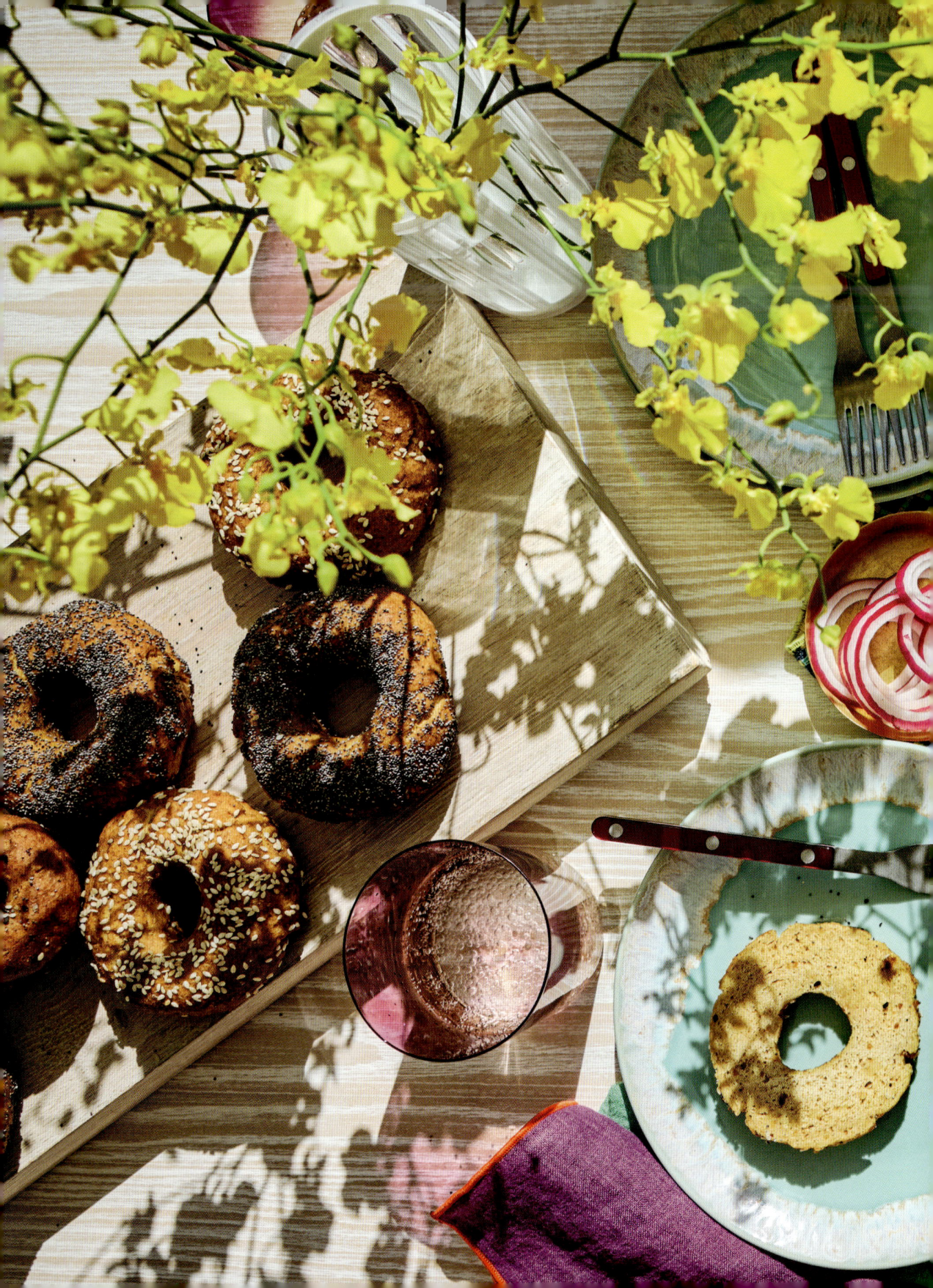

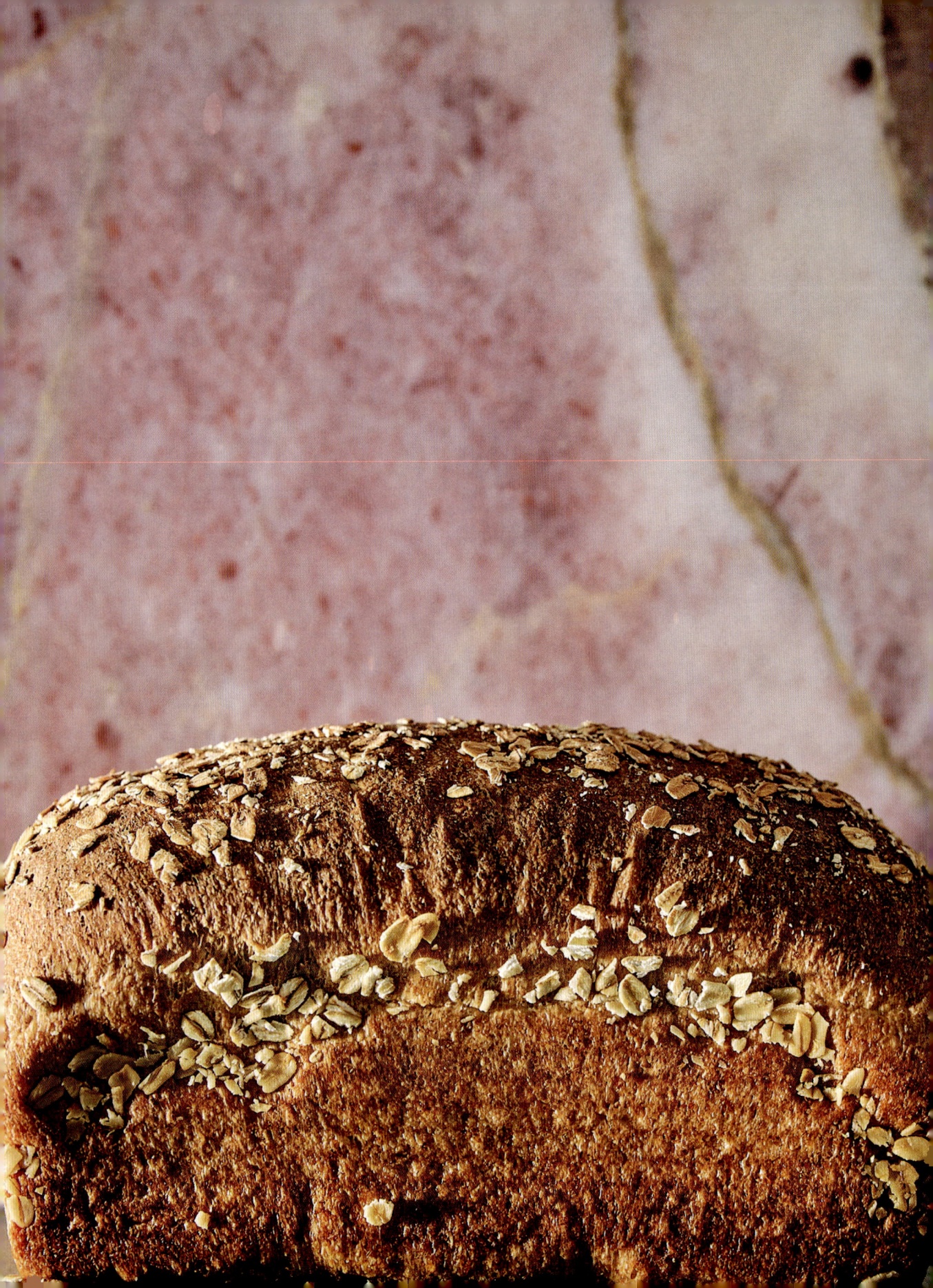

If bread had a training montage, this would be the final, triumphant run up the stairs. There's the fiber-rich whole wheat flour, a protein boost from vital wheat gluten, and soy milk to keep it light and fluffy. I love making my own bread because I get to control exactly what's in it — no hidden sugars, no weird additives — which is huge for me as someone who's mindful of blood sugar and fueling smart. Slice it, toast it, slather it with vegan butter, or use it to make the sandwiches in the I ♥ Sandwiches chapter (page 83) — this is the everyday bread you'll keep coming back to.

MAKES 1 LOAF

BREAD OF CHAMPIONS

Microwave the soy milk in 30-second bursts until warm to the touch, but not hot. Pour into the bowl of a stand mixer and sprinkle in the yeast and coconut sugar. Whisk and let sit until the yeast is fragrant and blooms at the surface, about 5 minutes.

Fit the stand mixer with the hook attachment. Add the flour, vital wheat gluten, and avocado oil to the bowl. Mix on low just to combine, then increase the speed to medium. Mix until the dough is smooth, pulling away from the sides, and just barely sticky, about 10 minutes. (This can also be mixed in a bowl with a wooden spoon, then turned onto a lightly floured work surface to knead for 10 minutes.)

Lightly coat a large bowl with avocado oil. Transfer the dough to the bowl and cover the bowl with plastic wrap. Set in a warm, draft-free spot to proof until more than doubled in volume, about 1 hour.

- 1¼ cups unsweetened soy milk or other plant-based milk
- 1 (¼-ounce) packet active dry yeast
- 1 tablespoon coconut sugar
- 2 cups whole wheat flour, plus more as needed
- ½ cup vital wheat gluten flour
- 2 tablespoons avocado oil, plus more for greasing the bowl and loaf pan
- 1 teaspoon kosher salt
- Old-fashioned oats, for topping (optional)

🏋️🏋️ *Moderate Lift*

⏱️⏱️⏱️ *1 Hour +*

Per slice (based on 12 slices)

Calories: 131

Fat: 3g

Carbs: 14g

Fiber: 2g

Protein: 10g

Recipe continues...

Lightly coat an 8 by 4-inch loaf pan with avocado oil. Lightly punch the dough down and turn out onto a clean work surface. (It should be fine to work with, but if it feels overly tacky, lightly dust the surface with flour.) Gently press the dough into a roughly 10 by 12-inch rectangle. Fold the top of the dough into the center and press with the heel of your hand to seal. Stretch the top corners out, then pull into the center and seal. Fold the top of the dough into the center again and seal. Roll the dough to the bottom and seal. Transfer, seam side down, to the prepared loaf pan and sprinkle the top with oats, if using. Loosely cover with a kitchen towel and proof until the dough is riding over the sides of the pan, 30 to 45 minutes.

Meanwhile, preheat the oven 450°F. Remove the towel and bake the loaf for 10 minutes, then reduce the oven temperature to 350°F. Continue to bake until the loaf has a golden brown crust and feels firm to the touch, about another 20 minutes. Let cool in the pan for 1 hour, then transfer the loaf to a wire rack to finish cooling. The cooled loaf can be stored in a zip-top bag at room temperature for up to 3 days.

Note: If I know I have a busy few weeks coming up, I like to multiply this recipe to make an extra loaf or two. The cooled loaves can be wrapped tightly in layers of plastic wrap and aluminum foil and frozen for up to 3 months (it's nice to slice the bread before freezing so you can just take as many slices as you need). Thaw overnight in the refrigerator and have fresh bread waiting for you by morning!

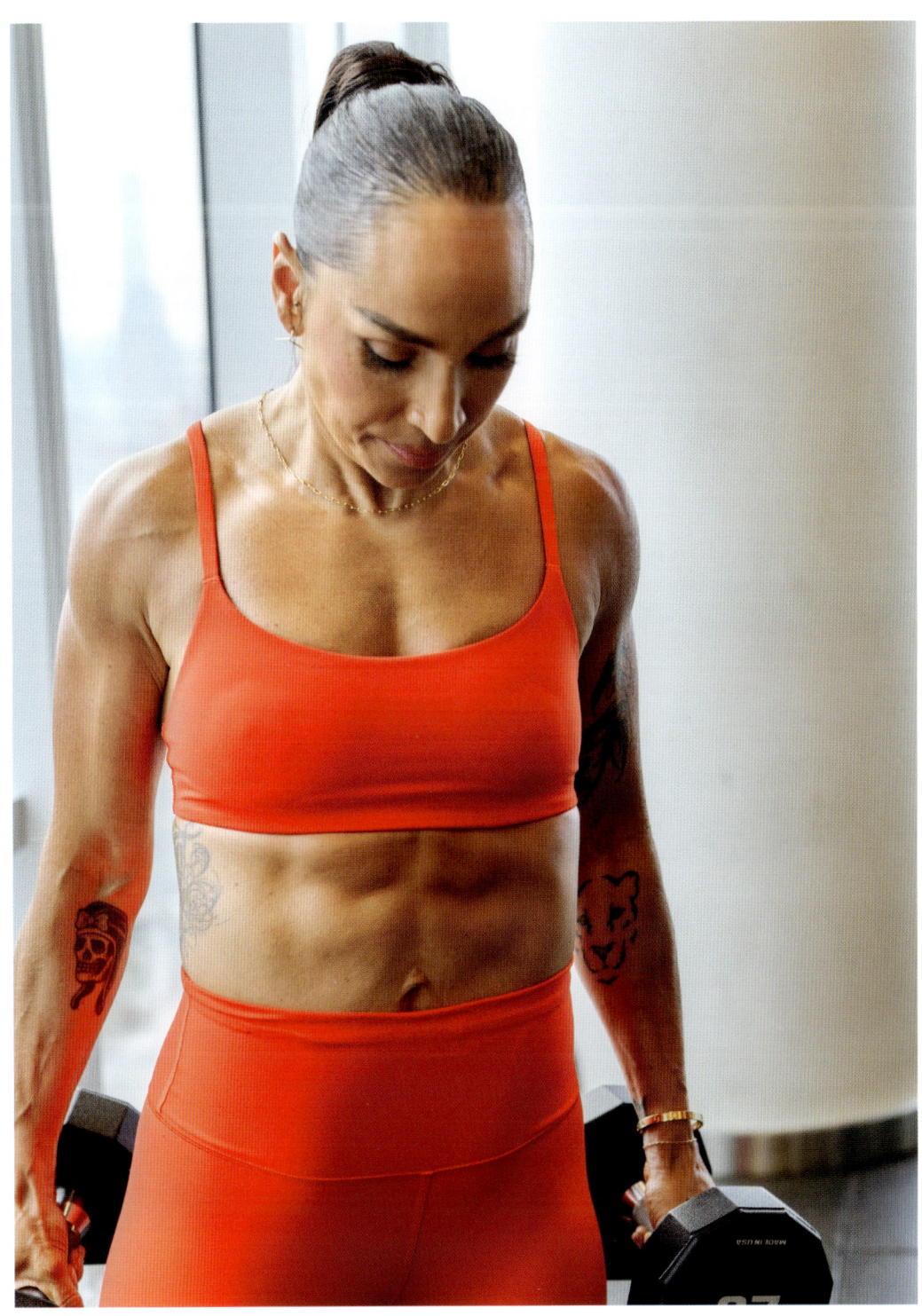

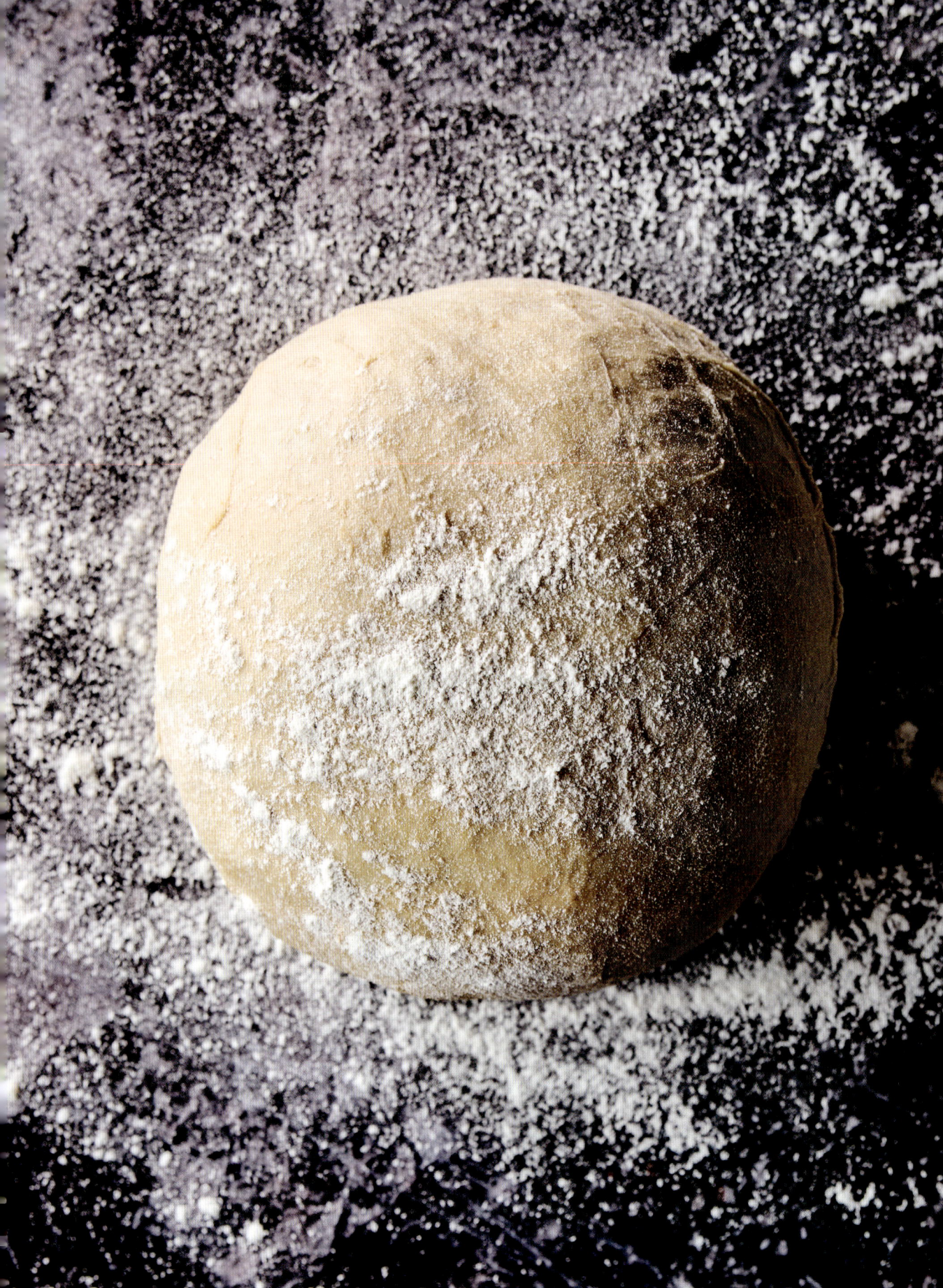

This dough is doing the absolute most. Between the Greek yogurt and the vital wheat gluten, you're getting a huge protein boost while still keeping the pizza crust soft, chewy, and perfectly crisp at the edges. No sad, floppy crusts here. It's a total game changer for pizza night with the kids — everyone can load up their own personal pie, and you know you're fueling them and making it fun. You can also roll the dough into Pizza Bites (page 170), twist it into garlic knots, or wrap it around vegan hot dogs for pigs in a blanket. Endless plays, all wins.

MAKES 2 PIZZA CRUSTS

PACKED PIZZA DOUGH

In a large bowl, whisk the flour, vital wheat gluten, baking powder, and salt together. Add the yogurt and stir into a shaggy dough. Knead the dough in the bowl until it's smooth and just slightly sticky, about 2 minutes. Cover the bowl with a kitchen towel and let the dough rest for 30 minutes.

Divide the dough into two halves. (If you want to save half for later, wrap tightly with plastic wrap and refrigerate for up to 3 days, then bring to room temperature before rolling. Or freeze for up to 3 months, thaw in the refrigerator overnight, then bring to room temperature before rolling.) Lightly flour a clean work surface. Turn out the dough and roll into a 12-inch round or any shape you need, about ½ inch thick. From here the toppings are up to you! The finished pizza can be baked on a rimmed baking sheet at 400°F until the crust is golden brown, 20 to 25 minutes.

- 2 cups all-purpose flour, plus more as needed
- ½ cup vital wheat gluten flour
- 1 tablespoon baking powder
- 1 teaspoon kosher salt
- 1½ cups plain vegan Greek yogurt

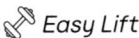 *Easy Lift*

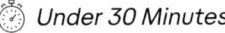 *Under 30 Minutes*

Per pizza (makes 6 slices)
Calories: 404
Fat: 8g
Carbs: 28g
Fiber: <1g
Protein: 56g

This salty, cheesy, herby "parm" is ready to take anything from meh to chef's kiss. Toss it on pasta, pizza, salads, roasted veggies, or even popcorn. It's so good, I've caught myself eating it straight from the jar.

MAKES 1 CUP

CASHEW PARM

In a blender or food processor, combine the cashews, nutritional yeast, salt, oregano, garlic powder, basil, and red pepper flakes. Pulse 6 to 8 times to make a fine powder. Transfer the parm to an airtight container and refrigerate for up to 2 weeks or freeze for up to 1 month.

1 cup raw cashews
1 tablespoon nutritional yeast
2 teaspoons kosher salt
1 teaspoon dried oregano
1 teaspoon garlic powder
½ teaspoon dried basil
¼ teaspoon red pepper flakes

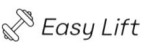 *Easy Lift*

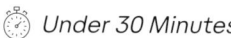 *Under 30 Minutes*

Per 1 tablespoon | Calories: 42 | Fat: 3g | Carbs: 2g | Fiber: <1 g | Protein: 1g

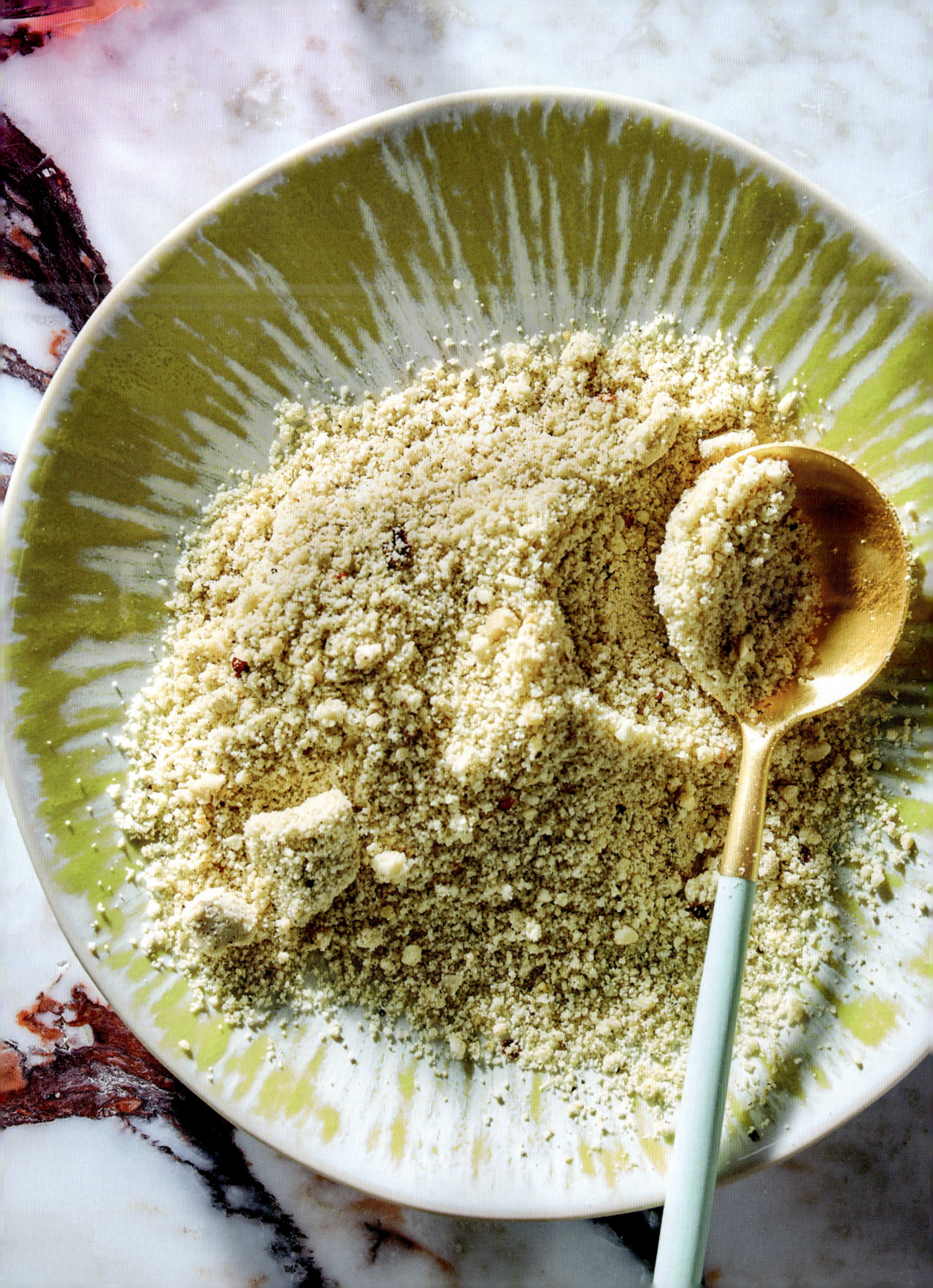

Protein: 31g | Calories: 165 | Fat: 1g | Carbs: 9g | Per ¼ pound

Seitan is a champion plant protein with 31 grams of protein per serving. You can grab it from most supermarkets (usually found near the tofu), but making seitan from scratch is not only way cheaper — it also lets you dial in the texture exactly how you want it. When it's marinated, it's tender and meaty (perfect for dishes like the Seitan Reuben Bowl on page 79), and when it's simmered or roasted (like in the Vegan Pernil Plate on page 149), it becomes juicy, chewy, and seriously hearty. Making your own might sound like a chore, but it's way easier than you think. This is your shortcut to plant-based cutlets, shredded "meat," or whatever shape your heart desires.

MAKES 1 POUND

DIY SEITAN

In a large bowl, whisk together the vital wheat gluten flour, nutritional yeast, baking powder, and salt. In a small bowl, whisk together the stock and soy sauce, then pour into the flour mixture and use a wooden spoon to stir. When the dough starts to get too firm, switch to your hands and start kneading the dough in the bowl. Knead for 3 to 4 minutes until the dough is completely combined, but still a little ragged. Cover the bowl with a damp kitchen towel and let rest for 30 minutes to allow the gluten to relax and develop.

Fill a large pot halfway with salted water. Set over high heat and bring to a boil. Press the dough into a large round and carefully lower it into the boiling water. The dough will puff up and expand as it cooks. Boil for about 30 minutes, using tongs to flip the dough occasionally, until the seitan is hydrated and tender (the center and edges will look uniform). Use tongs to transfer it to paper towels to drain and cool completely, about 1 hour.

The seitan can be patted dry and used immediately. Cut into any shape and cook according to the recipe directions. Or transfer to an airtight container and refrigerate for up to 3 days. Drain and pat dry before using. To freeze, place the cooled seitan in a freezer-safe bag. Freeze for up to 3 months. Transfer frozen seitan to the refrigerator and thaw overnight. Drain and pat dry before using.

Note: If you want to speed things up, you can skip the 30-minute rest and boil right away. But if you allow that extra time for the gluten to relax and develop, your seitan will have a much denser, meatier texture.

- 1 cup vital wheat gluten flour
- 6 tablespoons nutritional yeast
- ½ teaspoon baking powder
- ½ teaspoon kosher salt, plus more for boiling
- ¾ cup vegetable stock or Liquid Gold (page 235)
- 1 tablespoon soy sauce or tamari

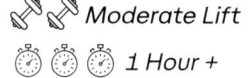 *Moderate Lift*

🕐🕐🕐 *1 Hour +*

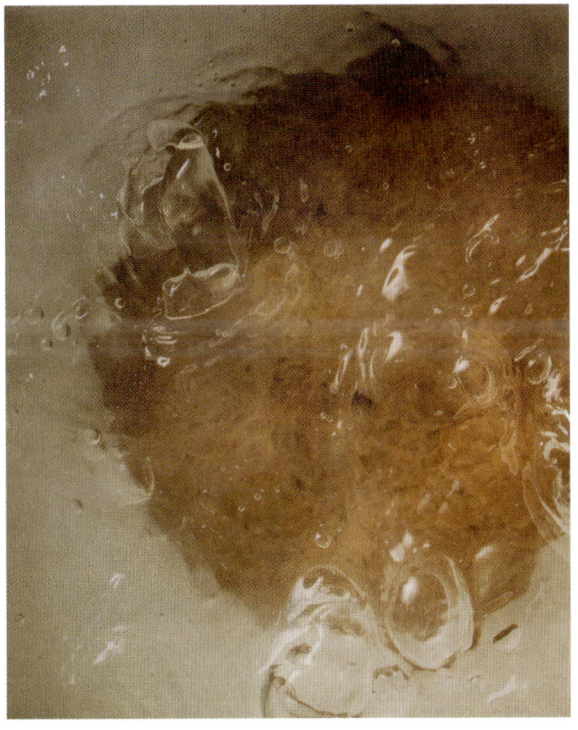
The seitan dough sinks at first.

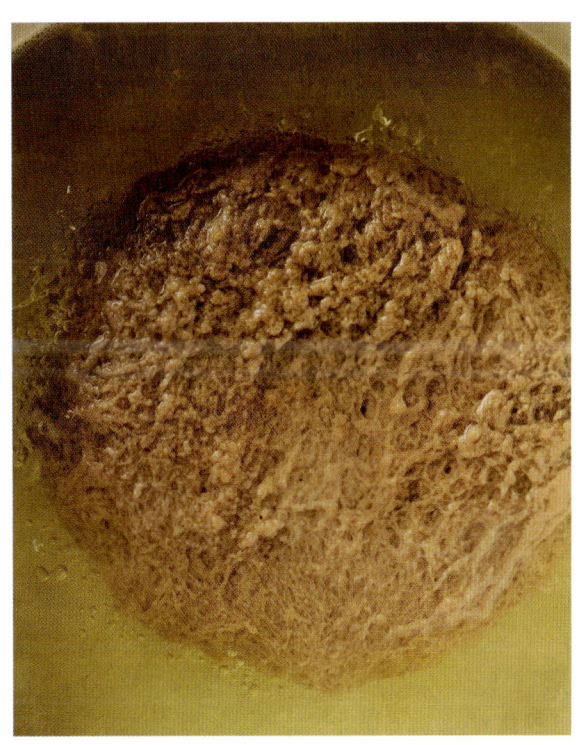
It will puff up and expand as it cooks.

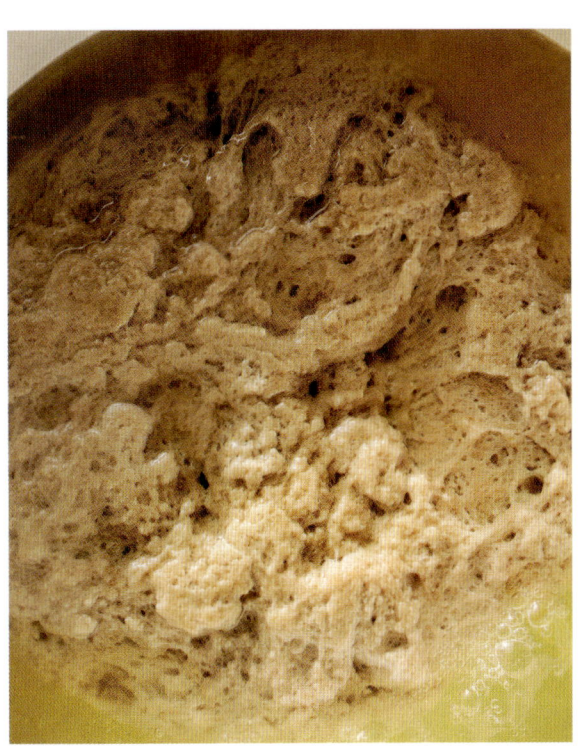
Cook until it expands and looks uniformly solid.

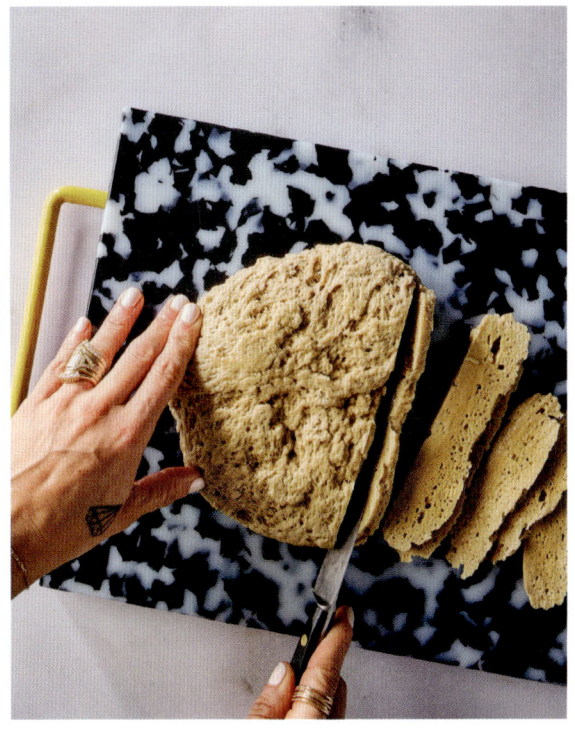
Drain, pat dry, slice, and use.

TVP (textured vegetable protein) doesn't sound sexy, but hear me out: This stuff is a workhorse. Made from soy flour, it's a plant-based protein that soaks up all the smoky, savory flavors you throw at it while it hydrates into a ground meat–like texture. It also packs a solid protein punch, making it the best base for taco meat, Bolognese-y pasta sauce, or chili. It's the meal prep MVP you didn't know you needed.

MAKES 1 POUND

TVP MVP

In a medium bowl, stir together the TVP, paprika, cumin, and salt. In a small saucepan, bring the stock and soy sauce to a boil over high heat. Pour the liquid over the TVP mixture and stir to incorporate. Let soak for 10 minutes.

Transfer the TVP to an airtight container and refrigerate until ready to use or up to 3 days. You can also portion into smaller containers and freeze for up to 1 month.

1½ cups dry TVP
1 teaspoon smoked paprika
1 teaspoon ground cumin
¼ teaspoon kosher salt
1 cup vegetable stock or Liquid Gold (page 235)
2 tablespoons soy sauce or tamari

 Easy Lift

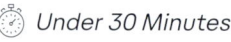 *Under 30 Minutes*

Per ¼ pound — Protein: 23g | Calories: 134 | Fat: 1g | Carbs: 15g | Fiber: 7g

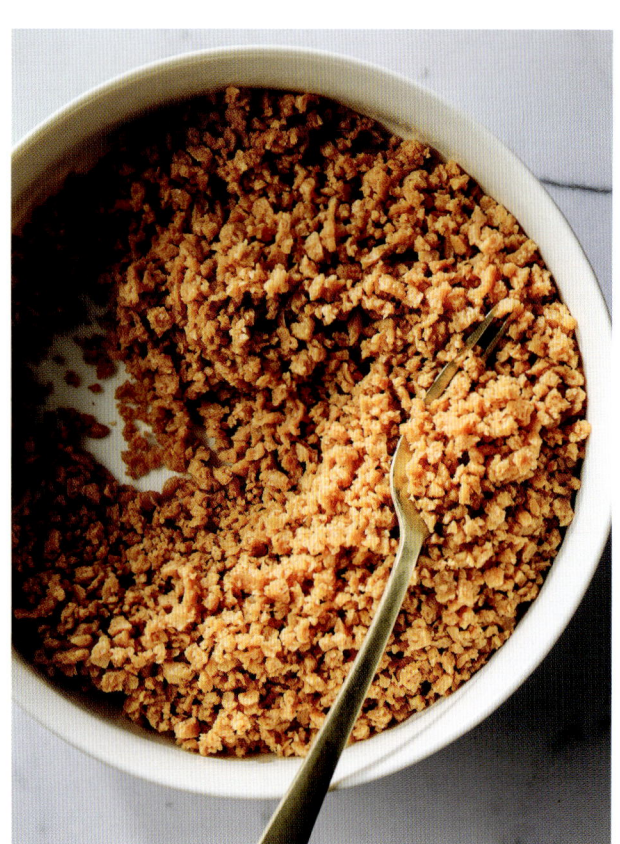

Let's be honest, everything tastes better roasted, and vegetables are no exception. Luckily, roasting couldn't be easier. Get into the practice of roasting veggies over the weekend and stock your fridge for fast salads, protein bowls, and even sandwich fixings! Four cups of raw vegetables generally yield about 2 cups roasted, or 2 servings. For nutrition details on specific vegetables, consult your favorite trusted nutrition-tracking app.

FIRE VEGGIES

Toss your veggies on a sheet pan with just enough olive oil to coat them lightly, then hit them with a generous pinch of salt and a few cracks of black pepper. Spread them out, taking care not to crowd them — those veggies need their space to get golden and crispy! And don't forget to rotate the baking sheet and give the veggies a quick toss halfway through so they roast evenly. Use the chart on page 226 for temperature and timing.

Notes:
Leftovers roasted vegetables can be refrigerated in an airtight container for up to 1 week. Reheat as needed in a 400°F oven for about 10 minutes. Vegetables that roast at the same temperature can be roasted on the same sheet pan — if one is listed as needing less time than another, divide the sheet pan into sections so you can easily remove the veg that's done before the one that isn't.

Vegetables prepped for roasting (page 226)
Extra-virgin olive oil

Easy Lift
Under 30 Minutes
30 to 60 Minutes

```
Dalina Says...
Meal prep doesn't have to be complicated—and
roasting a pan (or a few pans) of veggies can
make your week way easier. Fiber-rich options
like carrots, cauliflower, and sweet potatoes can
be added to salads, wraps, bowls, or eaten as
quick snacks. A little olive oil helps bring out
flavor and boosts absorption of key nutrients.
It's less about perfection and more about set-
ting yourself up to feel good.
```

VEGETABLE	TEMPERATURE	PREP	MINUTES
Asparagus	400°F	Whole, ends trimmed	10 to 15
Beets	400°F	Whole, wrapped in aluminum foil (peel and cut once cooled)	50 to 60
Bell Peppers	450°F	Strips or whole (after roasting, cover tightly with plastic wrap until skin peels easily)	20 to 30
Broccoli	400°F	Florets	20 to 30
Broccolini	400°F	Whole, ends trimmed	15 to 20
Brussels Sprouts	450°F	Trimmed, halved (or quartered if large), cleaned	20 to 30
Carrots	450°F 450°F	Whole 1-inch pieces	20 to 30 15 to 20
Cauliflower	425°F 450°F	Florets Whole	20 to 30 50 to 60
Eggplant	400°F 400°F 350°F	Peeled and cubed 1-inch-thick steaks, skin on Whole, about 1 pound (poked with a fork prior to roasting)	30 to 40 30 to 40 50 to 60
Fennel	425°F	Fronds removed, cored and cut into wedges	20 to 30
Garlic	375°F	¼ inch cut off the top of the head to expose the cloves, wrapped tightly in foil	40 to 50
Leeks	400°F	Halved, washed, tough tops removed, cut into 1-inch pieces	20 to 30
Onions	400°F	Peeled and cut into wedges	30 to 40
Parsnips	425°F	Peeled and cut into 1-inch cubes	30 to 40

Potatoes	400°F 400°F 425°F	Peeled and cut into 1-inch cubes Wedges, skin on Whole, pierced with a fork	25 to 30 25 to 30 40 to 50
Rutabagas	425°F	Peeled and cubed	30 to 40
Shallots	400°F 425°F	Peeled and halved Whole, skin on	30 to 40 50 to 60

MUSHROOMS

Chanterelle	400°F	Whole, cleaned	10 to 15
Cremini	400°F	Halved, cleaned	10 to 15
Morel	400°F	Whole, cleaned	10 to 15
Oyster	425°F	Whole or shredded, cleaned	40 to 50
Portobello	450°F	Whole, stems removed, cleaned	10 to 15
Shiitake	400°F	Whole, stems removed, cleaned	20 to 30

SQUASH

Acorn	450°F	Halved, seeds scooped out, cut into wedges	30 to 40
Butternut	450°F	Peeled, halved, seeds scooped out, cut into cubes	20 to 30
Delicata	450°F	Halved, seeds scooped out, cut into rings	20 to 30
Kabocha	450°F	Halved, seeds scooped out, cut into wedges	30 to 40
Spaghetti	450°F	Halved, seeds scooped out, roast cut side down	30 to 40

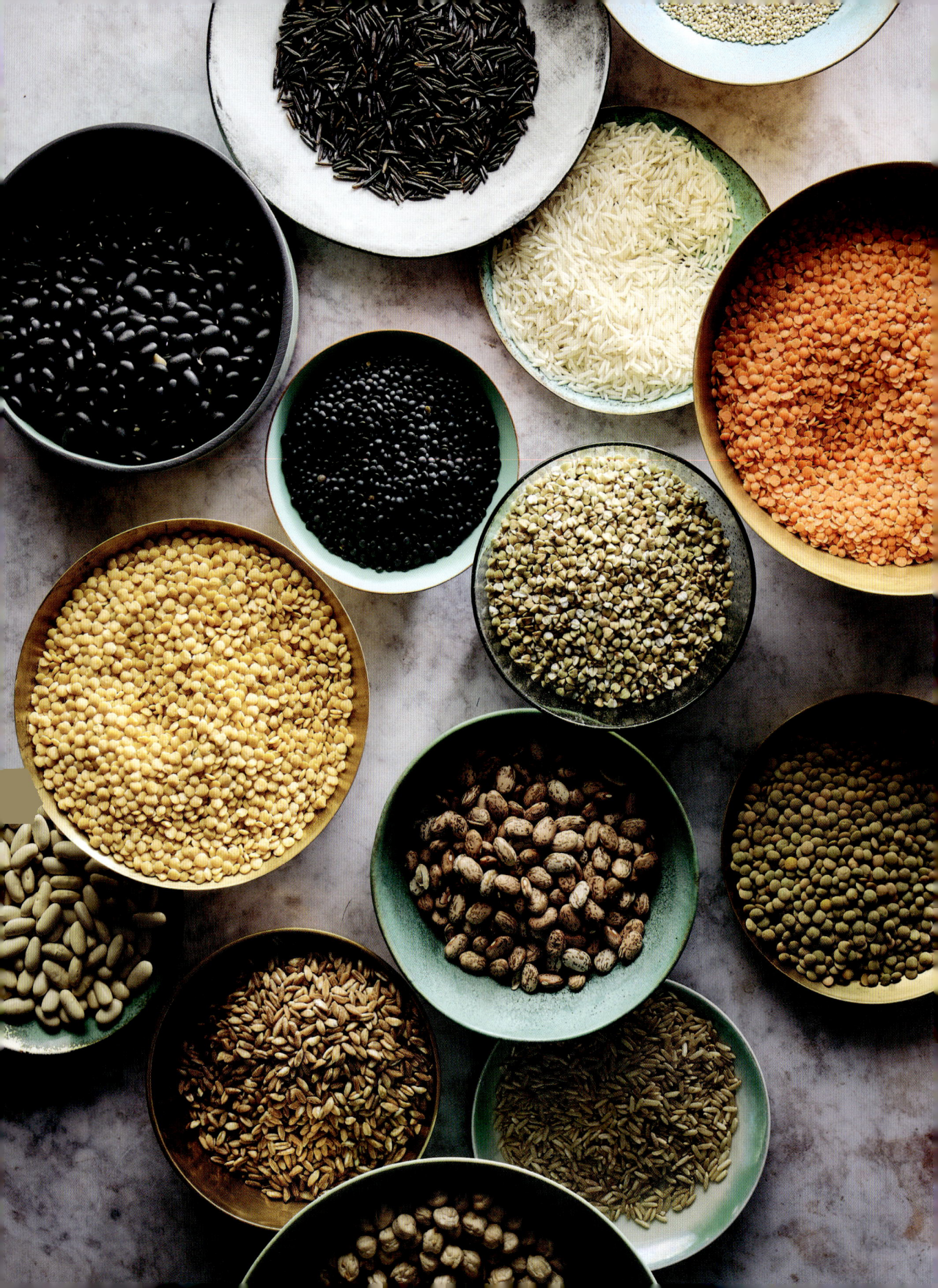

Having precooked grains ready to go in the fridge is an absolute game changer — like winning the meal prep lottery. Not only do they make throwing together a quick meal effortless, they are also a fantastic source of complex carbs, fiber, and essential nutrients like B vitamins and iron — and in the case of quinoa, farro, and wild rice, a great protein source too. Grains are a key part of a balanced diet, providing energy and pairing perfectly with plant-based protein sources to create complete proteins. Treat yourself to a weekly fridge full of grains, and you'll have a rainbow of flavors and textures to keep things exciting.

MAKES 3 CUPS

GRAINS FOR DAYS

Start by swishing your grains in a bowl of cold water. Wash and drain a few times until the water runs clear — this will remove any residue and excess starch. Follow the chart on page 230 for specific cooking guidance for each type of grain. After cooking and cooling, transfer to an airtight container to refrigerate for up to 5 days or freeze for up to 6 months. Let frozen grains thaw in the refrigerator overnight before using.

1 cup grains of your choice (page 230)
½ teaspoon salt

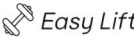 *Easy Lift*

Under 30 Minutes

30 to 60 Minutes, depending on the grain

GRAINS	WATER	SALT (KOSHER)	NOTES	PROTEIN (PER 1 CUP)
1 cup basmati rice or jasmine rice	1½ cups	½ teaspoon	Add the rice, water, and salt to a saucepan over high heat. Bring to a boil, then cover and reduce the heat to low. Simmer for 15 minutes. Remove from the heat and let it steam, still covered, for 10 minutes. Fluff with a fork.	4g
1 cup brown rice	2 cups	½ teaspoon	Add the rice, water, and salt to a saucepan over high heat. Bring to a boil, then cover and reduce the heat to low. Simmer for 45 minutes. Remove from the heat and let it steam, still covered, for 10 minutes. Fluff with a fork.	5g
1 cup wild rice	4 cups	½ teaspoon	Add the rice, water, and salt to a saucepan over high heat. Bring to a boil, then reduce the heat to medium-low. Simmer, uncovered, for 30 to 40 minutes, adding more water as needed, until tender. Drain thoroughly.	7g
1 cup buckwheat	2 cups	½ teaspoon	Bring the water to a boil over high heat. Stir in the buckwheat and salt. Reduce the heat to medium-low and simmer, uncovered, about 10 minutes, until tender. Drain thoroughly.	6g

GRAINS	WATER	SALT (KOSHER)	NOTES	PROTEIN (PER 1 CUP)
1 cup bulgur	2 cups	½ teaspoon	Bring the water to a boil over high heat. Stir in the bulgur and salt. Cover and remove from the heat. Steam for 20 to 30 minutes, until tender and fluffy. Drain any excess water and fluff with a fork.	6g
¾ cup couscous	¾ cup	½ teaspoon	Bring the water to a boil over high heat. Stir in the couscous and salt. Cover and remove from the heat. Steam for about 10 minutes, until tender and the liquid is absorbed. Fluff with a fork.	6g
1 cup farro	4 cups	½ teaspoon	Add the farro, water, and salt to a saucepan over high heat. Bring to a boil, then reduce the heat to medium-low. Simmer, uncovered, for 30 to 40 minutes, adding more water as needed, until tender. Drain thoroughly.	15g
1 cup quinoa	1¾ cups	½ teaspoon	Add the quinoa, water, and salt to a saucepan over high heat. Bring to a boil over high heat, then cover and reduce the heat to low. Simmer for 15 minutes. Remove from the heat and let steam, still covered, for 10 minutes. Fluff with a fork.	6g

Beans are hands-down my favorite protein source — they're affordable, versatile, and packed with fiber and nutrients that keep you full and energized. Canned beans are a lifesaver in a pinch, but when I have the time, I love cooking them from scratch. My secret ingredient is a piece of dried kombu (seaweed) — it helps soften the beans and makes them easier on your digestion (yes, less gas!). I like to cook big batches to stash in the fridge or freezer, so I'm always ready to throw them into whatever I'm making.

MAKES 3 CUPS

BEST BASIC BEANS

Rinse the beans well in a mesh strainer, picking out any little stones or broken pieces.

Add the beans, 1 tablespoon of the salt, and 2 quarts water to a Dutch oven. Bring to a boil over high heat, then remove from the heat and soak, uncovered, for 1 hour.

Preheat the oven to 375°F and set a rack in the center.

Drain and rinse the soaked beans, then return them to the pot with 2 quarts of fresh water. Add the aromatics and remaining ½ teaspoon salt. Bring to a boil over high heat, then cover and transfer to the oven. Bake until a few tester beans are all tender, 40 to 60 minutes.

Drain and cool the cooked beans, then transfer to an airtight container to refrigerate for up to 5 days or freeze for up to 6 months. Let frozen beans thaw in the refrigerator overnight.

- 1 cup dry beans (black, cannellini, pinto, kidney, chickpea)
- 1 tablespoon plus ½ teaspoon kosher salt
- 1 medium piece kombu
- 1 small carrot, diced
- 1 celery stalk, diced
- ½ white onion
- 4 garlic cloves, smashed
- 2 sprigs fresh rosemary

Moderate Lift

🕐🕐🕐
1 Hour +

Per 1 cup cooked

	Calories	Fat	Carbs	Fiber	Protein
Black	218	1g	40g	17g	15g
Cannellini	200	0g	36g	8g	14g
Pinto	206	2g	37g	11g	12g

Lentils are a staple in my kitchen. They're quick to cook and a powerhouse of plant-based protein, iron, and fiber. Unlike beans, lentils don't need to soak, and they're ready in under an hour, so they're perfect for last-minute meals. While green, brown, and black lentils hold their shape beautifully for salads, soups, or grain bowls, red and yellow lentils shine as thickeners in soups, stews, or curries. (They're not included here because they practically melt into dishes! And note that if brown lentils are overcooked, they will lose their shape.)

MAKES 2 CUPS

LENTILS ON LOCK

Rinse the lentils well in a mesh strainer, picking out any little stones or broken pieces.

In a medium saucepan, combine the lentils, salt, aromatics, and 3 cups water. Set over high heat and bring to a boil. Cover, reduce the heat to low, and simmer until a few tester lentils are all tender, about 15 minutes.

Once they're cooked, drain and discard the aromatics. Cool, then transfer to an airtight container to refrigerate for up to 5 days or freeze for up to 6 months. Let frozen lentils thaw in the refrigerator overnight.

- 1 cup dry lentils (black, brown, green, or French green)
- ½ teaspoon kosher salt
- ½ leek, rinsed and cut into quarters
- 2 garlic cloves, smashed
- 2 sprigs fresh rosemary

Easy Lift

Under 30 Minutes

Per 1 cup cooked

	Calories	Fat	Carbs	Fiber	Protein
Lentils	230	1g	40g	17g	18g
Kidney	207	1g	38g	11g	13g
Chickpea	211	2g	32g	11g	12g

Protein: 1g | Fiber: 0g | Carbs: 5g | Fat: 14g | Calories: 144 | Per ¼ cup

Whipped cream, but make it plant based and foolproof. Mixing soy milk and coconut oil basically makes a fat-rich cream that whips up into sweet, fluffy clouds. It's the perfect finishing touch for everything from desserts to hot chocolate (page 53) to fruit to sneaking spoonsful straight from the bowl. I use refined coconut oil so my whip doesn't taste like coconut — but if you prefer a coconut flavor, use unrefined oil.

MAKES 4 CUPS

VEGAN WHIP

In a small saucepan, combine the coconut oil and soy milk. Set over low heat until the coconut oil is melted and the soy milk is barely starting to bubble under the oil, about 3 minutes. (This can also be done in the microwave in 30-second bursts.) Pour the mixture into a blender and blend on high until emulsified, about 1 minute.

Pour into an airtight container and refrigerate until well chilled or up to 3 days.

Transfer the cream to the bowl of a stand mixer fitted with a whisk attachment (or a large bowl with a handheld mixer). Add the powdered sugar and vanilla. Beat on medium until the mixture transforms into a fluffy whipped cream with stiff peaks, about 6 minutes. Leftover whip can be refrigerated in an airtight container for up to 5 days.

1 cup refined coconut oil
1 cup unsweetened soy milk or other plant-based milk
½ cup powdered sugar
1 teaspoon pure vanilla extract

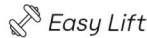 *Easy Lift*

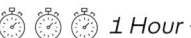 *1 Hour +*

This miso and nutritional yeast broth is a star all on its own — ready to rock any pot. Think of it as the Beyoncé of broths: irreplaceable.

MAKES 2 QUARTS

LIQUID GOLD

In a large pot, whisk 8 cups water with the nutritional yeast, miso, salt, and pepper. Set over low heat and whisk occasionally until it comes to a slow simmer. (Boiling miso knocks out its gut-healthy probiotics, so keep it low and slow.) Use immediately or refrigerate for up to 5 days before gently reheating.

⅓ cup nutritional yeast
2½ tablespoons white miso
1½ tablespoons kosher salt
2 teaspoons freshly ground black pepper

🏋 *Easy Lift*
⏱ *Under 30 Minutes*

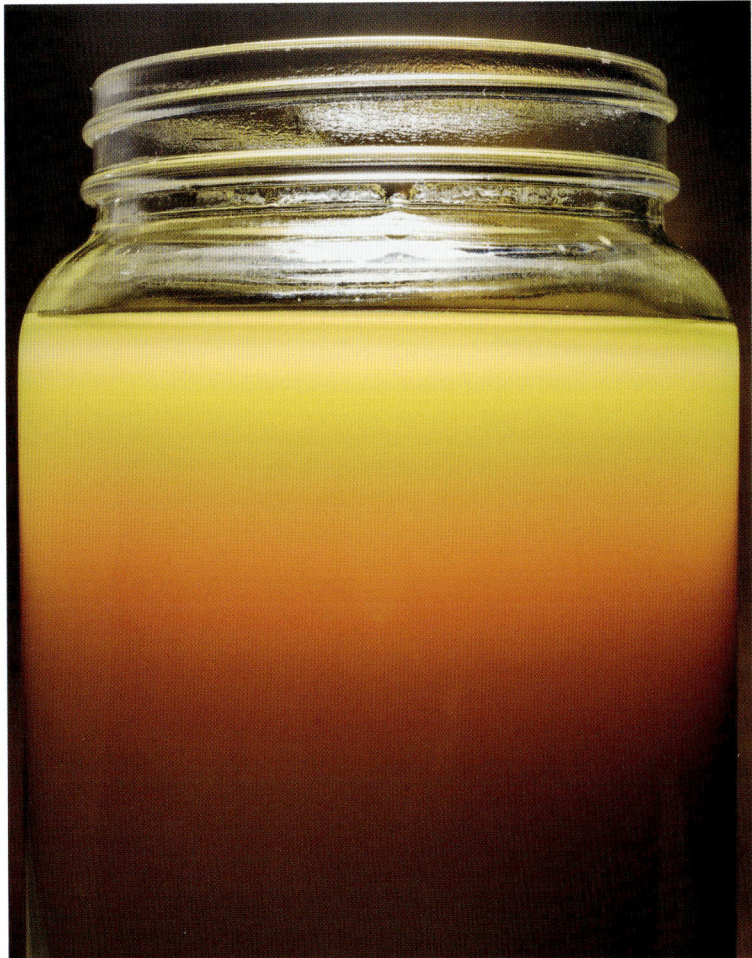

Per 1 cup | Calories: 60 | Fat: 2g | Carbs: 8g | Fiber: 4g | Protein: 6g

RECIPES BY EFFORT

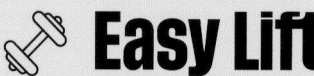 Easy Lift

- Acorn Squash Breakfast Bowls
- Anything-But-Basic Avo Toast
- Buckwheat & Berry Parfaits
- Drew's Famous Smoothie
- Lentil Waffle Mix (and Pancakes, Too!)
- Peppermint Hot Chocolate
- Protein Matcha Latte
- Savory Oats & Lentil Porridge
- Shakshuka-Style Tofu Scramble
- Chickpea Pozole
- Creamy Alfredo Pasta
- Classic Chi*ken Salad
- Lentil Sloppy Joes
- Kimchi Ginger Poke Bowl
- The Big (Kale) Salad with Tempeh "Croutons"
- Sriracha Mayo
- Vegan Hand Rolls
- Creamy Ziti & Broccoli
- Seitan Fajitas
- Vegan Sour Cream
- Sweet Crispy Treats
- Mini Energy Muffins
- Seasoned Kale Chips
- Tofu Chicharrones
- Crispy Air-Fried Tofu Nuggets
- Stacked Nacho Fries
- Tempeh Buffalo Dip
- Apple Chocolate "Nachos"
- Black Bean Brownies
- Chickpea Choco-Chip Cookies
- Oatmeal-Raisin Power Cookies
- PB&J Swirl Nice Cream
- Power-Packed Rice Pudding
- Sweet Potato Pie Bars
- Packed Pizza Dough
- Cashew Parm
- TVP MVP
- Fire Veggies
- Grains for Days
- Lentils on Lock
- Vegan Whip
- Liquid Gold

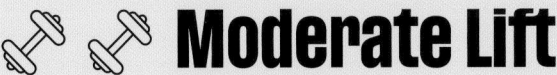
Moderate Lift

- A Weekend Jewish Deli Breakfast
- Sweet Bean–Stuffed French Toast
- Veggie & Pesto Frittata
- Chorizo Burrito Bowl
- Creamy Mac and Cheese
- Mushroom & Lentil Bolognese
- Red Lentil Curry
- Seitan Reuben Bowl
- Three-Bean Chili
- Bodega Chopped Cheese
- I'm from Philly Cheesesteak
- Plant-Powered Bean & Chile Burritos
- Fully Loaded Crunchy Wrap
- Loaded Cobb Salad
- Med Chopped Salad
- Lentil Shepherd's Pie
- Lupini Pot Pie
- Vegan Candy Bar Bites
- Air Fryer Artichoke Wings with Lemony Hummus Dip
- Pizza Bites
- Gooey Cinnamon Rolls
- Pumpkin Spice Mousse with Maple Brittle
- Silky Caramel Flan
- Strawberry Protein Pops
- Bagels with a Boost
- Bread of Champions
- DIY Seitan
- Best Basic Beans

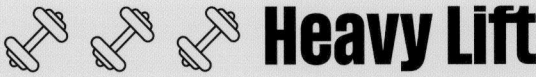
Heavy Lift

- Fried No-Chick Deluxe
- Vegan Big Stack
- Protein-Packed Lasagna
- Vegan Pernil Plate
- Coco-licious Cream Pie
- Chocolate Silk Pie

RECIPES BY TIME

⏱ Under 30 Minutes

Anything-But-Basic Avo Toast
Buckwheat & Berry Parfaits
Drew's Famous Smoothie
Peppermint Hot Chocolate
Protein Matcha Latte
Savory Oats & Lentil Porridge
Shakshuka-Style Tofu Scramble
Chickpea Pozole
Chorizo Burrito Bowl
Creamy Alfredo Pasta
Creamy Mac and Cheese
Red Lentil Curry
Three-Bean Chili
Bodega Chopped Cheese
Classic Chi*ken Salad
I'm from Philly Cheesesteak
Lentil Sloppy Joes
Fully Loaded Crunchy Wrap
Loaded Cobb Salad
Med Chopped Salad
The Big (Kale) Salad with Tempeh "Croutons"
Vegan Hand Rolls

Sriracha Mayo
Seitan Fajitas
Vegan Sour Cream
Sweet Crispy Treats
Mini Energy Muffins
Seasoned Kale Chips
Air Fryer Artichoke Wings with Lemony Hummus Dip
Crispy Air-Fried Tofu Nuggets
Stacked Nacho Fries
Tempeh Buffalo Dip
Apple Chocolate "Nachos"
Black Bean Brownies
Chickpea Choco-Chip Cookies
Oatmeal-Raisin Power Cookies
Packed Pizza Dough
Cashew Parm
TVP MVP
Fire Veggies
Grains for Days
Lentils on Lock
Vegan Whip
Liquid Gold

238 Eat to Hustle

30 to 60 minutes

Sweet Bean–Stuffed French Toast
Veggie & Pesto Frittata
Mushroom & Lentil Bolegnese
Plant-Powered Bean & Chile Burritos
Vegan Big Stack
Lentil Shepherd's Pie
Lupini Pot Pie

Protein-Packed Lasagna
Vegan Pernil Plate
Pizza Bites
Sweet Potato Pie Bars
Bagels with a Boost
Fire Veggies
Grains for Days

   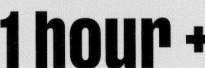

A Weekend Jewish Deli Breakfast
Acorn Squash Breakfast Bowls
Lentil Waffle Mix (and Pancakes, Too!)
Seitan Reuben Bowl
Fried No-Chick Deluxe
Kimchi Ginger Poke Bowl
Creamy Ziti & Broccoli
Tofu Chicharrones
Vegan Candy Bar Bites
Coco-licious Cream Pie
Gooey Cinnamon Rolls

PB&J Swirl Nice Cream
Power-Packed Rice Pudding
Pumpkin Spice Mousse with Maple Brittle
Chocolate Silk Pie
Silky Caramel Flan
Strawberry Protein Pops
Bread of Champions
DIY Seitan
Best Basic Beans
Vegan Whip

SOURCES

Understanding Macros (page 14)

Protein

Cintineo, Harry P., et al. "Effects of Protein Supplementation on Performance and Recovery in Resistance and Endurance Training." *Frontiers in Nutrition,* vol. 5, no. 83, 11 Sept. 2018, https://pmc.ncbi.nlm.nih.gov/articles/PMC6142015.

Escobar, Kurt A., et al. "Protein Applications in Sports Nutrition — Part II." *Strength & Conditioning Journal,* vol. 37, no. 3, June 2015, pp. 22–34, https://journals.lww.com/nsca-scj/fulltext/2015/06000/protein_applications_in_sports_nutrition_part_ii_.3.aspx.

Torre-Villalvazo, Iván, et al. "Protein Intake and Amino Acid Supplementation Regulate Exercise Recovery and Performance through the Modulation of MTOR, AMPK, FGF21, and Immunity." *Nutrition Research,* vol. 72, Dec. 2019, pp. 1–17, https://doi.org/10.1016/j.nutres.2019.06.006.

Carbohydrates

International Society of Sports Nutrition. "International Society of Sports Nutrition Position Stand: Nutrient Timing." *Journal of the International Society of Sports Nutrition,* vol. 14, no. 1, 2017, https://pubmed.ncbi.nlm.nih.gov/28919842.

Jeukendrup, A. E. "Carbohydrate intake during exercise and performance." *Nutrition,* vol. 21, no. 3, 2005, pp. 315–318. https://pubmed.ncbi.nlm.nih.gov/15212750.

Kanter, Mitch. "High-Quality Carbohydrates and Physical Performance." *Nutrition Today,* vol. 53, no. 1, 2018, pp. 35–39, https://pmc.ncbi.nlm.nih.gov/articles/PMC5794245.

Fats

Chianese, Rosanna, et al. "Impact of Dietary Fats on Brain Functions." *Current Neuropharmacology,* vol. 16, no. 7, 1 Aug. 2018, p. 1059, https://pmc.ncbi.nlm.nih.gov/articles/PMC6120115.

Clarke, Lionele. "Health Benefits of Incorporating Unsaturated Fats in Diet." *African Journal of Food Science and Technology,* vol. 14, no. 7, 2023, p. 4, https://www.interesjournals.org/articles/health-benefits-of-incorporating-unsaturated-fats-in-diet-101179.html.

Meijaard, Erik, et al. "Dietary Fats, Human Nutrition and the Environment: Balance and Sustainability." *Frontiers in Nutrition,* vol. 9, no. 1, 25 Apr. 2022, p. 878644, https://pubmed.ncbi.nlm.nih.gov/35548568.

Fiber

Barber, Thomas M., et al. "The Health Benefits of Dietary Fibre." *Nutrients,* vol. 12, no. 10, 21 Oct. 2020, p. 3209, https://pmc.ncbi.nlm.nih.gov/articles/PMC7589116.

Fu, Jiongxing, et al. "Dietary Fiber Intake and Gut Microbiota in Human Health." *Microorganisms,* vol. 10, no. 12, 18 Dec. 2022, p. 2507, https://pmc.ncbi.nlm.nih.gov/articles/PMC9787832.

Harvard T.H. Chan School of Public Health. "Fiber." The Nutrition Source, 2023, https://nutritionsource.hsph.harvard.edu/carbohydrates/fiber.

How to Read a Nutrition Label (page 15)

Protein

Nunes, Everson A., et al. "Systematic Review and Meta-Analysis of Protein Intake to Support Muscle Mass and Function in Healthy Adults." *Journal of Cachexia, Sarcopenia and Muscle,* vol. 13, no. 2, 20 Feb. 2022, pp. 795– 810, https://pubmed.ncbi.nlm.nih.gov/35187864.

Wempen, Kristi. "Are You Getting Too Much Protein?" www.mayoclinichealthsystem.org, 29 Apr. 2022, https://www.mayoclinichealthsystem.org/hometown-health/speaking-of-health/are-you-getting-too-much-protein.

Carbs & Fiber

American Heart Association. "Get to Know Grains: Why You Need Them, and What to Look For." www.heart.org, 2016, https://www.heart.org/en/healthy-living/healthy-eating/eat-smart/nutrition-basics/whole-grains-refined-grains-and-dietary-fiber.

Corliss, Julie. "How a Fiber-Rich Diet Promotes Heart Health." Harvard Health, 1 Aug. 2022, https://www.health.harvard.edu/heart-health/how-a-fiber-rich-diet-promotes-heart-health.

Benisi-Kohansal, Sanaz, et al. "Whole-Grain Intake and Mortality from All Causes, Cardiovascular Disease, and Cancer: A Systematic Review and Dose-Response Meta-Analysis of Prospective Cohort Studies." *Advances in Nutrition,* vol. 7, no. 6, 15 Nov. 2016, pp. 1052–1065, https://pubmed.ncbi.nlm.nih.gov/28140323.

Pandey, Manorama, et al. "Effectiveness of High-Fiber, Plant-Based Diets in Reducing Cardiovascular Risk Factors among Middle-Aged and Older Adults: A Systematic Review." Cureus, 24 Aug. 2024, https://pubmed.ncbi.nlm.nih.gov/39314563.

Fats

Harvard Health Publishing. "The Truth about Fats: The Good, the Bad, and the In-Between." Harvard Health, Harvard Medical School, 12 Apr. 2022, https://www.health.harvard.edu/staying-healthy/the-truth-about-fats-bad-and-good.

Juul, Filippa, et al. "Ultra-Processed Foods and Cardiovascular Diseases: Potential Mechanisms of Action." *Advances in Nutrition,* vol. 12, no. 5, 2021, https://www.sciencedirect.com/science/article/pii/S2161831322004628.

World Health Organization. "Trans Fat." www.who.int, 24 Jan. 2024, https://www.who.int/news-room/fact-sheets/detail/trans-fat.

The Protein Principle (page 16)

Morton, Robert W., et al. "A Systematic Review, Meta-Analysis and Meta-Regression of the Effect of Protein Supplementation on Resistance Training-Induced Gains in Muscle Mass and Strength in Healthy Adults." *Nutrition Reviews,* vol. 78, no. 7, 1 July 2020, pp. 524– 539. https://pubmed.ncbi.nlm.nih.gov/28698222.

Phillips, Stuart M., et al. "Dietary Protein for Athletes: From Requirements to Metabolic Advantage." *Applied Physiology, Nutrition, and Metabolism,* vol. 44, no. 6, June 2019, pp. 715– 722. https://pubmed.ncbi.nlm.nih.gov/17213878.

Landi, Francesco, et al. "Protein Intake and Muscle Health in Old Age: From Biological Plausibility to Clinical Evidence." *Nutrients,* vol. 8, no. 5, 14 May 2016, article 295, https://pubmed.ncbi.nlm.nih.gov/27187465.

Witard, Oliver C., et al. "Protein Considerations for Optimising Skeletal Muscle Mass in Healthy Young and Older Adults." *Nutrients,* vol. 12, no. 10, 18 Oct. 2020, 3109. https://pubmed.ncbi.nlm.nih.gov/27023595.

Mayo Clinic Health System. "Are You Getting Too Much Protein?" *Hometown Health: Speaking of Health*, 27 Nov. 2024, www.mayoclinichealthsystem.org/hometown-health/speaking-of-health/are-you-getting-too-much-protein.

Layman, Donald K. "Impacts of Protein Quantity and Distribution on Body Composition." *Frontiers in Nutrition,* vol. 11, 3 May 2024, article 1388986, https://pmc.ncbi.nlm.nih.gov/articles/PMC11099237.

Fact Check: Vegan Myths Busted (page 24)

MYTH: Vegans Don't Get Enough Protein

Askow, Andrew T, et al. "Impact of Vegan Diets on Resistance Exercise-Mediated Myofibrillar Protein Synthesis in Healthy Young Males and Females: A Randomized Controlled Trial." Medicine & Science in Sports & Exercise, 4 Apr. 2025, https://pubmed.ncbi.nlm.nih.gov/40197715.

Hevia-Larraín, Victoria, et al. "High-Protein Plant-Based Diet versus a Protein-Matched Omnivorous Diet to Support Resistance Training Adaptations: A Comparison between Habitual Vegans and Omnivores." Sports Medicine, vol. 51, no. 6, 18 Feb. 2021, https://pubmed.ncbi.nlm.nih.gov/33599941.

Monteyne, Alistair J., et al. "Vegan and Omnivorous High Protein Diets Support Comparable Daily Myofibrillar Protein Synthesis Rates and Skeletal Muscle Hypertrophy in Young Adults." The Journal of Nutrition, vol. 153, no. 6, Feb. 2023, https://pubmed.ncbi.nlm.nih.gov/36822394.

MYTH: Soy Will Mess with Your Hormones

Reed, Katharine E., et al. "Neither Soy nor Isoflavone Intake Affects Male Reproductive Hormones: An Expanded and Updated Meta-Analysis of Clinical Studies." Reproductive Toxicology, vol. 100, Mar. 2021, pp. 60–67, https://pubmed.ncbi.nlm.nih.gov/33383165.

MYTH: Carbs Are the Enemy

Martinez, Taylor M., et al. "Therapeutic Potential of Various Plant-Based Fibers to Improve Energy Homeostasis via the Gut Microbiota." Nutrients, vol. 13, no. 10, 29 Sept. 2021, p. 3470, https://pubmed.ncbi.nlm.nih.gov/34684471.

Tan, Denise, et al. "New Metrics of Dietary Carbohydrate Quality." Current Opinion in Clinical Nutrition and Metabolic Care, vol. 26, no. 4, 19 May 2023, pp. 358–363, https://pubmed.ncbi.nlm.nih.gov/37249917.

MYTH: Vegans Can't Get Enough Nutrients

B_{12}

Fernandes, Sávio, et al. "Exploring Vitamin B_{12} Supplementation in the Vegan Population: A Scoping Review of the Evidence." Nutrients, vol. 16, no. 10, 1 Jan. 2024, p. 1442, https://pubmed.ncbi.nlm.nih.gov/38794680.

Hannibal, Luciana, et al. "Vitamin B_{12} Status and Supplementation in Plant-Based Diets." Food and Nutrition Bulletin, vol. 45, no. 1_suppl, 1 June 2024, pp. S58–S66, https://pubmed.ncbi.nlm.nih.gov/38987876.

Vitamin D

Cui, A., Zhang, T., Xiao, P., Fan, Z., Wang, H., and Zhuang, Y. "Prevalence, Trend, and Predictor Analyses of Vitamin D Deficiency in the U.S. Population, 2001–2018." Frontiers in Nutrition, vol. 10, 2023, article 1070808, https://pubmed.ncbi.nlm.nih.gov/36263304.

Lee, Yu-Mi, et al. "Can Current Recommendations on Sun Exposure Sufficiently Increase Serum Vitamin D Level?: One-Month Randomized Clinical Trial." Journal of Korean Medical Science, vol. 35, no. 8, 22 Jan. 2020, https://pubmed.ncbi.nlm.nih.gov/32103645.

Creatine

Chilibeck, Philip, et al. "Effect of Creatine Supplementation during Resistance Training on Lean Tissue Mass and Muscular Strength in Older Adults: A Meta-Analysis." Open Access Journal of Sports Medicine, vol. Volume 8, Nov. 2017, pp. 213–226, https://pubmed.ncbi.nlm.nih.gov/29138605.

dos Santos, Ellem Eduarda Pinheiro, et al. "Efficacy of Creatine Supplementation Combined with Resistance Training on Muscle Strength and Muscle Mass in Older Females: A Systematic Review and Meta-Analysis." Nutrients, vol. 13, no. 11, 24 Oct. 2021, p. 3757, https://pmc.ncbi.nlm.nih.gov/articles/PMC8619193.

Gualano, Bruno, et al. "Creatine Supplementation in the Aging Population: Effects on Skeletal Muscle, Bone and Brain." Amino Acids, vol. 48, no. 8, 23 Apr. 2016, pp. 1793–1805, https://pubmed.ncbi.nlm.nih.gov/27108136.

Other Nutrients

Neufingerl, Nicole, and Ans Eilander. "Nutrient Intake and Status in Adults Consuming Plant-Based Diets Compared to Meat-Eaters: A Systematic Review." Nutrients, vol. 14, no. 1, 23 Dec. 2021, p. 29, https://pubmed.ncbi.nlm.nih.gov/35010904.

Vitale, Kenneth, and Shawn Hueglin. "Update on Vegetarian and Vegan Athletes: A Review." The Journal of Physical Fitness and Sports Medicine, vol. 10, no. 1, 25 Jan. 2021, pp. 1–11, https://doaj.org/article/2d7f20027f644c52bc14e82309e8fb65.

Health Matters (page 30)

Type 1 Diabetes

Bronczek, Gabriela Alves, et al. "Resistance Training Improves Beta Cell Glucose Sensing and Survival in Diabetic Models." *International Journal of Molecular Sciences,* vol. 23, no. 16, 2022, article 9427, https://doi.org/10.3390/ijms23169427.

Li, Jiahao, et al. "Effects of Resistance Training on Insulin Sensitivity in the Elderly: A Meta-Analysis of Randomized Controlled Trials." *Journal of Exercise Science & Fitness,* vol. 19, no. 4, 2021, pp. 241–251, https://doi.org/10.1016/j.jesf.2021.08.002.

Perimenopausal/Menopausal

Ouyang, Y., Huang, F., Zhang, X., Li, L., Zhang, B., Wang, Z., and Wang, H. "Association of Dietary Protein Intake with Muscle Mass in Elderly Chinese: A Cross-Sectional Study." *Nutrients,* vol. 14, no. 23, 2022, article 5130, https://pubmed.ncbi.nlm.nih.gov/36501159.

Kędzia, Gabriela, et al. "Impact of Dietary Protein on Osteoporosis Development." *Nutrients,* vol. 15, no. 21, 28 Oct. 2023, pp. 4581– 4581, https://pmc.ncbi.nlm.nih.gov/articles/PMC10649897.

Weaver, Ashley A, et al. "Effect of Dietary Protein Intake on Bone Mineral Density and Fracture Incidence in Older Adults in the Health, Aging, and Body Composition Study." *The Journals of Gerontology: Series A,* vol. 76, no. 12, 3 Mar. 2021, pp. 2213–2222, https://pubmed.ncbi.nlm.nih.gov/33677533/.

Inflammation and Recovery

Escalante-Araiza, Fabiola, et al. "The Effect of Plant-Based Diets on Meta-Inflammation and Associated Cardiometabolic Disorders: A Review." Nutrition Reviews, 27 Apr. 2022, https://pubmed.ncbi.nlm.nih.gov/35475468.

Kostovcikova, Klara, et al. "Diet Rich in Animal Protein Promotes Pro-Inflammatory Macrophage Response and Exacerbates Colitis in Mice." *Frontiers in Immunology,* vol. 10, 2019, p. 919, https://pubmed.ncbi.nlm.nih.gov/31105710.

Pourreza, Sanaz, et al. "Association of Plant-Based Diet Index with Inflammatory Markers and Sleep Quality in Overweight and Obese Female Adults: A Cross-Sectional Study." *International Journal of Clinical Practice,* vol. 75, no. 9, 26 June 2021, https://pubmed.ncbi.nlm.nih.gov/34081826.

ACKNOW-
LEDG-
MENTS

Writing a cookbook is a team sport — and luckily, I've got an all-star roster.

To Casey Elsass: Thank you for bringing big ideas and bold flavor to every part of this process. From dreaming up vegan twists to showing up with taste-test treats in hand, you made my kitchen a canvas for creativity. You challenged me to push the boundaries and stay rooted in joy. This book is better because of your spark.

To Dalina Soto: Thank you for grounding this book in science and no-nonsense clarity. You're a constant reminder that fueling smart doesn't mean abandoning where we come from or what we love to eat.

To my editor, Raquel Pelzel: Thank you for believing in this book from day one! Your editorial guidance made the pages sharper, the stories more personal, and the recipes even stronger. Thank you for pushing this vision across the finish line with love and precision.

To the dream team behind the camera: Johnny Miller, Rebecca Jurkevich, and Sarah Smart — you brought this book to life with incredible energy, talent, and vision. Every photo, every spread, every bite looks the way it does because of your brilliance. And huge thanks to Debbie Kim, Brett Statman, and Vicky Novak for keeping the wheels turning on set and making it all look easy.

To my chief of staff, Sydney Scherer: Thank you for being the center that keeps everything moving. From logistics to launch plans, your fingerprints are on every part of this project — and I couldn't have done it without you!

To Tiffanie Garrett-Reid: From shoot days to set days, your creativity has been part of this journey for over a decade. Thank you for always knowing when I needed a touch-up, a cat-eye, or just a breath. This book wouldn't shine the same without you.

To Karlee Rotoly: Thank you for stress-testing these recipes like a pro. If it made it into this book, it passed the Karlee test — and that says everything.

To the amazing team at Voracious: Mike Szczerban, thank you for your leadership and vision. Morgan James, you are an editorial rockstar. Jules Horbachevsky and Jess Chun, thank you for getting this book out into the world with heart and hustle. Rad Works and Kirin Diemont, this book looks so good because of you. And Sally Kim: I'll see you on the bike!

To my community: Thank you for trusting me to be part of your wellness journey. You fuel up so you can move through the world with power — and I'm honored to be part of that ritual. Whether you are new to the wolfpack, or an OG, I'm glad you're rocking with me. Your stories, your resilience, and your joy are what keep me pushing forward. This book is for you, baby.

To my incredible colleagues and friends at Peloton: Thank you for letting me bring my full self to work every day. I'm deeply proud of what we've built together. You remind me constantly that superheroes are real.

To the farmers and farm workers: The stewards of the earth, your labor, often unseen and underappreciated, is the foundation upon which wellness begins.

And most of all, to my family:

To my mom: Thank you for filling our home with Cuban flavor and showing me how to trust my intuition in the kitchen. I'll never forget how you cooked dinner at 7 a.m. before a full day as a doctor helping patients and raising two babies.

To my dad: My rhythm in kitchen dance parties and love of Puerto Rican sazón — it all started with you.

To my sister, Margaret: Thank you for inspiring my love of plant-based food — and proving just how good it can be.

To my husband, Drew: Thank you for taste-testing, cheering, and holding it down at home while I built this thing. You're my ride-or-die, always. Keeping me fed is a full time job.

And to Athena and Atlas: This book is a love letter to all the kitchen memories we've already had — and the many more to come.

Fuel with purpose. Hustle with heart.

INDEX

A

acorn squash
   Acorn Squash Breakfast Bowls, 40–41
   roasting, 227
agave syrup, 20, 45
Air Fryer Artichoke Wings with Lemony Hummus Dip, 166–167
Air-Fried Tofu Nuggets, 168–169
alcaparrado, 150
Alfredo sauce, 70–71
amino acids, 25, 68
Anything-but-Basic Avo Toast, 42–45
Apple Chocolate "Nachos," 178–179
Arroz Con Gandules (Rice with Pigeon Peas), 150
artichokes, 166–167
asparagus, 226
avocado oil, 20
avocados
   Anything-but-Basic Avo Toast, 42–45
   Chorizo Burrito Bowl, 68–69

B

bagels
   Bagels with a Boost, 211–213
   Weekend Jewish Deli Breakfast, 37–39
baking, 20
baking sheets, 23
bananas
   Acorn Squash Breakfast Bowls, 40–41
   PB&J Swirl Nice Cream, 190–191
bars
   Sweet Potato Pie Bars, 204–205
   Vegan Candy Bar Bites, 162–163
basil pesto, 62–63
basmati rice, 230
Bast Basic Beans, 232
batters, 23
beans, 232
   Bagels with a Boost, 211–213
   Black Bean Brownies, 180–181
   cannellini beans, 232
   Chickpea Pozole, 67
   Chorizo Burrito Bowl, 68–69
   Creamy Alfredo Pasta, 70–71
   kidney beans, 232
   Loaded Cobb Salad, 118–120
   Med Chopped Salad, 123
   Oatmeal-Raisin Power Cookies, 188–189
   overview, 19
   pinto beans, 80–81, 232
   Plant-Powered Bean & Chile Burritos, 100–103
   refried, 100–103
   as source of protein, 25
   soy beans, 27, 88–89
   Sweet Bean–Stuffed French Toast, 60–61
   Three-Bean Chili, 80–81
béchamel, 141
beets, 226
bell peppers, 226
berries, 46–47, 156–157, 202–203
Best Basic Beans, 232
beverages
   Drew's Famous Smoothie, 48–49
   Peppermint Hot Chocolate, 52–53
   Protein Matcha Latte, 54–55
   protein powder and, 20
Big (Kale) Salad with Tempeh "Croutons', 124–127
bites
   Pizza Bites, 170–171
   Vegan Candy Bar Bites, 162–163
black beans
   Black Bean Brownies, 180–181
   Three-Bean Chili, 80–81
black lentils, 233
blenders, 23
blood sugar
   controlling, 14
   spikes in, 11, 30
   type 1 diabetes and, 30
blueberries, 156–157
Bodega Chopped Cheese, 86–87
bowls
   Acorn Squash Breakfast Bowls, 40–41
   Chorizo Burrito Bowl, 68–69
   Kimchi Ginger Poke Bowl, 114–117
   as kitchen utensil, 23
   Seitan Reuben Bowl, 78–79
braises, Dutch oven and, 23

breads
- Anything-but-Basic Avo Toast, 42–45
- Bagels with a Boost, 211–213
- Bodega Chopped Cheese, 86–87
- Bread of Champions, 214–216
- Classic Chi*ken Salad, 88–89
- Fried No-chick Deluxe, 90–93
- I'm From Philly Cheesesteak, 94–97
- Lentil Sloppy Joes, 98–99
- rye, 78–79
- Seitan Reuben Bowl, 78–79
- Sweet Bean–Stuffed French Toast, 60–61
- Weekend Jewish Deli Breakfast, 37–39

breakfast recipes
- Acorn Squash Breakfast Bowls, 40–41
- Anything-but-Basic Avo Toast, 42–45
- Buckwheat & Berry Parfaits, 46–47
- Drew's Famous Smoothie, 48–49
- Lentil Waffle Mix (and Pancakes, Too!), 50–51
- overview, 33
- Peppermint Hot Chocolate, 52–53
- Protein Matcha Latte, 54–55
- Savory Oats & Lentil Porridge, 56–57
- Shakshuka-style Tofu Scramble, 58–59
- Sweet Bean–Stuffed French Toast, 60–61
- Vegan Whitefish Salad, 38–39
- Veggie & Pesto Frittata, 62–63
- Weekend Jewish Deli Breakfast, 37–39

brittle, 194–195

broccoli
- Creamy Ziti & Broccoli, 134–135
- roasting, 226

brown lentils, 233
brown rice, 68, 230
brownies, 180–181
Brussel sprouts, 226

buckwheat
- Buckwheat & Berry Parfaits, 46–47
- cooking time, 230

Buffalo sauce, 174
bulgur, 231

burgers
- Bodega Chopped Cheese, 86–87
- Fried No-chick Deluxe, 90–93
- Lentil Sloppy Joes, 98–99
- Vegan Big Stack, 104–107

burritos
- Chorizo Burrito Bowl, 68–69
- Plant-Powered Bean & Chile Burritos, 100–103

butter, 20
butternut squash, roasting, 227

C

calories, 15
candy bars, 162–163
cannellini beans, 232
- Creamy Alfredo Pasta, 70–71
- Oatmeal-Raisin Power Cookies, 188–189

caramel
- Silky Caramel Flan, 200–201
- Vegan Candy Bar Bites, 162–163

carbohydrates
- myth regarding, 27
- in nutrition labels, 15
- overview, 14

carrots
- carrot lox, 37
- roasting, 226

cashews
- Cashew Parm, 220–221
- cheese whiz, 96
- Creamy Mac And Cheese, 72–73
- vegan queso, 100

cast-iron skillets, 23

cauliflower
- Lentil Shepherd's Pie, 136–137
- roasting, 226

Chanterelle mushrooms, roasting, 226

cheese
- Bodega Chopped Cheese, 86–87
- cheese whiz, 96
- Fully Loaded Crunchy Wrap, 108–111
- I'm From Philly Cheesesteak, 94–97
- Protein-Packed Lasagna, 140–143
- Tempeh Buffalo Dip, 174
- Vegan Big Stack, 104–107
- vegan queso, 100

chef's knives, 23
chicharron, 160–161
chickpeas, 232
- Air Fryer Artichoke Wings with Lemony Hummus Dip, 166–167
- Anything-but-Basic Avo Toast, 45
- breadcrumbs, 134–135
- Chickpea Choco-Chip Cookies, 182–183
- Chickpea Pozole, 67
- Classic Chi*ken Salad, 88–89
- Creamy Ziti & Broccoli, 134–135
- Veggie & Pesto Frittata, 62–63

chili, 80–81
chilies, 100–103
chips, 158–159

chocolate
- Apple Chocolate "Nachos," 178–179
- Black Bean Brownies, 180–181
- Chickpea Choco-Chip Cookies, 182–183

Chocolate
  Silk Pie, 196, 198–199
  Mini Energy Muffins, 156–157
  Peppermint Hot Chocolate, 52–53
  Vegan
    Candy Bar Bites, 162–163
Chorizo Burrito Bowl, 68–69
cinnamon rolls, 186–187
Classic Chi*ken Salad, 88–89
cobb salad, 118–120
Coco-licious Cream Pie, 184–185
coconut milk, 202–203
coconut oil, 20, 234
coconut sugar, 20
complicated recipes, 13, 237
cookies
  Chickpea Choco-Chip Cookies, 182–183
  Oatmeal-Raisin Power Cookies, 188–189
cooking, 231
  grains, 228
  listening to music while, 13
  oils and, 20
  recipe features, 13
  vegetables, 226–227
couscous, 231
crackers, graham, 204–205
cream pie, 184–185
Creamy Alfredo Pasta, 70–71
Creamy Mac And Cheese, 72–73
Creamy Ziti & Broccoli, 134–135
creatine, 28
Cremini mushrooms, roasting, 227
Crispy Air-Fried Tofu Nuggets, 168–169
croutons, 124–127
crust
  Chocolate Silk Pie, 198–199
  Lupini Pot Pie, 138–139
  Sweet
    Potato Pie Bars, 204–205
cumin, 20
curry, 76–77

D

dairy, plant-based, 20
dates
  Lentil Waffle Mix (and Pancakes, Too!), 50–51
  Vegan
    Candy Bar Bites, 162–163
delicata squash, roasting, 227
desserts
  Apple Chocolate "Nachos," 178–179
  Black Bean Brownies, 180–181
  Buckwheat & Berry Parfaits, 46–47
  Chickpea Choco-Chip Cookies, 182–183
  Chocolate
    Silk Pie, 196, 198–199
  Coco-licious Cream Pie, 184–185
  Gooey
    Cinnamon Rolls, 186–187
  Mini Energy Muffins, 156–157
  Oatmeal-Raisin Power Cookies, 188–189
  PB&J
    Swirl Nice Cream, 190–191
  Power-Packed Rice Pudding, 192–193
  Pumpkin Spice Mousse with Maple Brittle, 194–195
  Silky Caramel Flan, 200–201
  Strawberry
    Protein Pops, 202–203
  Sweet Crispy Treats, 154–155
  Sweet
    Potato Pie Bars, 204–205
  Vegan
    Candy Bar Bites, 162–163
diabetes, type 1, 30
dinner recipes
  Arroz Con Gandules (Rice with Pigeon Peas), 150
  Big (Kale) Salad with Tempeh "Croutons', 124–127
  Creamy
    Ziti & Broccoli, 134–135
  Kimchi Ginger Poke Bowl, 114–117
  Lentil Shepherd's Pie, 136–137
  Loaded Cobb Salad, 118–120
  Lupini Pot Pie, 138–139
  Maduros (Fried Sweet Plantains), 151
  Med Chopped Salad, 123
  Protein-Packed Lasagna, 140–143
  Seitan Fajitas, 144–147
  Vegan Hand Rolls, 128–129
  Vegan Pernil Plate, 148–150
dips
  Air Fryer Artichoke Wings with Lemony
    Hummus Dip, 166–167
  Tempeh Buffalo Dip, 174
DIY Seitan, 222–223
dough
  Chocolate Silk Pie, 198–199
  Gooey
    Cinnamon Rolls, 186–187
  Packed Pizza Dough, 218–219
  Sweet
    Potato Pie Bars, 204–205
dressings
  edamame, 114, 116
  ginger, 114, 116
  hummus, 123
  Sriracha Mayo, 130–131
  tahini, 124–127
  Thousand Island dressing, 78
  Tofu Ranch dressing, 121–122
Drew's Famous Smoothie, 48–49
drinks. *See* beverages
Dumbbell Scores, 13
Dutch ovens, 23

E

easy recipes, 13, 236
eating with intention, 11
edamame

Anything-but-Basic Avo Toast, 42–45
dressing, 114, 116
eggplant, 226
environmental impact, reducing with plant-based diets, 13
exercise, 30–31
extra-firm tofu, 19
    Crispy Air-Fried Tofu Nuggets, 168–169
    Kimchi Ginger Poke Bowl, 114–117
    Protein-Packed Lasagna, 140–143
    Red Lentil Curry, 76–77
    Tofu Chicharrones, 160–161

F

fajitas, 144–147
farro, 231
fats, 14–15, 20
fennel, 226
fiber
    complex carbohydrates and, 27
    in nutrition labels, 15
    overview, 14
    in rice, 68
Fire Veggies, 225–227
firm tofu, 19
flan, 200–201
food processors, 23
French green lentils, 233
French toast, 60–61
Fried No-chick Deluxe, 90–93
Fried Sweet Plantains, 151
fries, 172–173
frittata, 62–63
Fully Loaded Crunchy Wrap, 108–111

G

garlic, 226
ginger
    dressings, 114, 116
    Kimchi Ginger Poke Bowl, 114–117
glazes, 186–187
Gooey Cinnamon Rolls, 186–187
graham crackers, 204–205
grains, 229–231
Grains for Days, 229
granola, 40–41
Greek yogurt, 20
    Acorn Squash Breakfast Bowls, 40–41
    Apple Chocolate "Nachos," 178–179
    Buckwheat & Berry Parfaits, 46–47
    Classic Chi*ken Salad, 88–89
    Creamy Ziti & Broccoli, 134–135
    Gooey Cinnamon Rolls, 186–187
    Lentil Shepherd's Pie, 136–137
    Med Chopped Salad, 123
    Pumpkin Spice Mousse with Maple Brittle, 194–195
    Silky Caramel Flan, 200–201
    Tempeh Buffalo Dip, 174
    tofu cream cheese, 37–39
grocery shopping, 25

H

health conditions
    exercise, recovering from, 31
    inflammation, 31
    menopause, 31
    overview, 30–31
    perimenopause, 31
    type 1 diabetes, 30
hearts of palms, 38
hoagie rolls
    Bodega Chopped Cheese, 86–87
    I'm From Philly Cheesesteak, 94–97
honey, 20
hormones, myth regarding, 27
hot chocolate, 52–53
hummus
    Air Fryer Artichoke Wings with Lemony Hummus Dip, 166–167
    Med Chopped Salad, 123

I

ice cream
    PB&J Swirl Nice Cream, 190–191
    Strawberry Protein Pops, 202–203
I'm From Philly Cheesesteak, 94–97
inflammation, 31
ingredients, 19–20
insulin insensitivity, 30
intentional eating, 11

J

jasmine rice, 230

K

kabocha squash, 227
kale
    Big (Kale) Salad with Tempeh "Croutons', 124–127
    Drew's Famous Smoothie, 48–49
    Seasoned Kale Chips, 158–159
kidney beans, 232
    Sweet Bean–Stuffed French Toast, 60–61
    Three-Bean Chili, 80–81
Kimchi
    Ginger Poke Bowl, 114–117
Kitchen Dance Party music playlist, 13
kitchen utensils, 23
knives, 23
kombu, 232
kosher salt, 20

L

lacinato kale, 124–127
lasagna, 140–143
latte, 54–55
leeks, 226
legumes. *See* beans; chickpeas; lentils
Lemony Hummus Dip, 166–167
lentils, 19
   Big (Kale) Salad with Tempeh "Croutons", 124–127
   black lentils, 233
   brown lentils, 233
   Creamy Mac And Cheese, 72–73
   French green lentils, 233
   Lentil Shepherd's Pie, 136–137
   Lentil Sloppy Joes, 98–99
   Lentil Waffle Mix (and Pancakes, Too!), 50–51
   Lentils on Lock, 233
   Mushroom & Lentil Bolognese, 74–75
   Pizza Bites, 170–171
   Red Lentil Curry, 76–77
   Savory Oats & Lentil Porridge, 56–57
   as source of protein, 25
linguine pasta, 70–71
Liquid Gold, 235
   Arroz Con Gandules (Rice with Pigeon Peas), 150
   Chickpea Pozole, 67
   DIY Seitan, 222–223
   Lentil Shepherd's Pie, 136–137
   Lupini Pot Pie, 138
   Mushroom & Lentil Bolognese, 74–75
   Red Lentil Curry, 76–77
   Savory Oats & Lentil Porridge, 57
   Three-Bean Chili, 80–81
   TVP MVP, 224
liquid sweeteners, 20
Loaded Cobb Salad, 118–120
lunch recipes
   Bodega Chopped Cheese, 86–87
   Chickpea Pozole, 67
   Chorizo Burrito Bowl, 68–69
   Classic Chi*ken Salad, 88–89
   Creamy Alfredo Pasta, 70–71
   Creamy Mac And Cheese, 72–73
   Fried No-chick Deluxe, 90–93
   Fully Loaded Crunchy Wrap, 108–111
   I'm From Philly Cheesesteak, 94–97
   Lentil Sloppy Joes, 98–99
   Mushroom & Lentil Bolognese, 74–75
   Plant-Powered Bean & Chile Burritos, 100–103
   Red Lentil Curry, 76–77
   Seitan Reuben Bowl, 78–79
   Three-Bean Chili, 80–81
   Vegan Big Stack, 104–107
lupini beans, 19
   Chickpea Pozole, 67
   Lupini Pot Pie, 138–139
   Med Chopped Salad, 123

M

mac and cheese, 72–73
macronutrients
   benefits of, 14
   carbohydrates, 14
   fats, 14
   nutrition labels and, 15
   overview, 14–15
   proteins, 14
   in recipes, 13
   tracking, 15
Maduros (Fried Sweet Plantains), 151
mangoes, 48–49
Maple Brittle, 194–195
maple syrup, 20
marshmallows, 154–155
matcha, 54–55
meal planning, 30
measuring cups, 23
Med Chopped Salad, 123
Medjool dates
   Lentil Waffle Mix (and Pancakes, Too!), 50–51
   Vegan Candy Bar Bites, 162–163
menopause, 31
Mini Energy Muffins, 156–157
mixing bowls, 23
moderate recipes, 13, 237
Morel mushrooms, roasting, 227
mousse, 194–195
muffins, 156–157
muscle mass, 30–31
mushrooms
   Mushroom & Lentil Bolognese, 74–75
   roasting, 226–227
music playlists, 13

N

nachos
   Apple Chocolate "Nachos," 178–179
   cheese, 108–111
   Stacked Nacho Fries, 172–173
nonstick skillets, 23
nori sheets, 128–129
nuggets, 168–169
nutrition labels, 15
nutritional yeast, 20
   Bodega Chopped Cheese, 87
   Cashew Parm, 220
   Creamy Alfredo Pasta, 71
   Creamy Mac and Cheese, 72
   Creamy Ziti & Broccoli, 134
   Crispy Air-Fried Tofu Nuggets, 168–169
   DIY Seitan, 222–223
   Liquid Gold, 235
   Seasoned Kale Chips, 158
   Shakshuka-style Tofu Scramble, 58–59
   Tahini Dressing, 125
   tofu ricotta, 142

Veggie & Pesto Frittata, 62
nutritionists, 12, 15
nuts, 220–221

O

oats
   Oatmeal-Raisin Power Cookies, 188–189
   Savory Oats & Lentil Porridge, 56–57
oils, 20
1-hour recipes, 239
onions, 227
oranges, 148–150
oregano, 20
oyster mushrooms, roasting, 227

P

Packed Pizza Dough, 218–219
pancakes, 50–51
paprika, 20
parfait, 28, 46–47
parsnips, 227
pasta, 19
   Creamy Alfredo Pasta, 70–71
   Creamy Mac And Cheese, 72–73
   Creamy Ziti & Broccoli, 134–135
   linguine, 70–71
   Mushroom & Lentil Bolognese, 74–75
   Protein-Packed Lasagna, 140–143
patties, vegan, 104–107
PB&J Swirl Nice Cream, 190–191
Peppermint Hot Chocolate, 52–53
peppers, 226
perimenopause, 31
pernil plate, 148–150
pesto sauce, 62–63
pies
   Chocolate Silk Pie, 198–199
   Coco-licious Cream Pie, 184–185
   Sweet Potato Pie Bars, 204–205
pigeon peas, 150
pinto beans, 80–81, 232
pizza
   Packed Pizza Dough, 218–219
   Pizza Bites, 170–171
plantains, 151
plant-based diets
   benefits of, 11, 25
   environmental impact, reducing with, 13
   myths regarding, 25, 27–28
   protein and, 8, 19
   transitioning into, 8, 11
plant-based milk, 20
   Air Fryer Artichoke Wings with Lemony Hummus Dip, 166–167
   Bagels with a Boost, 211–213
   Bread of Champions, 214–216
   Buckwheat & Berry Parfaits, 46–47
   Coco-licious Cream Pie, 184–185
   Creamy Mac And Cheese, 72–73
   Fried No-chick Deluxe, 90–93
   Fully Loaded Crunchy Wrap, 108–111
   I'm From Philly Cheesesteak, 94–97
   Lentil Waffle Mix (and Pancakes, Too!), 50–51
   Lupini Pot Pie, 138–139
   Mini Energy Muffins, 156–157
   Oatmeal-Raisin Power Cookies, 188–189
   PB&J Swirl Nice Cream, 190–191
   Peppermint Hot Chocolate, 52–53
   Power-Packed Rice Pudding, 192–193
   Protein Matcha Latte, 54–55
   Sweet Bean-Stuffed French Toast, 60–61
   Vegan Whip, 234
plant-based protein powder. *See* protein powder
Plant-Powered Bean & Chile Burritos, 100–103
poke bowl, 114–117
pops, 202–203
porridge, 56–57
Portobello mushrooms, 227
pot pie, 138–139
potatoes
   Lentil Shepherd's Pie, 136–137
   roasting, 227
   Power-Packed Rice Pudding, 192–193
pozole, 67
Protein Matcha Latte, 54–55
protein pops, 202–203
protein powder, 20, 48–49
   Black Bean Brownies, 180–181
   Chickpea Choco-Chip Cookies, 182–183
   Chocolate Silk Pie, 198–199
   Gooey Cinnamon Rolls, 186–187
   Mini Energy Muffins, 156–157
   Oatmeal-Raisin Power Cookies, 188–189
   PB&J Swirl Nice Cream, 190–191
   Peppermint Hot Chocolate, 52–53
   Power-Packed Rice Pudding, 192–193
   Strawberry Protein Pops, 202–203
   Sweet Crispy Treats, 154–155
   Sweet Potato Pie Bars, 204–205
Protein-Packed Lasagna, 140–143
proteins
   legumes as source of, 19, 25

muscle mass, preserving and building, 31
myth regarding vegans and, 25
in nutrition labels, 15
overview, 14
pastas, 19
plant-based diets and, 8
tracking intake of, 15
pudding, 192–193
puff pastry, 138–139
Pumpkin Spice Mousse with Maple Brittle, 194–195

Q

quinoa, 231
   Air Fryer Artichoke Wings with Lemony Hummus Dip, 166–167
   Big (Kale) Salad with Tempeh "Croutons', 124–127
   Three-Bean Chili, 80–81

R

raisins, 188–189
ranch dressing, 121–122
recipes. *See also specific recipes by name*
   complicated, 237
   by cooking time, 238–239
   Dumbbell Scores feature, 13
   easy, 236
   environmental impact, reducing and, 13
   flexibility and, 12
   macronutrient breakdown in, 13
   meal prep and, 12
   moderate, 237
   music playlist and, 13
   Start the Clock feature, 13
Red Lentil Curry, 76–77
refried beans, 100–103
rice
   Arroz Con Gandules (Rice with Pigeon Peas), 150
   basmati rice, 230
   brown rice, 68, 230
   Chorizo Burrito Bowl, 68–69
   cooking, 228
   fiber in, 68
rice (cont.)
   jasmine rice, 230
   Red Lentil Curry, 76–77
   Rice with Pigeon Peas, 150
   Vegan Hand Rolls, 128–129
   wild rice, 230
rice cereal, 154–155
rice pudding, 192–193
ricotta, 141
rigatoni pasta, 74–75
roasting vegetables, 226–227
rutabagas, 227
rye bread, 78–79

S

salads. *See also* dressings
   Big (Kale) Salad with Tempeh "Croutons', 124–127
   Classic Chi*ken Salad, 88–89
   Kimchi Ginger Poke Bowl, 114–117
   Loaded Cobb Salad, 118–120
   Med Chopped Salad, 123
   Seitan Reuben Bowl, 78–79
   Vegan Whitefish Salad, 38–39
salsa, avocado, 68
salt, 20
sandwiches
   Bodega Chopped Cheese, 86–87
   Classic Chi*ken Salad, 88–89
   Fried No-chick Deluxe, 90–93
   Fully Loaded Crunchy Wrap, 108–111
   I'm From Philly Cheesesteak, 94–97
   Lentil Sloppy Joes, 98–99
   Plant-Powered Bean & Chile Burritos, 100–103
   Vegan Big Stack, 104–107
sauces
   Alfredo, 70–71
   béchamel, 141
   blenders and, 23
   bolognese, 74–75
   caramel, 200
   edamame, 114
   ginger, 114
   for hamburger, 104
   for lasagna, 140
   pesto, 62–63
   soy, 20
   tamari, 20
   Tempeh Buffalo Dip, 174
   tofu as base for, 19
Savory Oats & Lentil Porridge, 56–57
sazón, 20, 150
scrambles, 58–59
Seasoned Kale Chips, 158–159
seeds, 45
   Anything-but-Basic Avo Toast, 45
   brittle, 45
   Buckwheat & Berry Parfaits, 46
   Drew's Famous Smoothie, 49
   fats in, 15
   Pumpkin Spice Mouse with Maple Brittle, 194
   Savory Oats & Lentil Porridge, 57
seitan, 19
   DIY Seitan, 222–223
   Fried No-chick Deluxe, 90–93
   I'm From Philly Cheesesteak, 94–97
   making from scratch, 222–223
   pickling, 78
   Seitan Fajitas, 144–147
   Seitan Reuben Bowl, 78–79
   Vegan Pernil Plate, 148–150
serrano peppers, 68–69
Serving Size (nutrition labels), 15
Shakshuka-style Tofu Scramble, 58–59
shallots, 227

shepherd's pie, 136–137
Shiitake mushrooms, 227
silken tofu, 19
   Chocolate Silk Pie, 198–199
   Coco-licious Cream Pie, 184–185
   Creamy Alfredo Pasta, 70–71
   Lupini Pot Pie, 138–139
   Red Lentil Curry, 76–77
   Seitan Reuben Bowl, 78–79
   Silky Caramel Flan, 200–201
   Sriracha Mayo, 130–131
   Sweet
      Potato Pie Bars, 204–205
   Tofu Ranch Dressing, 121–122
   Vegan Sour Cream, 146–147
Silky Caramel Flan, 200–201
60-minute recipes, 239
skillets, 23
sloppy joes, 98–99
smoked paprika, 20
smoothies
   blenders and, 23
   Drew's
      Famous Smoothie, 48–49
snacks
   Air Fryer Artichoke Wings with Lemony
      Hummus Dip, 166–167
   Crispy Air-Fried Tofu Nuggets, 168–169
   Mini Energy Muffins, 156–157
   Pizza Bites, 170–171
   Seasoned Kale Chips, 158–159
   Stacked Nacho Fries, 172–173
   Sweet Crispy Treats, 154–155
   Tempeh Buffalo Dip, 174
   Tofu Chicharrones, 160–161
   Vegan
      Candy Bar Bites, 162–163
Soto, Dalina, 12
soups
   Chickpea Pozole, 67
   Dutch oven and, 23
sour cream, 146–147
soy beans, 27, 88–89
soy milk, 20

Air Fryer Artichoke Wings with Lemony
   Hummus Dip, 166–167
Bagels with a Boost, 211–213
Bread of Champions, 214–216
Buckwheat & Berry Parfaits, 46–47
Coco-licious Cream Pie, 184–185
Creamy Mac And Cheese, 72–73
Fried No-chick Deluxe, 90–93
Fully Loaded Crunchy Wrap, 108–111
I'm From Philly Cheesesteak, 94–97
Lentil Waffle Mix (and Pancakes, Too!), 50–51
Lupini Pot Pie, 138–139
Mini Energy Muffins, 156–157
Oatmeal-Raisin Power Cookies, 188–189
PB&J
   Swirl Nice Cream, 190–191
Peppermint Hot Chocolate, 52–53
Power-Packed Rice Pudding, 192–193
Protein Matcha Latte, 54–55
Sweet Bean-Stuffed French Toast, 60–61
Vegan Whip, 234
soy sauce, 20
spaghetti squash, roasting, 227
spatulas, 23
spice mousse, 194–195
spices, 20
spinach
   Loaded Cobb Salad, 118–120
   Shakshuka-style Tofu Scramble, 58–59
spoons, 23
squash
   Acorn Squash Breakfast Bowls, 40–41
   Chickpea Pozole, 67
   roasting, 227

Sriracha Mayo, 130–131
Stacked Nacho Fries, 172–173
Start the Clock, 13
steaks, vegan, 94–97
stews, 23
storage containers, 23
Strawberry
   Protein Pops, 202–203
sugar. *See* blood sugar
sushi, 128–129
Sweet Bean-Stuffed French Toast, 60–61
Sweet Crispy Treats, 154–155
Sweet Potato Pie Bars, 204–205
sweeteners, 20, 45

T

tahini
   Air Fryer Artichoke Wings with Lemony
      Hummus Dip, 166–167
   Big (Kale) Salad with Tempeh "Croutons', 124–127
tamari sauce, 20
tempeh
   Big (Kale) Salad with Tempeh "Croutons', 124–127
   Loaded Cobb Salad, 118–120
   Tempeh Buffalo Dip, 174
   Veggie & Pesto Frittata, 62–63
textured vegetable protein (TVP).
   See TVP (textured vegetable protein)
30-minute recipes, 238–239
Thousand Island dressing, 78
Three-Bean Chili, 80–81
toasts
   Anything-but-Basic Avo Toast, 42–45
   Sweet Bean-Stuffed French Toast, 60–61
tofu, 19
   Chocolate Silk Pie, 198–199
   Coco-licious Cream Pie, 184–185
   cream cheese, 37

Creamy Alfredo Pasta, 70–71
Crispy Air-Fried Tofu Nuggets, 168–169
extra-firm, 19
firm, 19
Kimchi Ginger Poke Bowl, 114–117
Lupini Pot Pie, 138–139
Protein-Packed Lasagna, 140–143
Red Lentil Curry, 76–77
sauces, as base for, 19
scrambles, 58–59
Seitan Reuben Bowl, 78–79
Shakshuka-style Tofu Scramble, 58–59
silken, 19
Silky Caramel Flan, 200–201
Sriracha Mayo, 130–131
Sweet Potato Pie Bars, 204–205
Tempeh Buffalo Dip, 174
Tofu Chicharrones, 160–161
Tofu Ranch Dressing, 121–122
Vegan Hand Rolls, 128–129
Vegan Sour Cream, 146–147
Veggie & Pesto Frittata, 62–63
Weekend Jewish Deli Breakfast, 37–39
tomatillos, 68–69
tongs, 23
tortilla chips, 174
tortillas
　Fully Loaded Crunchy Wrap, 108–111
　Plant-Powered Bean & Chile Burritos, 100–103
　Seitan Fajitas, 144–147
tostadas, 108–111
TVP (textured vegetable protein), 19
　Bodega Chopped Cheese, 86–87
　Chorizo Burrito Bowl, 68–69
　Fully Loaded Crunchy Wrap, 108–111
　making from scratch, 224

Protein-Packed Lasagna, 140–143
Stacked Nacho Fries, 172–173
TVP MVP, 224
Vegan Big Stack, 104–107
type 1 diabetes, 30

V

Vegan Big Stack, 104–107
Vegan Candy Bar Bites, 162–163
Vegan Hand Rolls, 128–129
Vegan Pernil Plate, 148–150
vegan queso, 100
Vegan Sour Cream, 146–147
Vegan Whip, 234
Vegan Whitefish Salad, 38–39
vegans/veganism
　accessibility, 25
　ingredients, 20
　myths regarding, 25, 27–28
vegetables
　Fire Veggies, 225–229
　roasting, 226–227
　Veggie & Pesto Frittata, 62–63
vitamins, 28

W

waffle fries, 172–173
waffles, 50–51
watermelon, 114–117
Weekend Jewish Deli Breakfast, 37–39
wheat gluten flour, 222–223
whipped cream, 234
whisks, 23
Whitefish Salad, 38–39
wild rice, 230
wings, 166–167
wooden spoons, 23
wraps, 88–89, 108–111

Y

yogurt, 20
　Acorn Squash Breakfast Bowls, 40–41

Apple Chocolate "Nachos," 178–179
yogurt (cont.)
　Buckwheat & Berry Parfaits, 46–47
　Classic Chi*ken Salad, 88–89
　Creamy Ziti & Broccoli, 134–135
　Gooey Cinnamon Rolls, 186–187
　Lentil Shepherd's Pie, 136–137
　Med Chopped Salad, 123
　Pumpkin Spice Mousse with Maple Brittle, 194–195
　Silky Caramel Flan, 200–201
　Tempeh Buffalo Dip, 174
　Weekend Jewish Deli Breakfast, 37–39
Your Latina Nutritionist website, 12

Z

ziti pasta, 134–135

Copyright © 2026 by Robin Arzón

Hachette Book Group supports the right to free expression and the value of copyright. The purpose of copyright is to encourage writers and artists to produce the creative works that enrich our culture.

The scanning, uploading, and distribution of this book without permission is a theft of the author's intellectual property. If you would like permission to use material from the book (other than for review purposes), please contact permissions@hbgusa.com. Thank you for your support of the author's rights.

Voracious / Little, Brown and Company
Hachette Book Group
1290 Avenue of the Americas, New York, NY 10104
voraciousbooks.com

First Edition: March 2026

Voracious is an imprint of Little, Brown and Company, a division of Hachette Book Group, Inc. The Voracious name and logo are trademarks of Hachette Book Group, Inc.

The publisher is not responsible for websites (or their content) that are not owned by the publisher.

The Hachette Speakers Bureau provides a wide range of authors for speaking events. To find out more, go to hachettespeakersbureau.com or email HachetteSpeakers@hbgusa.com.

Little, Brown and Company books may be purchased in bulk for business, educational, or promotional use. For information, please contact your local bookseller or the Hachette Book Group Special Markets Department at special.markets@hbgusa.com.

Photography by Johnny Miller
Design by Rad Works
Food Styling by Rebecca Jurkevich, assisted by Brett Statman and Debbie Kim
Prop Styling by Sarah Smart

ISBN 9780316594271

Library of Congress Control Number: 2025944119

10 9 8 7 6 5 4 3 2 1

APS

Printed in China